What Exactly is Dandruff?

What Exactly is Dandruff?

Rama Murthy DVSB MD
Professor and Head
Department of Dermatology, Venereology, and Leprosy
Katuri Medical College
Chinakondrupadu
Guntur District, Andhra Pradesh, India

Foreword
IS Reddy

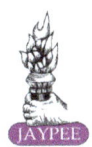

JAYPEE BROTHERS MEDICAL PUBLISHERS
The Health Sciences Publisher
New Delhi | London

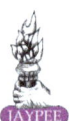 **Jaypee Brothers Medical Publishers (P) Ltd**

Headquarters

Jaypee Brothers Medical Publishers (P) Ltd
4838/24, Ansari Road, Daryaganj
New Delhi 110 002, India
Phone: +91-11-43574357
Fax: +91-11-43574314
Email: jaypee@jaypeebrothers.com

Overseas Office

J.P. Medical Ltd
83 Victoria Street, London
SW1H 0HW (UK)
Phone: +44 20 3170 8910
Fax: +44 (0)20 3008 6180
Email: info@jpmedpub.com

Website: www.jaypeebrothers.com
Website: www.jaypeedigital.com

© 2021, Jaypee Brothers Medical Publishers

The views and opinions expressed in this book are solely those of the original contributor(s)/author(s) and do not necessarily represent those of editor(s) of the book.

All rights reserved. No part of this publication may be reproduced, stored or transmitted in any form or by any means, electronic, mechanical, photocopying, recording or otherwise, without the prior permission in writing of the publishers.

All brand names and product names used in this book are trade names, service marks, trademarks or registered trademarks of their respective owners. The publisher is not associated with any product or vendor mentioned in this book.

Medical knowledge and practice change constantly. This book is designed to provide accurate, authoritative information about the subject matter in question. However, readers are advised to check the most current information available on procedures included and check information from the manufacturer of each product to be administered, to verify the recommended dose, formula, method and duration of administration, adverse effects and contraindications. It is the responsibility of the practitioner to take all appropriate safety precautions. Neither the publisher nor the author(s)/editor(s) assume any liability for any injury and/or damage to persons or property arising from or related to use of material in this book.

This book is sold on the understanding that the publisher is not engaged in providing professional medical services. If such advice or services are required, the services of a competent medical professional should be sought.

Every effort has been made where necessary to contact holders of copyright to obtain permission to reproduce copyright material. If any have been inadvertently overlooked, the publisher will be pleased to make the necessary arrangements at the first opportunity. The **CD/DVD-ROM** (if any) provided in the sealed envelope with this book is complimentary and free of cost. **Not meant for sale.**

Inquiries for bulk sales may be solicited at: jaypee@jaypeebrothers.com

What Exactly is Dandruff? / Rama Murthy DVSB

First Edition: **2021**

ISBN: 978-93-5152-237-9

The Supreme Biotechnologist
Lord *SHIRDI SAI BABA*

The Man behind Triggering Pathogenic Mechanism of Psoriasis
Heinrich Koebner
(1838–1904)

Foreword

The two in one monograph titled *"What Exactly is Dandruff?"* and *"South Indian's Foot: A Storehouse of Diagnostic Clues for Psoriasis"* authored by senior and eminent dermatologist Professor Rama Murthy DVSB, though a tad audacious, is very interesting and thought provoking. These monographs are the culmination of the focused and scholarly observations of the author extended well over the period of three decades.

The author's statement "Looking beyond the skin lesions and also looking beyond the patient" emphasizes the importance of the role of history taking and through clinical examination. The author's inference that pityriasis capitis, seborrheic dermatitis, and psoriasis belong to the same spectrum of a disease process, i.e., the first and second entities are nothing but psoriasis is debatable and may raise many eyebrows. The author made a sincere attempt to prove his point. The author's claim that lack of granular cell layer in psoriasis is the cause for the early skin changes that need further corroboration.

As it is mentioned in these monographs, the standard textbooks of dermatology include pitting, onycholysis, and salmon patches (oil drops) as the usual nail changes are observed in psoriasis. The author deserves a lot of accolades for bringing out so many hitherto unreported nail changes such as "angulation, overcurvature, melanonychia, etc." A special emphasis is laid to examine the toenails in addition to fingernails. The clinical photographs, especially that of various types of nail changes, are so vivid and of high quality. The references are extensive and up-to-date.

In these monographs, Professor Rama Murthy DVSB presented his clinical observations, newer concepts based on these observations, and his arguments to support these concepts. Most of these observations were supported by high quality images. Though the author presented his views, it is up to the reader to reflect, evaluate, and validate them. I am confident that these monographs will kindle lot of interest in both younger as well as senior dermatologists.

IS Reddy MD DD DNB
Consultant Dermatologist
Apollo Hospitals, Jubilee Hills
Hyderabad, Telangana, India

Preface

I would first like to pay my humble *pranam* to the creator of this universe and the supreme biotechnologist, Lord *Shirdi Sai Baba*, and to my beloved patients without whose blessings and co-operation this book would not have seen the light of the day.

This book titled *"What Exactly is Dandruff?"* is, in fact, a combination of two monographs. The title of second monograph is *"South Indian's Foot: A Storehouse of Diagnostic Clues for Psoriasis."* While the former deals with how the author identified the exact etiology of dandruff, while dealing with scaling scalps over the last 3.2 decades, the later deals with the amazing creation of *clues to psoriasis* which HE asked the feet to store and display when wanted by a dermatologist.

According to overseas literature, psoriasis is characterized by well-defined erythematous plaques covered with silvery white scales. Many variants have also been described with typical features; meaning that psoriasis and its variants can be diagnosed clinically itself with ease. Some fingernail changes have also been described which enable a dermatologist to diagnose nail psoriasis (only) in unequivocal terms. In case of any doubt, biopsy is recommended which may either confirm or rule out psoriasis.

Against this backdrop, why Rama Murthy DVSB, a nonentity in the world's arena of dermatology including in his own country, ventures to author a book titled *"What Exactly is Dandruff?"*

The first reason is that psoriasis in this region does not generally conform to the Western literature including those who are as fair as Caucasians; it is in winter that occasionally does one present with so-called "typical morphology."

The second reason is psoriasis expresses itself in different morphological forms at different locations in the same individual; these expressions include excoriated papules, miliaria rubra-like lesions, subacute eczematous to lichenoid plaques, lichenoid papules, prurigo nodularis-like lesions, keratolysis exfoliativa-like lesions, pompholyx-like picture, autosensitization dermatitis, and may present as various forms of dermatitis, involving any part of the body, which do not fit into any known endogenous eczema, or may mimic any known eczema either exogenous or endogenous and may mimic even scabies by presenting as acute prurigo, in particular, in winter season.

This is my experience/clinical observation over the last 3.2 decades. Hence, my hunt for clues began. In the process, *what I realized is the beauty of art of examining a skin patient lies in looking beyond the lesions* that are initially shown to the dermatologist by the patient. After some time, I also realized that psoriasis being a genetically inherited disease, *one (dermatologist) must look beyond the patient*, i.e., any genetically-related individual accompanying the patient. If any member of the pedigree accompanying the patient displays psoriasis or gives history of psoriasis or gives history of psoriasis in his family, the patient's clinical presentation should be interpreted against this backdrop.

Thus, I learned many lessons from many patients who include patients from all Southern states of India (Guntur is almost a small cosmopolitan city).

Another invaluable lesson I learnt is not to expect our histopathologists to come to our rescue for diagnosing puzzling presentations of common dermatoses (which should be diagnosed clinically by the dermatologist himself or herself). Perhaps, it is not nice to depend upon/trouble our histopathologists, in this regard, and finally throw blame on them that they have failed to come to our rescue. What I mean to say is that a histopathologist can be relied upon in respect of rare dermatoses such as tumors, etc.

The creator is mischievous in the sense that HE creates a tricky presentation and HE, being very generous and kind to the mankind, keeps clues in hidden or far away regions. The feet are the most distant acral parts of the human body. These clues should be relied upon, only when no other etiology is found for the presenting, tricky dermatitis, in question.

HE has been kind to me; therefore, I could focus on feet for the last 1.5 decades and on scaling scalp, hence this book.

I have touched upon a part of the body that has been, hitherto, missed by Caucasian researchers/authors. I am given to understand that the dermatologists in cosmopolitan cities and in peripheries too of my country are simply at all rather blindly getting carried away by (in spite of our huge patient bank as against the Caucasian's patient bank) overseas literature that emerges from a small volume of clinical material that forces them to depend on various investigations, perhaps, which are more of commercial value.

I hope this book would inspire practicing dermatologists with rich clinical experience across the country, to speak out their mind in their respective areas of interest, and, thus, contribute to enriching clinical dermatology—Indian perspective.

Rama Murthy DVSB MD
Email: dvsbrm@gmail.com

Acknowledgments

Patients, undoubtedly, constitute the backbone for clinical research. I am fortunate that I am an Indian and teaching/practicing dermatologist in a country like India, wherein, even today, doctors are considered equal to God by the patients to whom I am indebted and I bow my head as a mark of respect to all of them.

There is a big list of individuals who helped me technically and otherwise, to whom I should extend my sincere gratitude. Some of them whom I can never forget in my lifetime include Mr Debasish Haldar, Mr Tanuja Prasad, Mr Srinivas (Medical Photographer), Mr Durga Prasad, Mr Venugopal, and the medical team at Jaypee Brothers Medical Publishers (P) Ltd, New Delhi.

My thanksgiving will not be complete without mentioning Shri Jitendar P Vij (Group Chairman), Dr Richa Saxena (Associate Director, Professional Publishing) and Himani Pandey (Development Editor) at Jaypee Brothers Medical Publishers (P) Ltd, New Delhi, who helped me in publishing this book so nicely.

I am thrilled by the dynamism of the CAPTAIN and his team of CANIXA, for sponsoring this book, and I am indebted to CANIXA.

I cannot but express my sincere gratitude to Dr IS Reddy for having written a 'book review' like foreword, sparing his invaluable time for this.

Contents

Preface ix
Acknowledgments xi
List of Abbreviations xv

What Exactly is Dandruff?

1. Impetus — 3
2. What Dandruff Means to a Patient? — 4
3. What Dandruff Meant to me till 14th January 2003? — 6
4. What Happened on 14th January 2003 and Thereafter? — 8
5. Now, the Question is — 12
6. Spongiosis: Found only in Seborrheic Dermatitis but not in Psoriasis!? — 15
7. Mycobiome — 17
8. Role of Yeasts in Dandruff and Seborrheic Dermatitis — 18
9. When does a Commensal Turn Pathogenic? — 19
10. How a Genius Succeeds in Putting an End to the Long Drawn Controversy Shrouding Dandruff versus Yeasts? — 20
11. The Author's Viewpoint Rather Counterargument — 23
12. Author's Final Word — 27
13. Color Atlas of Dandruff — 29
    - (I) Dandruff in Adults — 29
    - (II) Dandruff in Children — 44
    - (III) Subclinical Psoriasis Capitis — 53
    - (IV) Sebopsoriasis Masquerading as Seborrheic Dermatitis — 74
    - (V) Patients Complaining of Dandruff with Scaly Plaques on Scalp — 114

South Indian's Foot: A Storehouse of Diagnostic Clues for Psoriasis

1. The "Program" Underlying Epidermis   125
2. Anatomy of Normal Nail and Toenail in Psoriasis   137
3. (I) Color Atlas: Abnormalities Involving the Epidermis   149
    (II) Color Atlas: Nail Abnormalities   164

Index   187

List of Abbreviations

What Exactly is Dandruff?

V Dsq	: Visible Desquamation		(L) RETRO. AUR.AREA	: Left Retroauricular Area
(R) GTN	: Right Great Toenail		SUHK	: Subungual Hyperkeratosis
(L) GTN	: Left Great Toenail		ABCD	: Airborne Contact Dermatitis
HK	: Hyperkeratosis		G Father	: Grandfather
APMCE	: As Per My Clinical Experience		MG Father	: Maternal Grandfather
SD	: Seborrheic Dermatitis		MA	: Masquerading As
Psv	: Psoriasis Vulgaris		PPP	: Palmoplantar Psoriasis
RSL	: Robust Scientific Logic		EAC	: External Auditory Canal
TNs	: Toenails		SM Region	: Submental Region
SCPC	: Subclinical Psoriasis Capitis		RN Fold	: Retronasal Fold
RAN	: Retro Ala Nasi		PD	: Photodistribution
(R) RETRO. AUR.AREA	: Right Retroauricular Area			

South Indian's Foot: A Storehouse of Diagnostic Clues For Psoriasis

TDP	: Terminal Differentiation Program		PNF	: Proximal Nail Folds
CE	: Cornified Envelope		LNF	: Lateral Nail Fold
CLE	: Cornified Lipid Envelope		ONL	: Onycholysis
PKC	: Protein Kinase C Family		KLN	: Koilonychia
BMZ	: Basement Membrane Zone		MLN	: Melanonychia
DEJ	: Dermoepidermal Junction		SUHK	: Subungual Hyperkeratosis
TASC	: Transit-amplifying Stem Cells		LND	: Lateral Nail Dystrophy
Dsg	: Desmoglein		CLC	: Cave-like Curvature
Dsc	: Desmocollin		LTN	: Little Toenail
Pkp	: Plakophilin		TN	: Toenail
HK	: Hyperkeratosis/Hyperkeratotic		GTN	: Great Toenail
GT/s	: Great Toe/s		DSE	: Dome-shaped Elevation

What Exactly is Dandruff?

1

Impetus

It is neither far from truth, nor, a hyperbole, if somebody, perhaps, opines that there had been no dermatological disorder other than dandruff that enjoyed the privilege of the honor of unabated research, by a few dozens of researchers, that went on and on for nearly 110 years, till a Genius, in early 1990s, proved that dandruff was not primarily a hyperproliferative disorder and *Pityrosporum ovale* plays the key role in the etiopathogenesis of dandruff. The dermatological community across the globe took for granted what the Genius said and since then it has been observing quietism.

What appears to have been resolved forever should not become an issue of debate once again, had it been flawlessly resolved or had it been accomplished with sanctity of heart.

Otherwise, time (the most powerful and influential factor that has command over the entire universe) cannot keep quiet and waits till it finds an appropriate soul to ignite it and thus re-open the case that was seemingly shutdown forever about 35 years ago.

What Dandruff Means to a Patient?

The conversations between me and the patients who consult me for their dandruff go like this.

A

Patient: "Sir! I have dandruff."

Doctor: "Do you mean scales come off from your scalp?"

The 19-year-old female patient offers a puzzled look for a few seconds and answers.

Patient: "No sir! It is actually… when I scratch my scalp, some kind of dirt, black in color, comes off."

B

Patient: "Sir! My problem is dandruff."

Doctor: "Ok! Does that mean scales come off from your scalp?"

Patient: "No sir! I take shower three to four times a week, so my scalp never scales…"

Doctor: "Then… what exactly is your problem!?"

Patient: "Sir! I finished my B. Tech recently and joined a software company in Bengaluru. Perhaps, the water there does not suit me…"

Doctor: "Oh! No Miss Anita, please give a straightforward answer to my question. What exactly is your problem that you are consulting me?"

Patient: "Sir! Actually… I am losing my hair in very large numbers these days. Look at my scalp… how thin my hair has become!"

Doctor: "So, your actual problem is hair loss, not dandruff! Am I right?"

Patient: "Absolutely sir!"

C

Patient: "Sir! I have dandruff. My scalp itches a lot these days."

Doctor: "What about scales…?"

Patient: "No scaling sir! It just itches horribly."

D

Patient: "Sir! I am suffering from dandruff for the last 3 years. It becomes worse, particularly, during winter. My sister, studying her MBBS, also suffers from this, but she stays away from me in a hostel. When I use a shampoo regularly, it goes off, but soon it recurs!"

I look at his scalp and the skin along frontal hairline. I find no scales on hair or any cutaneous lesions along frontal hairline or scaly erythema on facial sites.

Doctor: "Ok! From which region of the scalp, scales come off in large numbers!"

Patient: "Entire scalp sir!"

Doctor: "That is Ok! From which part of the scalp usually?"

Patient: "From this region sir!" He puts his hand on his occiput.

I look at his occiput, later entire scalp; skin is found normal and no scales on hair!

Doctor: "What man! Your scalp is absolutely normal. I find no scales at all."

Patient: "That is because, before coming to you, I had a thorough shower with a shampoo sir! Otherwise, there would have been scales."

Doctor: "Did you ever see the scales really?"

Patient: "What sir! Scales fall on my shirt whenever, I comb my hair!"

So, dandruff means to lay people either black material on scalp or hair loss or scalp pruritus or scaling scalp. Thus, most of them seem to have no clear idea about dandruff. At least, do we dermatologists have?

What Dandruff Meant to me till 14th January 2003?

I started (had to) my private clinical practice on 25th January, 1988 in a nearby small town, which I used to visit on Sundays regularly. The consultation fee was ₹30/- per patient per month. I was also working as Assistant Professor of Dermatology for Guntur Medical College and Government General Hospital, drawing a meager salary of ₹3,500/- per month. Thus, both the incomes were just adequate enough to make both ends meet.

Therefore, I ventured (because there was prohibition on private clinical practice by government doctors) to start my clinic in Guntur, risking serious consequences, on 12th May, 1988, with the fond hope that I could earn a little more money. The point I had that enabled me to venture to start private practice was our, the then, Chief Minister himself was acting in films while being the head of Andhra Pradesh Government (the actor whom I still regard as the best that India has ever produced). So, why I cannot start private practice when government was paying a meager salary? Have I pursued such a tough, time taking medical curriculum to run around people begging hand loans, if any contingency arises at the age of 30 years heading a family of three adults and a small kid?

Alas, 2 years gone, not able to pick up good practice in Guntur. As usual, prices were going up. Then, a friend of mine (rather my godfather) encouraged me to start a clinic at another town. Yes, in no time, I picked up good practice. I heaved a sigh of relief. Luck started turning in my favor in Guntur also from 1991 onwards. Thus, I was doing well at all my three clinics.

Coming to the point, I was diagnosing pityriasis capitis (dandruff) in every postpubertal patient of either sex approaching me for their dandruff after making sure that scaling was confined to scalp and that they had no scaly patches elsewhere. I used to take it for granted their dandruff and never bothered to look at their scalps. I just used to look at the skin along frontal hairline only to find no lesions.

But, I used to get puzzled to the extent of getting frustrated whenever, a prepubertal child (though rarely) was brought to me by their parents reporting a history that their child was suffering from dandruff.

I was curiously examining the child's hair and scalp to find any scales. Alas, no visible desquamation! Whenever I used to declare that I was not convinced with their history and argue with them that dandruff does not occur at that age, there used to be one of the two following responses from the parents.

A

Parent: "Sir! Today morning my son has been given a shower."

B

Parent: One of the parents used to scratch their child's scalp with one of their fingernails and thus demonstrate scaling to give me a shocking surprise.

After returning home from my clinic, I used to eagerly refer to our major textbooks to find any such line that reads as "dandruff can rarely occur in prepubertal children" only to get disappointed and remain perplexed.

While this was the experience with dandruff, which was described as the mild form of seborrheic dermatitis, my curiosity and enthusiasm to diagnose seborrheic dermatitis were being hampered by confusion as the scaly plaques in seborrheic distribution were not displaying textbook described greasy yellowish scales or crusts.

Yet, I used to label some elderly patients in their 60s or 70s, when they presented with scaly plaques on face typically involving the medial eyebrows, nasolabial furrows, upper lips with or without moustaches, beard region, and retroauricular areas as seborrheic dermatitis, even in the absence of greasy yellowish scales or crusts. Some of them used to display scaly plaques in their intermammary areas, but not in the midposterior chest region. I could readily visualize very thin scaly plaques on some of their tonsured scalps or bald scalps.

After few months, some patients used to report "Sir! In my previous visits, your medicines worked very well sir! I brought those old prescriptions along with me, but this time, I have developed terribly itchy patches on my legs sir!"

Those lesions on their dorsae of feet and shins were typically psoriatic. I used to immediately take away the old prescriptions from their hands; my previous diagnosis was seborrheic eczema of face. Then, my eyes focus on their face; I find some scales in their medial eyebrows and in moustache. Some of their bald scalps were displaying inconspicuous scaly patches. Then, I make use of a glass slide only to elicit profuse silvery white scales from their scalp lesions.

I used to introspect; did I go wrong!? I got answer after a few years. Yes! I was wrong; I happened to mistake sebopsoriasis to seborrheic eczema, out of overenthusiasm to diagnose the later condition. I was sure about my wrong labeling. Then, what about seborrheic eczema!? Does it not occur in this region or is it extremely rare?

I got answer for this too; seborrheic eczema in this region does not conform to textbook description. It presents as dense eruption of flesh-colored follicular papules involving face, extensive involvement of posterior trunk and anterior chest, predominantly the midchest region.

Perhaps, there is no change in the 32 years of my clinical experience with regard to seborrheic dermatitis (i.e., pre- and post-2003). The year 2003 was a landmark year in my carrier as a practicing dermatologist, in particular 14th January of 2003.

What Happened on 14th January 2003 and Thereafter?

The 13th, 14th, 15th, and 16th of January of every year are the dates fixed for celebrating a festival called Makar Sankranti (Pongal) in this region. At villages, it is celebrated with lot of enthusiasm and religious fervor as most of the peasants get back their money from their harvest by that time. That was the right time, I thought for me to go on holidaying with my family in one or the other major city of India. But, in 2003, just a couple of days before our scheduled tour, my 81-year-old, otherwise, healthy mother was struck by a viral fever. Therefore, I could not move out of the station. On 13th, I stayed back at home looking after my mother and spending time with my kids. But on 14th, I grew restless, sitting idle at home, and made up my mind at 11 AM to go to my clinic against the wish of my wife and kids.

I knew there would be, at least, a dozen patients, but contrary to my expectations I could hardly see six patients and it was 3 PM; so I decided to leave the clinic for home and informed the same to my receptionist. I was feeling hungry and I grew eager to enjoy the special festival items in my lunch. I got up from my chair and suddenly I heard some kind of commotion outside my chamber. I hear a lady's voice loudly shouting at my receptionist. Some altercation was going on between the two and suddenly a lady intruded into my chamber with her two daughters. I shouted at her in anger and said to her "it is not nice on your part to trouble me like this at this hour that too on a festival day." "Sir! Please! Only one patient!" she was literally begging me.

Being a villager and on a festival day, I did not want to disappoint her, after all, just one patient. I sat down in my chair and when I raised my head to look at her she was in tears, but started thanking me profusely.

Mother: "Sir! With great difficulty, I could bring my daughters today sir! I would have come earlier, but it seems there is some minister in the town, so there was traffic jam everywhere."

Doctor: "Ok ok! Who is the patient?" I was growing restless.

Mother: "Sir! My younger daughter!" She directed her daughter to sit on the stool near my chair.

Doctor: "So, what is your problem?"

Mother: "Dandruff and hair fall sir!" Her mother intervened and replied.

Doctor: "Do scales fall off from your head?"

Mother: "Yes sir! Yesterday I noticed her whole scalp studded with scales; today, of course, yesterday also I gave her thorough shower with a shampoo, these being festival days."

Doctor: "Please! Let her answer!" suppressing my anger and trying my best to keep my cool I said to her, unable to bear her loud, irritant, and arrogant voice.

Doctor: "Now tell me from which part of your scalp scales come off more profusely?"

Daughter: "Entire scalp doctor."

Doctor: "That is okay, but from which region more exactly?"
She was in dilemma. "Ok ok! Let me examine your scalp."
I thoroughly searched her scalp only to find no scales. I could understand; because of having shower on two consecutive days with a shampoo, scales are gone. I started penning my prescription for her dandruff; while doing so, I heard some murmurs.

Mother: "Sir! Please be kind to us. This time our crops failed to fetch us profits. In fact, we incurred heavy losses. Today morning, I had to borrow money from my neighbor. Their father is a drunkard; he does not take care of us."

Doctor: "Ok ok! What do you want me to do?"

Mother: "Sir! She is my eldest daughter and very mild in nature. In fact, she has more problem. Please see her also. Sir! I will definitely pay your fees in our next visit!"
I became softer and started pitying them for their plight.

Doctor: "Ok! You may sit! Tell me what is your problem?"

Daughter: "Same thing sir! Dandruff."

Doctor: "You also took shower?"

Patient: "No sir! I am running temperature so I did not!"
She leaned toward me. I started examining her scalp skin by pushing apart the hair. I could see many discrete, well-elevated plaques covered with silvery white scales all over her scalp.

Doctor: "Do you have any patches on your body?"

Patient: "Yes sir! I have one on my (right) foot."
The dorsum of her (right) foot displayed a plaque of psoriasis.

Doctor: "Ok! Anywhere else?"

Patient: "No sir!"
I started writing prescription for her scalp psoriasis. I heard the mother asking the daughter to get up and she sat on the stool.

Mother: Sir! Please! I have terribly itchy patches for quite some time on my soles; I stopped my pen and looked at her sole. I looked at the other sole and then her palms. She was a case of palmoplantar psoriasis!

Doctor: "Ok! I will give prescription to you also. Keep quiet! But you are going to pay my fees in your next visit. Not after reaping a good harvest!"

Mother: "Sure sir!" She was all smiles. While penning prescription for her, she volunteered to report!

Mother: "Sir! Even my mother also suffered from same problem for many years, but she died recently."
Thank God! I heaved a sigh of relief. I disposed them off and got into my car. While driving back home, though, feeling very hungry, my mind could not help plunging into action.
I started analyzing; the younger daughter was reported to have heavy scaling of scalp, but, because of shampooing her scalp on two consecutive days, her scalp displayed no scales. But I should have stroked her scalp, which I failed to do as I was in a hurry to get back home.
The elder daughter had well-evolved, psoriatic plaques on her scalp plus a typical plaque on her (right) foot; a clear case of psoriasis.

Their mother had palmoplantar psoriasis and their grandmother too seems to have suffered from palmoplantar psoriasis. It is natural; after all, psoriasis is a genetic disease. In this family, mode of inheritance appears to be autosomal dominant.

One question suddenly appeared on the wind screen of my car, making road a bit invisible; I slowed down and the question I was facing read as: "Had only the younger daughter alone, without scales on her scalp, come to consult you for her dandruff?"

I thought for a while; well, I would have never thought of psoriasis capitis in her. Nor I would have tried to elicit family history as dandruff is not known to be a genetic disorder.

That means the road is now clearly visible as a big cloud vanished from my brain and the clear road led me to the psoriatic origin of dandruff.

From the very next day onward, I started thoroughly examining the scalp and rest of the skin in every patient who sought my intervention for their dandruff; I used to try to obtain a thorough history as to psoriasis in their pedigrees.

While doing so, some of the patients volunteered to report that their heels were fissured, causing severe pain and discomfort, and they were not able to go to their fields. I used to look at their hindfeet also to find extensive deep fissuring along the borders of their foot. In some, fissured areas were infected, discharging purulent fluid adding to their discomfort and causing morbidity and some were seeking medicine for their candidal intertrigo of their feet, particularly females.

I used to tell them "after all, this is a common happening among you guys working in fields and indulging in wet work."

Patient: "That is true sir! But this winter, it is worse!"

Some patients, finding me talkative, used to go on complaining that their soles itch a lot, occasionally entire body (which readily used to respond to a tablet of cetirizine or levocetirizine), adding further that their under toes also feel rough and get cracked causing pain and insist that I examine their soles thoroughly; I used to oblige them only to find what they complained was true. That time, I did not have the clinical acumen required to correlate various findings and interpret them. That was the story before 2003.

In some seasons, it used to appear as though palmoplantar psoriasis (PPP) was more common than psoriasis vulgaris (PsV). I started examining the soles, borders of feet in every case of psoriasis including PPP (unlike in pre-2003 period). I gained the impression that while intertriginous hyperkeratosis (HK) and under toe HK are frequent components of PPP, they were not uncommon in PsV.

Hyperkeratosis and fissuring of borders of feet, in particular, heel borders, appeared to be more common than under toe or intertriginous HK of feet. Nevertheless, as I made it a point to enquire about their dandruff since 15th January 2003, in every case of PPP or PsV, I used to get a positive answer not infrequently.

From these positive answers, I cannot, but draw the following conclusions about their dandruff: (1) Severity of their dandruff (scaling) varies from mild to moderate to severe, (2) Mild and moderate cases of dandruff used to respond to regular showers with a shampoo of their choice, (3) Dandruff could be a single episode story, which the patient may not readily recollect or of recurrent episodes or persistent with seasonal exacerbation, (4) Itching of scalp was more frequently associated with moderate-to-severe cases of dandruff, (5) Dandruff need not be present in their parents or siblings or genetically-related uncles or aunts or in first cousins, implying that psoriasis could be present elsewhere on the body, and (6) At the time of consultation, the patient may not be suffering from dandruff. Then why should he/she consult? On the eve of leaving for overseas or on the eve of leaving the station for a far off place for higher studies or job purpose in India, he/she approaches a dermatologist lest his/her dandruff should recur.

A significant number of the patients who approach me for their dandruff do not display scales either on hair shafts or on scalp surface. The reason-the same story-before coming to me they take a shower with some shampoo.

Then, I used to stroke with a glass slide that part of the scalp, which was reported to be a heavy producer of scales, only to succeed.

In some, scalps were found to display frank psoriatic plaques. I used to try to elicit scales from the apparently normal skin in between the plaques. This act of mine is used to succeed in a fairly good number of patients. That means the so-called dandruff is nothing but subclinical scalp psoriasis, which causes scalp itching not uncommonly. Therefore, the act of scratching elicits scaling. Similarly, the act of combing hair and vigorous toweling of scalp after a shower. This was interpreted as visible desquamation and was given the name pityriasis capitis (dandruff) by our overseas Caucasian researchers.

That was because in a significant number of patients, the subclinical scalp psoriasis (i.e., devoid of plaques, apparently normal skin, and a few/no scales on scalp hair), there will not be any readily visible evidence of psoriasis elsewhere on the body.

Groin psoriasis is fairly common, but is usually asymptomatic; hence, the patient never volunteers to report that he/she has some problem in the groin. This is, perhaps, because of two reasons: One is—the patient is never aware of the presence of erythema—it being asymptomatic—the patient does not care to have a look at the groins and the second reason is unlike other animals, the human being feels shy to show his private parts until and unless it becomes an unbearable nuisance. Therefore, examining groins for the presence of psoriasis provide corroborative evidence in a tricky presentation of dermatitis.

We, the dermatologists, are taught by our textbooks and our professors to take cognizance of existence of four distinct entities: (1) Pityriasis capitis, (2) Seborrheic dermatitis, (3) Psoriasis capitis, and (4) Sebopsoriasis.

While some argue in favor of pityriasis capitis being a mild form of seborrheic dermatitis and there seems to be no one who does not consider sebopsoriasis as one of the variants of PsV.

When we strongly believe in this piece of our subject of dermatology, where is the question of looking for evidence of psoriasis elsewhere on the body in a patient with dandruff?

After all, the art of examining a skin patient lies in looking "beyond" the lesion/s exhibited by the patient and also looking "beyond the patient" when dealing with a genetically inherited disease like psoriasis, i.e., examining a genetically-related accompanying person like the patient's sibling or grandparent/s or father's siblings or mother's siblings or their progeny.

Examining beyond the lesion/s (psoriasis, in particular) means taking pains to examine all such areas as groins, external genitalia including glans penis, natal cleft, elbows, knees, feet, in particular, the intertriginous areas, heel borders, in steps of feet, under toes and toenails, and external auditory canal and retroauricular areas, paronychia, particularly of lateral nail folds of either fingers or toes, and last but not the least malleoli of feet and dorsae of great toes.

Apart from a thorough physical examination, a thorough pedigree history as to psoriasis is to be sought. This means fielding various questions to extract a history of psoriasis at least in one member of the pedigree. This exercise is more important and very useful, when the patient in question with dandruff does not display evidence of psoriasis elsewhere on his body or does not give a history of psoriasis in his family members.

I am, of course, thoroughly convinced that there is nothing like pityriasis capitis.

5

Now, the Question is

How the textbook literature (authored by Caucasians) and our teaching faculty on our soil made us believe that there exists a condition called pityriasis capitis.

To explore this, I happened to refer to some editions of the major textbooks that we follow in our day to day clinical practice and teaching including the older editions.

I did not find a chapter exclusively on pityriasis capitis. What I could find was only few lines amidst the text on seborrheic dermatitis (SD). The definition of dandruff goes like this—"If scaling isolates to the scalp with little or no overt inflammation, it is referred to as dandruff or pityriasis capitis, which is considered the mildest form of SD, although there is no conclusive evidence for this."[1]

This means, there are, at least, some Caucasian researchers (CR)/colleagues who do not believe in the concept/assumption of pityriasis capitis evolving into SD.

In another edition, how dandruff evolves into SD is described—"Dandruff (visible desquamation from the scalp surface) "appears" to be the precursor of SD and this may generally progress through redness, irritation, and increasing scaling of the scalp to true SD."[2]

There is no reference given for the above statement. Perhaps, it must be understood as the personal opinion of the contributing author or a collective opinion expressed by both the author and the editorial board.

In the name of honesty, how the Western literature thrusts its confusion, lack of clarity, and dilemma on the global community that become evident on reading the following texts.

"The condition known as SD of infancy is normally confined to the first few months of life, but it is not established that it is the same condition as SD of adolescence and adult life."[1,3]

We are given to understand that the onset of SD coincides with the maturity of sebaceous glands at the time of puberty under the influence of androgens.

"…….the role of seborrhea in the pathogenesis of the condition is debatable!"[1,2,4]

Me: Then why name it SD? I know what the answer is going to be!

Caucasian researcher: "No No! It is just a misnomer my friend!"

Me: "No! That is not the apt answer!"

Caucasian researcher: "See………it occurs in those areas, which are rich in sebaceous glands, hence that name!"

Me: "Oh I see! If that is the case, other diseases too should have been named based on their distribution."

Caucasian researcher: "No my friend! That is not the right argument! Wherever it is possible, we do so!"

Me: "Ok! But a young researcher may embark upon for decades together to explore the link between sebum and dermatitis producing 100s of papers!"

Caucasian researcher: "Yeah! You are right my friend! We cannot rule out that possibility."

I do not want to argue beyond this point, knowing pretty well, that it is their very way of living.

Coming to the pathology of SD.

"The histopathology is not diagnostic, but generally shows features of psoriasis and chronic dermatitis and much of the stratum is often lost in the process of fixation and most of its cells are parakeratotic."[2,3]

"It seems likely that the initial event is the "squirting papilla" described by Pinkus and Mehregan.[5] Capillary dilatation in the papillae is followed by migration of inflammatory cells through the vessel walls into the epidermis, where they incite spongiosis. This is similar to the burst of inflammation that sometimes occurs in psoriasis."

"As the inflammation subsides, there is an increase in the production of keratinocytes. Epidermal proliferation, as measured by the mitotic and labeling indices, is increased and desquamation is also increased."[6]

Capillary dilatation in the papillae, stratum corneum being composed of parakeratotic cells, increased epidermal proliferation, and desquamation; all these histopathological features except spongiosis (which is described as the only feature that distinguishes SD from psoriasis) very much match the clinical behavior of psoriasis including Auspitz's sign.

The histopathology of SD, thus, very much closely resembles that of psoriasis, the only distinguishing feature being spongiosis, any itchy disease of any etiology; it is well-known that the act of scratching can induce dermatitis and spongiosis.

Textbook literature, as to psoriasis, in 1980s, did not seem to have taken cognizance of pruritus associated with psoriasis. The present editions of textbooks describe psoriasis as an itchy disease, the severity of which may vary from individual to individual and it may not be as severe as in atopic eczema.[7] When a psoriatic plaque is scratched over a period of time, spongiosis is most likely to be observed on histopathological examination of that plaque. How our Western colleagues and histopathologists missed spongiosis in the biopsy specimens of psoriatic lesions?

Was it because they reposed robust confidence in spongiosis being exclusive to SD that can differentiate SD from psoriasis unequivocally or was it because psoriasis enjoys the privilege of striking any part of the skin. Involvement of some seborrheic areas also is not uncommon in psoriasis vulgaris. Involvement of seborrheic areas predominantly is a characteristic feature of sebopsoriasis. Presence of spongiosis in a biopsy specimen from a plaque located in one of the seborrheic areas in psoriasis vulgaris seems to have misled them to interpret it as SD. Similarly, perhaps, sebopsoriasis was also mistaken to SD for the same reason.

The overseas literature tries to define every disease in a terrific way. I very much adore those definitions (both as an undergraduate and as a postgraduate student in dermatology, I always tried to memorize those definitions. Now, at the age of 62 years, having obtained my MD 33 years ago, I admit, I have forgotten most of those definitions as there was no need to memorize anymore).

It is a pity that, even today, the Caucasian authors/researchers are somehow scared to define SD.

"This is a chronic dermatitis, which is difficult to define exactly," in spite of SD being described as a disease with a distinctive morphology and distribution, i.e., in seborrheic areas.[3]

With respect to the epidemiology of SD, "SD is a common dermatitis, but estimates of its true prevalence in different populations are hampered by lack of validated diagnostic criteria."[1]

Here, at this juncture, I cannot but put a question to my esteemed Caucasian authors and researchers: Why the above uncertainties and dilemmas initially expressed some decades ago, continue to be expressed even today, in spite of your laboratory, which you trust the most and keep in high esteem that has been upgraded beyond one's imagination, has not come to your rescue to drive away those uncertainties and dilemmas from your genius minds!?

After all, we, the semi-white Indians, perhaps, rest of the Caucasians and the dark-skinned lots hold you white-skinned Americans, Britishers, and other Europeans in high esteem with respect to your laboratory and your honest research.

When do you people realize that the actual reason behind this deplorable scenario is you are plagued by lack of adequate clinical material (we have been learning modern medical sciences from you people, i.e., the textbooks, the journals that you publish and market across the globe, and it is you people who taught us the clinics through your literature that stressed the importance of various clinical findings being the most important and they all have to be brought under one umbrella meaning that we should not group clinical features displayed by a given patient and thus stick different labels, i.e., different diagnosis to different groups of features displayed by a given patient).

In spite of having come out with a wonderful account on various diseases including genetic disease and various conditions that strike the human body across the globe, well-supported by laboratory data, wherever necessary, each member of the editorial board and each contributing author, I am sure, has some apprehension in one or the other corner of their minds lest they should be found at fault with regard to the literature that has been contributed or edited and is going to be published and, thus, made available to the international community.

"Why such apprehensions in your minds or why such uncertainties get published?" I think I can explain............I reiterate you are plagued by lack of adequate clinical material. In spite of exercising utmost caution while preparing/editing the text, you people do make some misleading statements. For example, "polymorphous light eruption (PMLE) is the most common photosensitivity across the globe!" Globe means to you only Americas and Europe! What about Asia, the largest continent? What about India, subcontinent of Asia!? Because of that statement, even today every dermatologist, irrespective of age and experience, labels every photoeruption as PMLE in India while that is not the ground reality. It is photosensitive psoriasis that is the most common etiology of a photoeruption in this part of India, i.e., personal experience.

Do not you people realize time has come for you to pick up such a country that provides the largest clinical material and call for such senior clinicians with vast clinical appearance and recruit them as helper guides to your researchers in laboratories and as helper guides to your editorial boards for different textbooks, leave alone asking them to contribute chapters to your textbooks so that you can gift the globe such literature that contains very few uncertainties and offers many warranted clarifications. I need not reiterate that a clinician grows confident day by day with regard to his clinical skills, as he picks up good practice and, thus, sees a good number of patients each day. For a clinician who attends to his duties at his clinic or hospital regularly, *time is not just money, but time is invaluable clinical knowledge.*

6

Spongiosis: Found only in Seborrheic Dermatitis but not in Psoriasis!?

Well, coming to spongiosis as a distinguishing feature of seborrheic dermatitis (SD) from psoriasis; way back in 1986, when I was on deputation to the Department of Dermatology and sexually transmitted diseases (STDs) at AIIMS, New Delhi, in the month of August and September, for a period of 6 weeks, I made the best use of two libraries, one in the campus of AIIMS and the other one nearby National Library. At the National Library, on one fine day in the evening, I found booklets of North American Dermatology Clinics lined up filling an entire rack. While I was rushing through various issues, in one of them, it appeared an article named "eczematous psoriasis," which interested me. I thoroughly read that report. To my utter surprise, no major Textbook on Dermatology has touched upon this particular clinical behavior of psoriasis. What gives relief to me, in this regard, is a report by Abramovits and others in 2007, which describes coexistence of psoriasis and eczema.[8]

Nor was there any article reported in any readily available issues, on this clinical aspect of psoriasis, such as Archives of Dermatology, American Academy of Dermatology, or British Journal of Dermatology, the most popular and leading journals, to the best of my knowledge. 34 years elapsed ever since I read that report, but there seems to have been no further talk of eczematous psoriasis in the international arena, I make a wild guess, leave alone my country, and its top dermatologists rather high profile dermatologists who play safe and thus tend to derive immense pleasure and satisfaction and deem it safer to toe the western line always, so that they can enjoy the fruits of such attitude.

This attitude reminds me of a melodious Hindi song, rendered by a great singer, called Mr Mukesh who used to render his voice for playback singing mostly for two legends (i.e., Raj Kapoor and Manoj Kumar), from a Hindi film "Safar"! The song goes like this *"Jo Tumko Ho Pasand Wohi Baat Kahenge Tum Din ko Agar Raat Kaho Raat Kahenge."*

"Hero to heroine: "Dear! Whatever you say about what you like, I too will; if you call a day a night, I too will call the day a night........"

In my 33 years of clinical practice, I have come across a number of hand eczema cases including so called pompholyx (dyshidrotic eczema) evolving into frank psoriasis of palms and soles sooner or later. Yes! Eczematous psoriasis exists, of course, beyond doubt! I confidently claim and ascertain. I have never believed in telling the audience what has been already written in our major textbooks, therefore I have never happened to shout at "public places" as I kept myself busy exploring Indian dermatology with the help of a wonderful hand lens bestowed on me by the almighty. This hand lens is made up of two things: One is the handle that represents the Western literature and the lens is made up of my Indian eyes.

I think and hope my exploration is almost complete; hence this long waits to speak through this book. Long wait……..yes! I wanted to be doubly sure that whatever I am saying is a fact. I am wise enough not to take my learned colleagues for a ride.

I understand that, overseas, there have been no takers for the eczematous behavior of psoriasis; I feel very sad and sorry about that researcher, who had his article "eczematous psoriasis", published in one of the issues of North American Dermatology Clinics more than three decades ago, had not received due attention. It is highly deplorable that somebody's published clinical experience was not only paid due respect, but also suppressed for such a long time, as it has not found place in any of our major textbooks (I come to know that in one of the latest editions of our major textbooks, there were hardly a few lines about this presentation of psoriasis). There are two reasons, I strongly believe for the failure on the part of Caucasian clinicians/researchers not to have paid due respect to eczematous behavior of psoriasis: (1) When psoriasis presents in eczematous form, the biopsy specimen on histopathological examination reads as acute or subacute or chronic eczema, and (2) The overseas clinicians/researchers have been not aware of one fact about psoriasis, i.e., like a killer, who always leaves behind a clue in the scene of a murder, so also psoriasis, but their blind trust in laboratory report does not seem to permit them to search various areas of the body, in puzzling or tricky dermatological presentations, to pickup other findings/clues, which may be not infrequently subtle yet highly significant and thus correlate all the clinical findings and arrive at a particular diagnosis with ease, confidence, and unequivocal specificity.

Their doubts and dilemmas with regard to dandruff and SD to be noted are:

- "Dandruff is said to be the mildest form of SD and yet there is no conclusive evidence for this."[1]
- "Seborrheic dermatitis is a chronic dermatitis that is difficult to define. Validate criteria have not been laid down because of which estimates of its prevalence in different populations are hampered";[1] this, in spite of SD, being described as a dermatitis which exhibits distinctive morphology and distinctive distribution.
- It is included in the chapters of both papulosquamous diseases and endogenous eczemas as well. Thus, it can be considered both as a papulosquamous disease and as an endogenous eczema.
- Though SD occurs in those areas of the skin that are rich in sebaceous glands, yet, the role of seborrhea in the pathogenesis of SD is debatable.
- Some clinicians believe that there is increased prevalence of SD among patients with acne vulgaris (AV) and rosacea, but there are no data to support this.[1-4,9]
- It is not yet established that SD of infancy is the same condition as SD of adolescence and adult life.[1,3,9]
- The histopathology of SD is not specific. It may closely resemble that of psoriasis or dermatitis.[2,3]
- Spongiosis is the only feature that helps discern SD and psoriasis.[2,3]

I cannot, but emphasize one point that their literature makes us stand at crossroads and we never realize this for the simple reason that we, Indians, remain slaves to the opinions/concepts of Caucasians. We never realize that they are clinically a confused lot because their Patient Bank is inadequate; their so-called highly humane laws force them to depend on laboratory for both diagnostic and therapeutic purposes.

At the end of the day, it is their laboratory that plays a key role in the discharge of their medical services to the ailing lot. On the whole, it is a machine-guided tackling of the human disease rather than the physician's clinical acumen and common sense.

But, it is clinical acumen and common sense that had been enabling Indian physicians and surgeons discharge their duties very effectively and thus save the lives of even poorest people in remotest areas of the country, where there was no power supply, anesthetists were not available with minimal routine blood and urine investigations and simple X-ray of the required part, of course, till three decades ago.

7

Mycobiome

It is a section of human skin microbiome. Obesity, graft-versus-host disease, hepatitis B infection, inflammatory bowel disease, etc., according to recent studies, are likely to influence the mycobiome in different sites of the human body. *Malassezia* species dominate most skin surfaces (50–80%).[10,11] Thus, they are found all over the body, predominantly the sebaceous areas that include face, scalp, and back, except feet.[12] It may be noted that the heel, toenails, and toe webs display remarkable diversity, harboring, but few, low voluminous fungi.

As *Malassezia* species are lipophilic yeasts, they are mainly found in the infundibulum of sebaceous gland which provides them the required energy source, i.e., lipids that are freely available in abundance.[13,14]

Among the *Malassezia* species, while in children it is *Malassezia globosa* (*M. globosa*) that is common whereas in adults it is *Malassezia sympodialis*, which is present in abundance. On the trunk, it is *M. globosa* that predominates, while on head and face it is *Malassezia restricta*. These variations can be attributed to the different lipid preferences of *Malassezia* species and also to the age factor that influences the composition of secreted lipids.

8

Role of Yeasts in Dandruff and Seborrheic Dermatitis

It was first Louis-Charles Malassez (1874)[15] who proposed the role of fungi in seborrheic dermatitis (SD) and therefore he was honored by giving his name to the genus of yeasts that have been isolated from the lesional skin in SD and dandruff. Prior to this, only *Pityrosporum ovale* and *Pityrosporum orbiculare* were thought to be part of the normal flora of the skin. Subsequently, these two yeasts were reclassified in the genus *Malassezia* as a single species *Malassezia furfur* (*M. furfur*). Later on, advances in genetic analysis demonstrated 13 separate species of lipophilic yeasts; of these, seven species are more common on human skin.[16]

What came to be known as *M. furfur* is probably a complex of species, in particular *Malassezia globosa* (*M. globosa*). This complex densely colonizes some particular areas of the skin that are rich in sebaceous glands such as scalp, the upper trunk, and flexures. While pityriasis versicolor is most commonly associated with *M. globosa* according to some researchers, according to some it is *Malassezia sympodialis* and *M. furfur*. Recent works suggest that *M. globosa* and *Malassezia restricta* are most commonly associated with SD and dandruff and few other species were also isolated from some patients.[16] Thus, it becomes evident that *M. globosa* plays a role in the pathogenesis of both pityriasis versicolor and SD and dandruff.[1,16]

9
When does a Commensal Turn Pathogenic?

It is well-known that some *Malassezia* exhibits more pathogenic potential, as they turn mycelial more readily. It need not be emphasized that the prevalence of pityriasis versicolor is fairly high among people living in warmer climates with high humidity and hot humid weather is a predisposing factor for pityriasis versicolor, apart from host factors, implying that *Malassezia* species, which are part of normal flora of the skin and which are not conventional pathogens, can turn pathogenic when a predisposing factor or factors exist. As *Malassezia globosa* is common to both pityriasis versicolor and seborrheic dermatitis (SD)/dandruff, that subclinical hyperkeratosis is the predisposing factor for increasing colonization by *Malassezia* species on scalp and other seborrheic areas is not a far-from-truth assumption, I opine.

How a Genius Succeeds in Putting an End to the Long Drawn Controversy Shrouding Dandruff versus Yeasts?

For many decades, role of yeasts in the pathogenesis of seborrheic dermatitis (SD)/dandruff was not established beyond doubt till a Genius, after undertaking an amazing and assiduous exercise of reviewing a vast literature, that had got piled up over more than a century, concluded very convincingly with his robust scientific logic (RSL) that yeasts play a primary role in the pathogenesis of dandruff and thus pulled the curtain down forever.[17] "That yeasts play a primary role" was somehow I could not digest. I thought I better go through his article that appeared in one of the issues of a popular journal published overseas. His English was something unusual and the sentence construction was very tough. I found it rather difficult to assimilate; hence, I went on reading the article umpteen numbers of times. At last, I could emerge victorious in understanding his arguments, his scathing attack on the researchers finding fault with the standard of literature, opining it is poor, with defects in design, methods, statistics, and interpretation.[17]

He frankly expresses his aversion toward the hypothesis that dandruff (pityriasis capitis) is primarily a hyperproliferative disorder and ruthlessly criticizes those researchers and authors who strongly favored this hypothesis.

He, similarly, strongly dislikes the promoters of the concept that emerges from the reports that describe cytostatic agents as being effective in ameliorating dandruff because such studies support the hypothesis that dandruff is primarily a hyperproliferative disorder.[18,19]

He, vested with RSL, does not hesitate to vehemently argue in favor of *Pityrosporum ovale* (*P. ovale*) being directly responsible for causing visible desquamation on scalp (i.e., dandruff) based on the experiments conducted by the researchers; this visible desquamation is due to the presence of *P. ovale* in large numbers on the scalps afflicted with dandruff, i.e., removing the *P. ovale* from scalp skin with the help of an antifungal agent such as selenium sulfide, nystatin, or a more effective agent such as ketoconazole that results in remission of the dandruff and on recolonization of the scalp with the yeast, dandruff relapses.[17]

He also refutes the published reports on the role of cytostatic agents in the management of dandruff; if cytostatic agents were to be effective in dandruff, it could be due to their inhibitory effect on one of the *P. ovale*-induced pathogenic mechanisms inciting secondary hyperproliferation of epidermis and not due to their effect on normal epidermopoiesis. He warns against the use of cytostatic agents in the management of dandruff as the role of *P. ovale* is obvious and more so in the light of such reports which promote the causative role of *P. ovale* in dandruff and he laments that such reports were buried under a huge rock of human error due to poor standard of the literature with defects in design, methods, etc.[17]

Nevertheless, one is bound to appreciate rather recognize this Genius as an honest professor to the core, if one goes through his article because he repeats the following lines at least four times in his article: "Mild psoriasis and SD cannot be differentiated from dandruff either clinically or histopathologically."[17]

Apart from his being an honest and an astute reviewer, he appears to exhibit his lack of adequate clinical experience by expressing/suggesting the following (perhaps, it is not nice on my part to pass this comment about him; after all, after reviewing such vast literature that is studded with meaningless, ridiculous, and funny research works, one's IQ levels are bound to scale down along a vertical axis at least transiently).

"Simple diagnostic studies allowing a panel of clinicians to examine only the scalp are required to validate diagnostic criteria."[17]

My simple question to him in a very humble manner—"Respected sir! You yourself admit that mild SD and psoriasis cannot be distinguished from dandruff. In clinical practice, whenever a patient presents with the condition of scaling scalp, a dermatologist tends to look for evidence of either SD or psoriasis by examining other areas of the skin. Then, how can a panel of clinicians examine only the scalp to validate diagnostic criteria for dandruff?"

His RSL continues to argue against the hypothesis that dandruff is primarily a proliferative disorder leading to visible desquamation and the alleged cytostatic action, i.e., of antidandruff agents, a decrease in dandruff (assessed clinically or measured as scale) has been found after the use of selenium sulfide, zinc pyrithione, nystatin, and econazole, was, because the common feature of all the agents employed in ameliorating dandruff, was their antifungal action and argues further that none of the studies, he reviewed, provided any concrete evidence in favor of the cytostatic action of the wide ranging agents that were employed.

Now the Genius applies his RSL further; if the cytostatic effect by antifungals was to be true, then how is it possible to justify the presence of heavy colonies of the fungus in scalps with dandruff, if the fungus had no causative role in the pathogenesis of dandruff and then how to accept dandruff being primarily a hyperproliferative disorder in the light of the evidence provided by various studies that after the use of antifungals, the fungal colonies drastically come down and on stopping antifungals, not only does dandruff recur, there is again heavy colonization of the scalp by the fungus.[20,21]

The Genius does not fail to admit, at the end of his article, a doubt, as to how *P. ovale* induces dandruff is not clear: Inflammation and desquamation with some increase in cell production (i.e., hyperproliferation or increased cell turnover is the end result, meaning that the cytostatic effect attributed to antidandruff agents could be because of indirect inhibition of one of the *P. ovale*-induced mechanisms that induce increased cell turnover, i.e., by their direct effect on the fungus).[17]

▇ THE MISTAKES/BLUNDERS

Which I committed in my three decades of clinical practice both as a faculty member and as a private practitioner, I strongly opine rather reiterate that a doctor working as a faculty should be allowed to do his/her private practice in the time available for him or her. It has two wonderful advantages; one is, he acquires excellent clinical and therapeutic skills which are very useful to OPD patients and private patients and the second is, it enables him/her to emerge as a highly skilled clinical teacher due to the fact that he sees a good number of patients in his private clinic on his own with no scope for obtaining clinical help whatsoever from other faculty. This results in escalation of the dermatologist's self-confidence levels day by day.

MISTAKES COMMITTED AND LESSONS LEARNT

Had I not committed these mistakes (thanks to the overseas literature), I would not have missed scalp psoriasis in all such cases till January 2003.

At the end of his pains taking review of a vast literature, piled up over 108 years, he frankly admits that there are some doubts rather questions that remain to be answered which include what exactly is the pathogenic role played by *P. ovale* in inducing scaling of scalp and the other is an individual's susceptibility to *P. ovale*-induced scaling of scalp remains obscure and the third is how dandruff evolves into SD and the fourth is, is dandruff, in fact, psoriasis, by any chance, representing pityrosporal Koebner phenomenon and lastly, there is no clarity obtained with regard to clinical and histopathological dissociation of dandruff from early SD and psoriasis.[17]

Respected Genius Sir! Hats off to you for your dedication and sincerity displayed by you in reviewing such a vast literature and also your honesty and frankness in expressing your doubts and for raising certain relevant questions in your article while forcing *P. ovale* into wedlock with dandruff, instead of psoriasis.

The Author's Viewpoint Rather Counterargument

Sir! It is a well-known fact that for a commensal like *Pityrosporum ovale* (*P. ovale*) to become pathogenic, there must be some predisposing factor and that is nothing but primary hyperproliferation of psoriatic origin which does not express clinically. Then you raise a question as to what makes an individual susceptible to *P. ovale* infection. It is the same genetic susceptibility that makes an individual susceptible to psoriasis.

You yourself justified my argument by expressing a doubt as to how much even of scalp psoriasis is a pityrosporal Koebner phenomenon and also by concluding that clinical and histopathological dissociation of dandruff from early seborrheic eczema and psoriasis has not been made by any of the research works that you happened to review.

God created 1,000s of microorganisms and bestowed on some of them the privilege of being part of inside of and the outer surface of human body and to live as commensals, symbionts, and pathogens. He permits the same commensals to become pathogenic whenever, there arises a predisposing factor in the human body (a commensal is defined as a microorganism that benefits from the host, but the host does not benefit from it, but it can become pathogenic when local factors favor it, though commensals are not regarded as conventional pathogens).

Thus, the creator proves himself mischievous and naughty like a kid.

The basis for my opinion that there exists psoriasis in a subclinical state:

- Not infrequently, a patient approaches me complaining of severe itching that initially began on lower legs and slowly progressed in a stepwise fashion to involve rest of the body; the skin over lower legs appears apparently normal. Then, my (right) upper limb involuntarily reaches the glass side box on my table and picks up one glass slide. Then, my (right) hand starts stroking the skin over both the shins; to my utter surprise, the skin that is apparently normal turns scaly, i.e., silvery white.
- Patients present to me with the history of dandruff; when I examine their scalps, typical, discrete, and scaly plaques are found. I do stroke the apparently normal looking skin in between the plaques. It turns scaly; not just scaly, my act of stroking elicits significant amount of silvery white scales. (Plewig G, Kligman AM. The effect of selenium sulfide on epidermal turnover of normal and dandruff scalps. J Soc Cosmet Chem. 1969;20:767-75)
- I do not understand why the Genius was so averse to the opinion of some of the researchers (whose publications he

reviewed) that dandruff could be primarily a hyperproliferative disorder, on the basis of, attributing the effectiveness of some cytostatic agents in ameliorating dandruff or the antifungals could be, because, of exerting a cytostatic effect rather than their antifungal property per se.

It is well-known rather does not need to be reiterated that for a commensal to turn pathogenic, it requires a predisposing factor and that is nothing but (as already mentioned above) subclinical hyperkeratosis (i.e., subclinical psoriasis). The fact that your robust scientific logic (RSL) proposes that the antifungals might be inhibiting a cytostatic mechanism, incited by the yeast as one of its pathogenic mechanisms, in ameliorating dandruff also speaks volumes in favor of the so-called dandruff, being a hyperproliferative disorder (irrespective of it being primary or secondary to *P. ovale*); hence, the researchers, at least a very few of them, might have successfully employed the cytostatic agents that were available those times, in the treatment of dandruff.

These three instances, I need not emphasize, are enough to suggest that there exists psoriasis in a subclinical state (subclinical histopathology of psoriasis is already reported and described). This subclinical psoriasis on scalp, acts as a predisposing factor, provides an otherwise conventionally nonpathologic commensal, i.e., *P. ovale* ample opportunity to multiply and produce a heavy colony of its species. Various agents/substances, I propose, elaborated by this yeast's colony, incite inflammatory changes, and thus result in visible desquamation initially followed by heavy scaling, during which process it evolves into frank psoriatic plaques.

This visible desquamation was mistaken to dandruff and its more inflammatory form to seborrheic dermatitis (SD) and this resulted in an unwarranted, 108-year-old long-drawn research concerning dandruff and SD as to their etiopathogenesis, because, the same mistakes that I committed before 2003, seem to have been committed by our Caucasian researchers and clinical dermatologists.

Their failure to define and find evidence in favor of seborrhea/sebum in the pathogenesis of so-called SD; their dilemmas as to whether infantile SD represents the same SD of adolescence and adults, the role of cytostatic effect in ameliorating dandruff rather than the antifungal action of various antifungals of different chemical nature becoming part of the debate as a result of published reports describing antifungal's cytostatic effect, though this was refuted by the Genius while he himself admitting that dandruff cannot be differentiated from early SD and psoriasis and authors/researchers/the Genius frankly admitting that there is lot of clinical and histopathological overlap between dandruff, SD, and psoriasis and these points keeping the minds of researchers and clinical dermatologists confused for decades together leading to unwarranted research and piling up of vast literature ever since Malassez authored (1874) his "Note sur le champignon du pityriasis simple" amply justify my argument that unless the dermatologist learns to look beyond the lesion exhibited by the patient and also look beyond the patient and thus pickup various clinical findings from the patient and a positive history of clinical features as to psoriasis from the accompanying genetically-related subject and/or pedigrees and unless finally correlate all of them, he cannot make an apt diagnosis. For common diseases, it is foolish to depend on a histopathology, as per my experience as a dermatologist practicing/teaching in India which provides me a vast patient bank.

All their mistakes/confusions/dilemmas leading to forwarding their so-called (ill-conceived) hypothesis which would be thrust on global community, resulting in, in particular, Indian dermatologists, unable to derive job satisfaction and at the end of the day returning home in a frustrated state. Perhaps, many sensitive dermatologists, I guess, indulge in cursing themselves for having become dermatologists: What a pity?

Dermatology, perhaps, is the most adorable of all the medical branches and provides immense job satisfaction. Thanks to the Western literature, which has killed the happiness of many dermatologists of my country and made them suffer from inferiority complex and it needs to be emphasized that, after some time, this inferiority complex transforms into superiority complex, which is bound to hurt the ego of fellow dermatologists and it is a vicious cycle into which finally all such dermatologists get entangled.

All cases of dandruff, I do not hesitate to reiterate, are nothing but psoriasis capitis; it initially remains in a subclinical state. This clinical observation of mine that there exists a state of subclinical hyperkeratosis is well-supported by the following studies: (1) Abnormal epidermal dynamics is observed in clinically normal skin in psoriasis patients.[22,23] (2) K16 expression is observed in nonlesional posiratic skin and may serve as a marker of preclinical psoriasis.[24] Many studies have shown that K6 and K16 represent hyperproliferative keratins.[25-27] The following lines found in overseas literature, also, seem to support my view that scalps with dandruff (devoid of frank psoriatic plaques) represent a very mild, psoriasis capitis (i.e., subclinical hyperkeratosis). This is the predisposing factor for colonization by the commensal *P. ovale*. As this progresses, the subclinical psoriasis becomes a little more inflammatory and causes itching.

Moderate-to-severe pruritus is a frequent complaint made by psoriatic patients in this region, while few patients flatly deny history of itching. The itching, by disturbing their sleep during nights,[28,29] causes impairment of quality of life, thus in turn, subjecting them to heightened stress. One report describes that itching caused by psoriasis is not as severe as itching in atopic eczema,[7] but, this is contrary to my personal experience. Thus, psoriasis, being a pruritic disease, the act of scratching, vigorous toweling of scalp after a shower, and frequent combing of hair, results in displacement of the loose parakeratotic cells which land on hair shafts, i.e., visible desquamation (which was mistaken to dandruff).

There appears to be a consensus among various contributing authors of different editions of a major textbook as to histopathology of SD (dandruff is said to be the mildest form of SD and yet there is no conclusive evidence for this).[1] The histopathology of SD is not diagnostic, but generally shows features of both psoriasis and chronic dermatitis.[1,3,9]

The Caucasians keep spongiosis in high esteem and deem it a crucial finding that helps discern psoriasis and SD. I have come across a remarkable number of patients with hand eczema evolving into frank psoriasis at a later date. A report[30] describes occurrence of spongiosis in 3 of 28 patients who developed SD-like picture on face, who were undergoing psoralen and ultraviolet A (PUVA) treatment for their psoriasis. It anguishes rather puzzles me why Caucasian colleagues tend to ignore, not infrequently, the Koebner phenomenon (perhaps to their convenience). I interpret those 28 patients of 402 patients, who were undergoing PUVA treatment for their psoriasis, developed sebopsoriasis as a result of Koebner phenomenon on their faces which was mistaken to SD.

It is time for the global community of dermatologists to accept spongiosis as a feature of not only SD but also psoriasis. I have already discussed about the eczematous behavior of psoriasis (see above) and I also consider it as the most common atypical presentation of psoriasis in this region. I have had noticed, not infrequently, the presence of flesh colored or erythematous, edematous papules amidst classical lesions of psoriasis in my patients in this region.

It has been very unfortunate and misleading that the overseas literature has not taken cognizance of various lesions produced by psoriasis. I give two reasons for their failure in this respect. Reason 1: Their failure to realize that a given cutaneous disease in a given patient may produce different morphological lesions at different locations of the body and Reason 2: Their robust trust (rather forced to trust) in histopathology report.

The Genius, in spite of having reviewed such a vast literature, could not understand what makes an individual susceptible to dandruff, even though, he expresses repeatedly his dilemma as to early SD and psoriasis cannot be distinguished either clinically or histopathologically.[17] The genetic/predisposing factors in acquiring SD have not found place in many editions of two popular textbooks, except in the editions of one of the same. While one of the two major textbooks makes a statement, a family history of SD is often available,[4] the following is described by those two textbooks.

An Israeli Jewish Moroccan family was found with an autosomal dominant "seborrhea-like dermatitis" with psoriasiform elements reported to have been caused by a mutation within the ZNF750 encoding a C2H2 zinc finger protein.[31] The latest edition of a major textbook, while describing the same report[31] as above, replaces ZNF750 with PSORS2 locus.[1] At least nine chromosomal loci with statistically significant evidence for linkage (PSORS1-PSORS9) in determining genetic susceptibility to psoriasis have been identified by classical genome-wide linkage analysis in pedigrees.[32]

Thus, the Israeli Jewish Moroccan family is described to have a "seborrhea-like dermatitis" with psoriatic elements, mediated by a mutation in a particular gene locus PSORS2 (which is also incriminated in determining genetic susceptibility to psoriasis). This report enables me to strongly opine that the "seborrhea-like dermatitis" with psoriatic elements described in the above family was, in fact, an atypical presentation of sebopsoriasis that was mistaken to SD by the authors.

Two more issues concerning SD are still debatable as per the overseas literature. First issue: SD in infancy and adulthood cannot be deemed as the same beyond doubt and Second issue: Even though SD occurs predominantly in sebaceous gland-rich areas of the skin, till date, researchers could not prove the exact role of sebum in the pathogenesis of SD. Let me keep aside this issue: Why should some psoriatics display predilection for seborrheic areas? Why should psoriasis confine only to seborrheic areas in some? The answer from my side is: When I argued in favour of *P. ovale* becoming pathogenic taking advantage of subclinical psoriatic state of scalp, the same should hold good for psoriasis preferring seborrheic areas elsewhere.

Author's Final Word

Should I still believe that there exist three separate entities, i.e., (1) Dandruff, (2) Seborrheic dermatitis (SD), and (3) Psoriasis vulgaris (PsV). In view of the clinical and histopathological overlap between dandruff, SD, and psoriasis, spongiosis being a feature of SD and PsV, and genetic predisposition determining gene locus for SD being PSORS2 which also determines genetic susceptibility to psoriasis (though PSORS1 is the predominant gene locus in determining genetic susceptibility to PsV; in fact, there are a total of nine loci, i.e., PSORS1-PSORS9), many issues concerning SD still remain unresolved/debatable and the fact that our Genius was wondering how to explain this increasing colonization by *Pityrosporum ovale* (*P. ovale*) of the scalps with dandruff, without *P. ovale* playing a primary pathogenic role in dandruff (it was because what failed to strike the mind of the Genius was that psoriasis can exist in a subclinical state); but, as he was obsessed with the idea that dandruff is not primarily a hyperproliferative disorder and the hyperproliferation seen in dandruff was secondary to some mechanism, induced and employed by *P. ovale*. The Genius expresses his extreme aversion toward such studies that promote the theory of dandruff as primarily a hyperproliferative disorder,[33-37] for reasons known to him only.[38]

Perhaps, because of a predisposing factor, commensal-turning pathogenic link slipping off his mind and the Genius failing to realize that a predisposing factor exists in the form of subclinical hyperproliferation of epidermis, he strongly refutes such studies (commenting that their study design is imprecise and poor) which describe that antidandruff agents exert a cytostatic effect and thus ameliorate dandruff; against this scenario of controversies, debatable issues, dilemmas in respect of dandruff, SD in infancy and adulthood, and sebopsoriasis being mistaken to SD, 100% clarity can be instantaneously achieved, if I do not escape to ascertain that all the four, i.e., (1) Pityriasis capitis, (2) SD, (3) PsV, and (4) Sebopsoriasis belong to the same spectrum of a disease process, i.e., psoriasis.

I might not be wrong in guessing that most of my esteemed colleagues find it very difficult to digest or find it highly unpalatable my above statement/conclusion because of the following facts: (1) My stature is confined to a localized region, (2) I have no identity either at national or international level as a speaker, and (3) Nor do I have many papers, published in reputed journals, to my credit. I would like to place before you one fact, i.e., I may sound dogmatic, but I ascertain that I do not believe in such an approach. But anybody who gets interested in proving me wrong one is most welcome to do so. In fact, I kept myself checking whether, my clinical experience/observations match the overseas literature or not and the result of my exercise is emergence of this book with two monograms.

I may also add that why SD in Caucasians produces greasy yellowish scales? The sebum composition and their dietary habits such as carrot consumption, etc., should be subjected to intensive research, so that the cause of yellowish and greasy character of the scale in SD (which kept the Caucasian community of dermatologists misleading them to mistake sebopsoriasis to SD) can be determined.

Color Atlas of Dandruff

I. Dandruff in Adults
(No. of Patients Depicted—14)

Patient 1

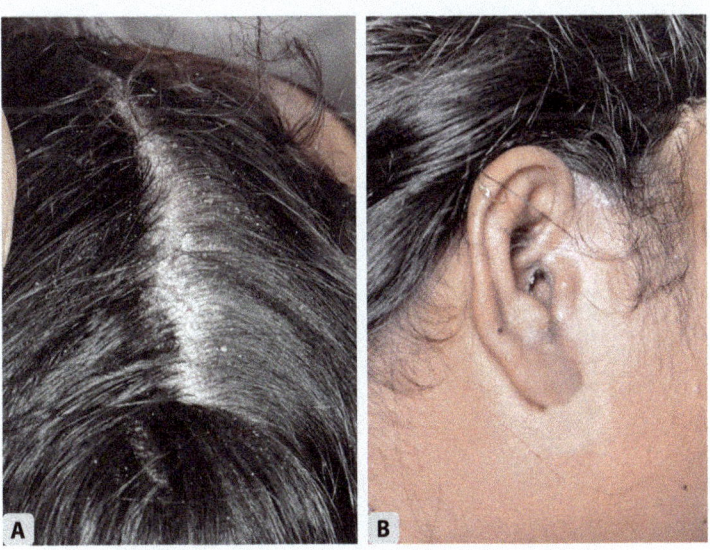

PATIENT 1: A 24-year-old housewife with 2 years history of dandruff. (A) Hair parting is significantly scaly. (B) (R) External earlobe-interior of the (R) ear and periauricular area scaly. A plaque of psoriasis may be noted adjoining the upper part of earlobe.

Patient 2

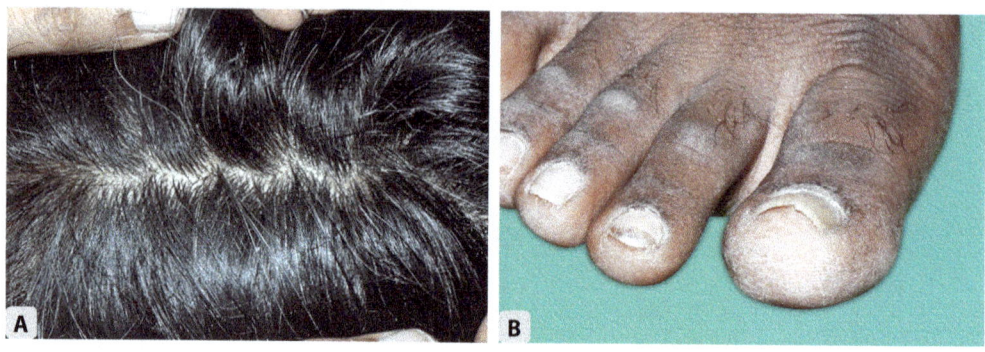

PATIENT 2: (A) A 20-year-old engineering student with 4 years history of dandruff; and (B) (Right) great toenail (GTN) displays angulation.

Patient 3A (father of the above patient)

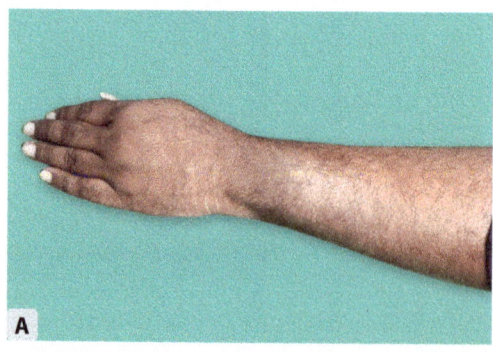

PATIENT 3A: A group of scaly papules in one of the sun-exposed areas, i.e., photodistribution (PD).

Color Atlas of Dandruff

Patient 3B (father of the patient 2)

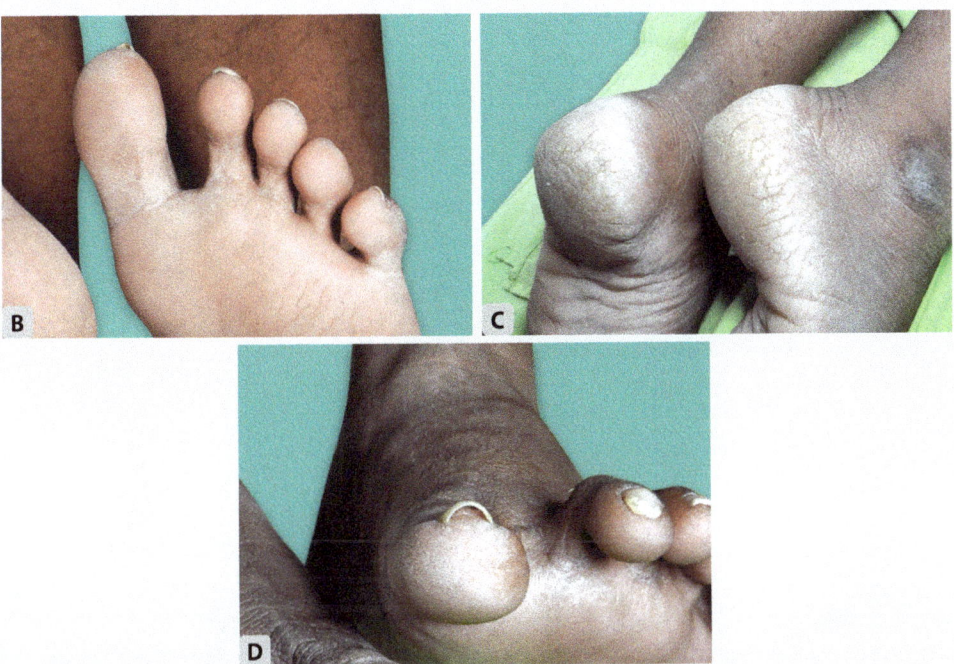

PATIENT 3B: (B) Under toe HK; (C) Heels: HK fissuring; and (D) (Left) GTN: Overcurvature.
(GTN: great toenail; HK: hyperkeratosis)

Patient 4

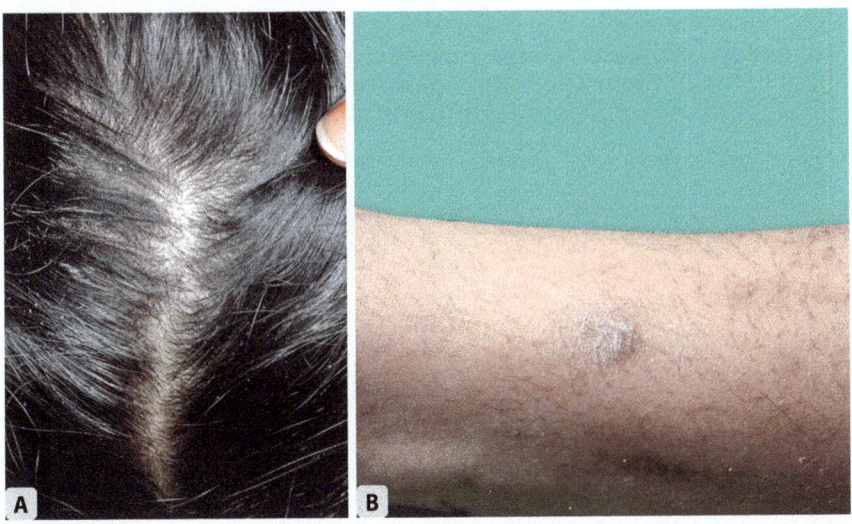

PATIENT 4: An 18-year-old (female)—a school dropout—2 years history of dandruff.
(A) Hair shafts—visible desquamation; and (B) (Left) lower leg—well-defined scaly plaque.

Patient 5

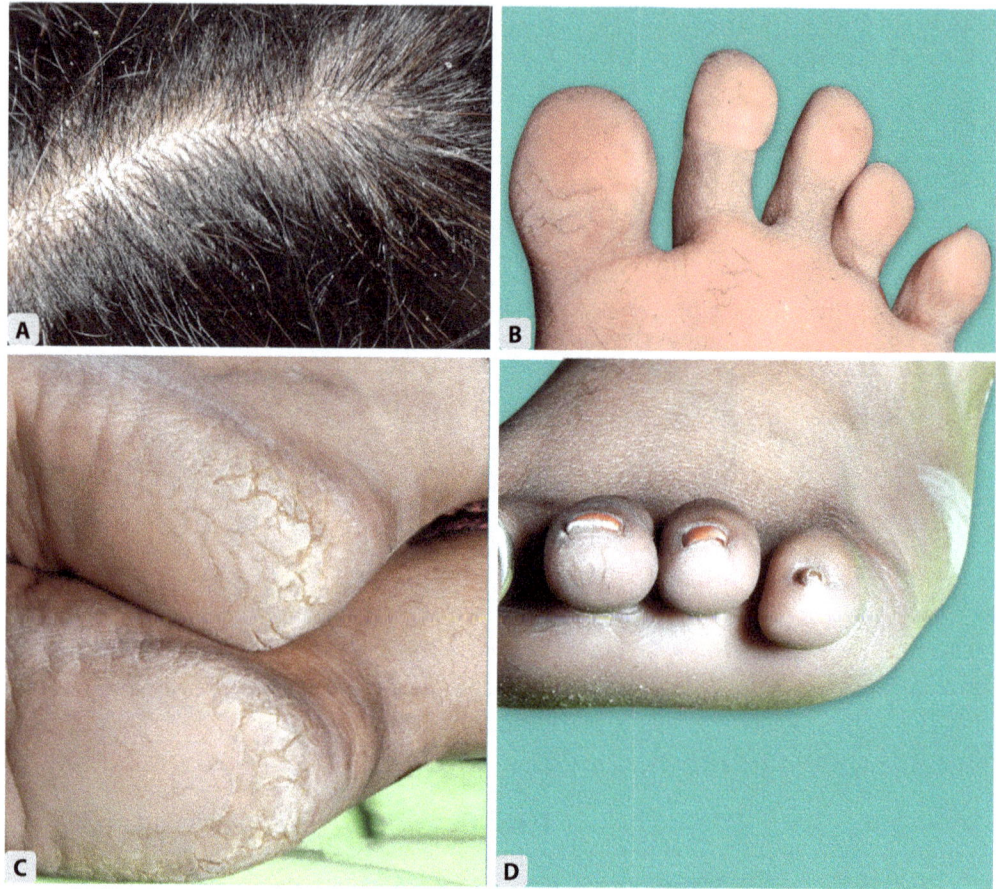

PATIENT 5: A 39-year-old housewife—2 years history of dandruff. (A) Visible desquamation; (B) Under toe—HK; (C) Heels—remarkable HK and fissuring; and (D) LTN—pincer nail.

(HK: hyperkeratosis; LTN: little toenail)

Patient 6A

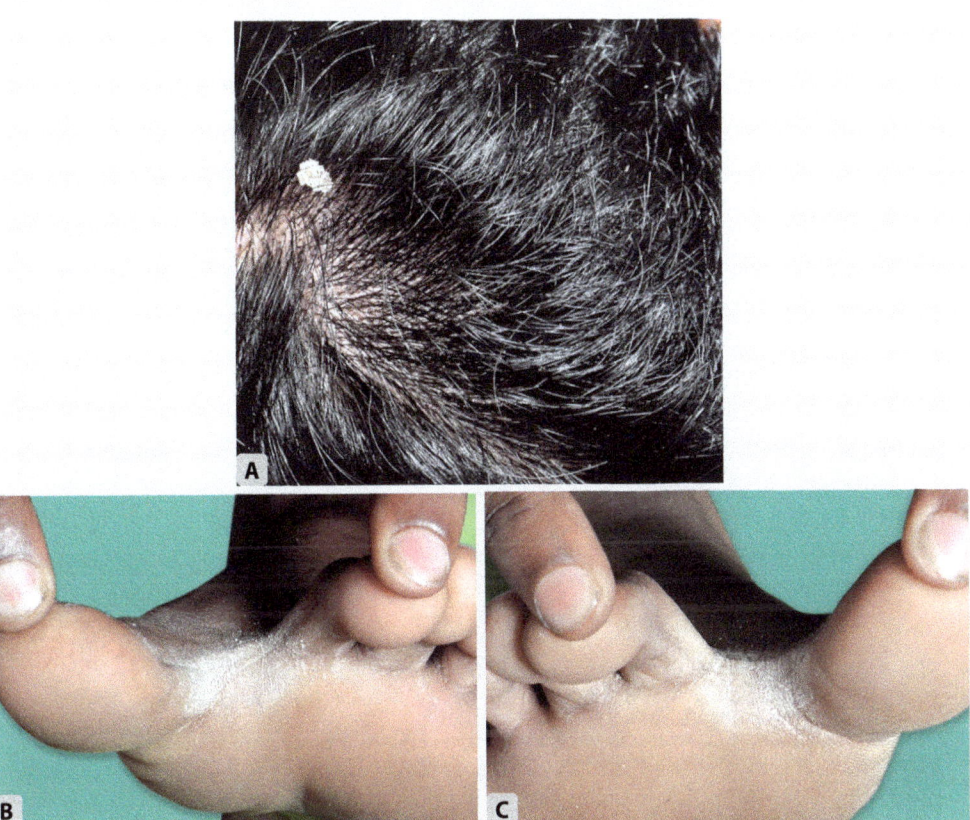

PATIENT 6A: A 23-year-old male—an engineering graduate—10 years history of dandruff. (A) Occiput area of scalp—visible desquamation; and (B and C) Toe webs—hyperkeratosis (HK) and scaling (after stroking).

Patient 6B

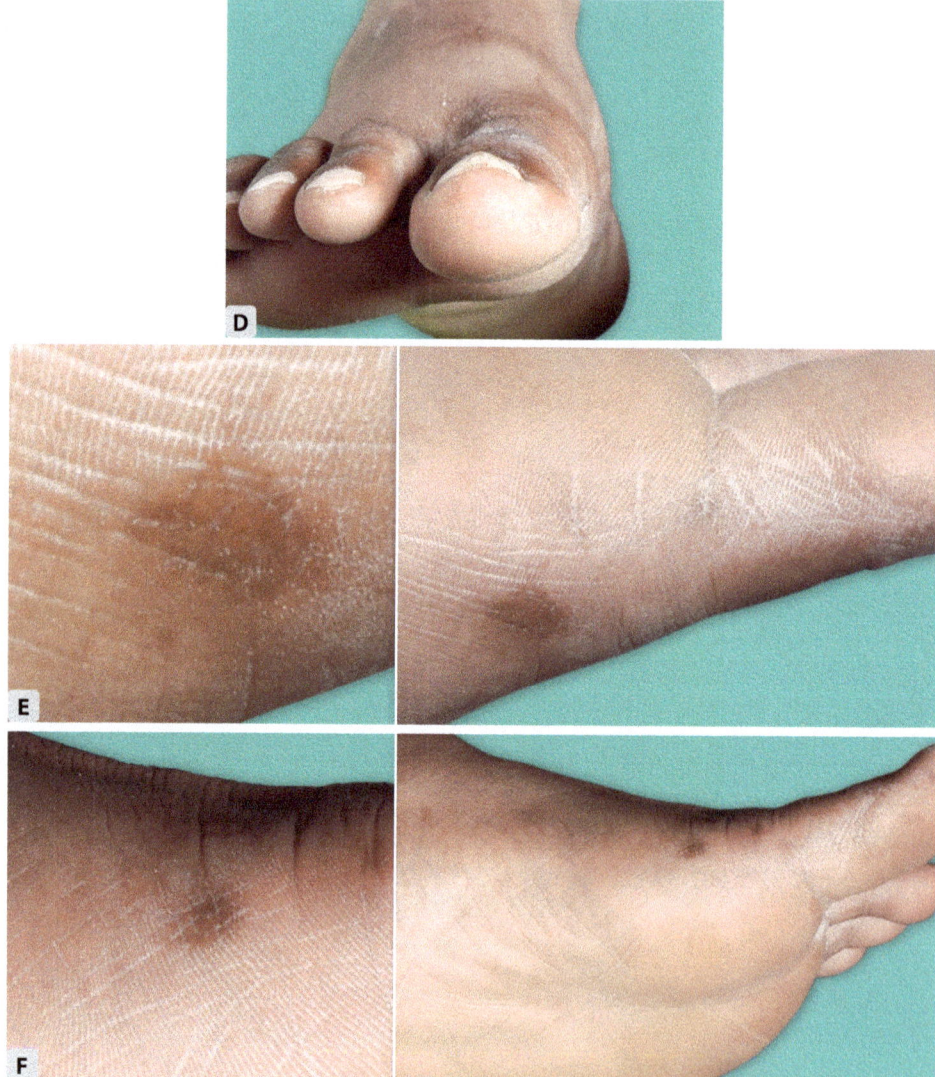

PATIENT 6B: (D) (Right) great toenail (GTN)—angulation; (E) Medial border of (right) forefoot—a group of vesicles; and (F) Same as in "E" but of the other foot.

Patient 7

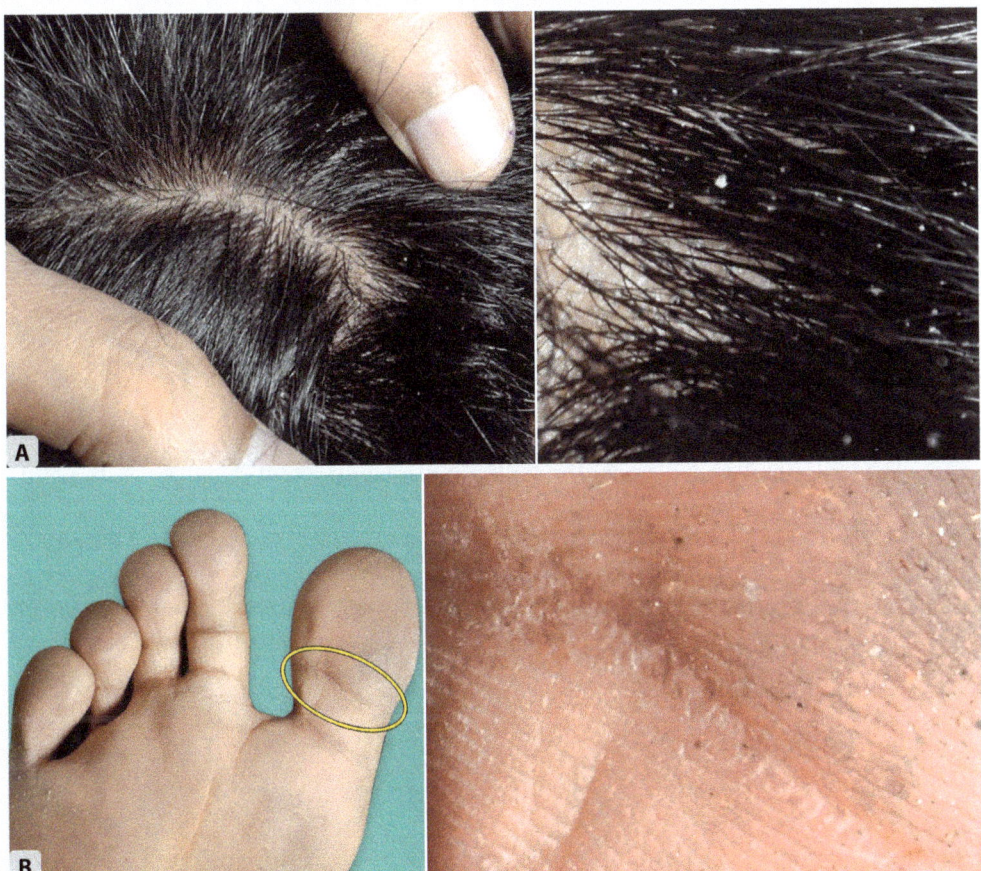

PATIENT 7: A 17-year-old student—2 years history of itching and scaling of scalp.
(A) Vertex—minimal scaling, enlarged image of (A)—more scales may be noted on hair shafts; and
(B) Undersurface of (right) great toe (GT)—an ill-formed scaly plaque across the surface of under toe (yellow circle).

Additional information: History of dandruff in his brother. Paternal grandfather is a known case of psoriasis vulgaris.

Patient 8

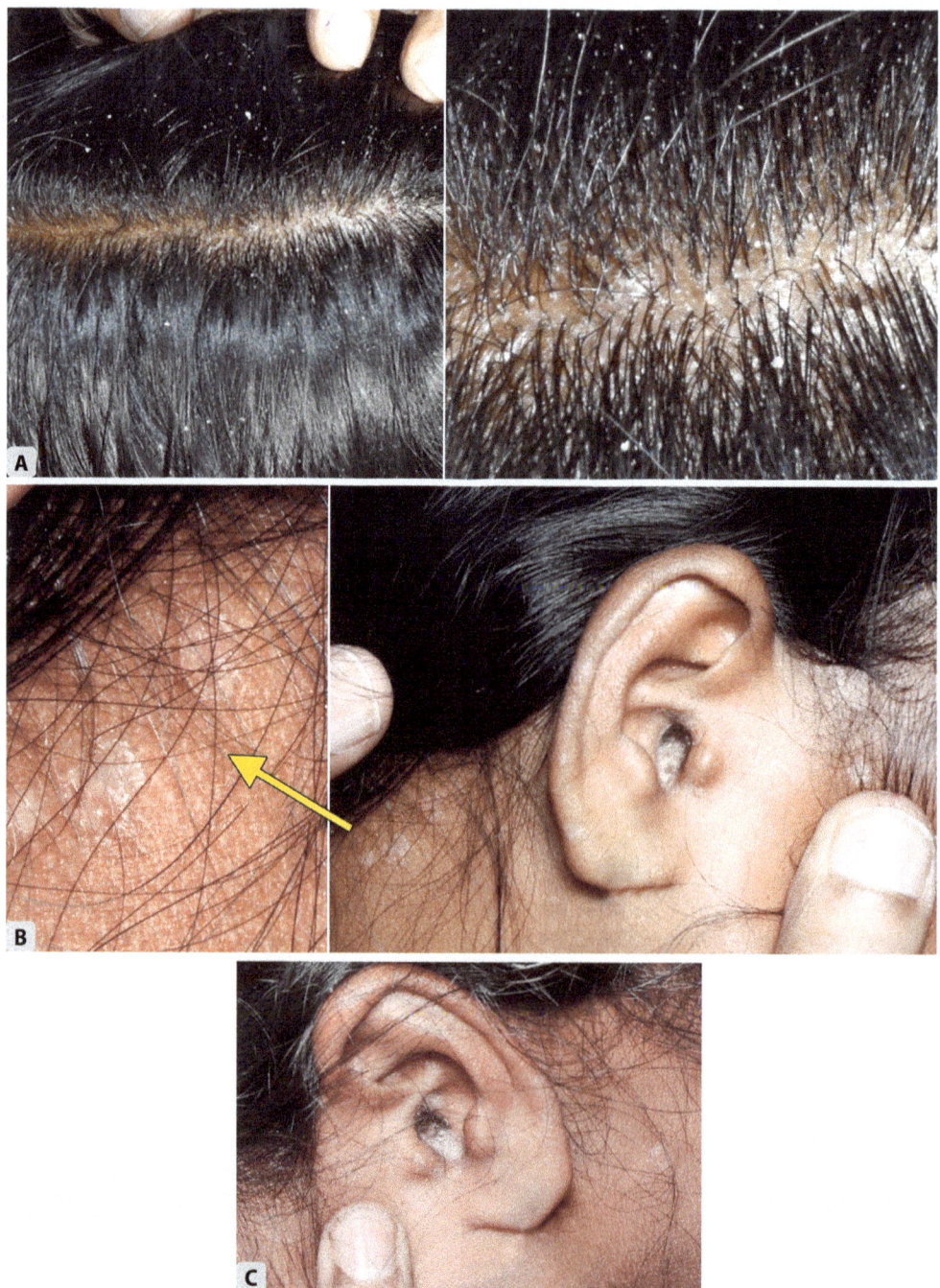

PATIENT 8: A 26-year-old employed engineer—1 month history of dandruff. (A) Scalp—visible desquamation; (B) (Right) external auditory canal—scaling (yellow arrow) and (right) posterior neck—discrete thin plaques of psoriasis; and (C) Same as in "B".

Patient 9

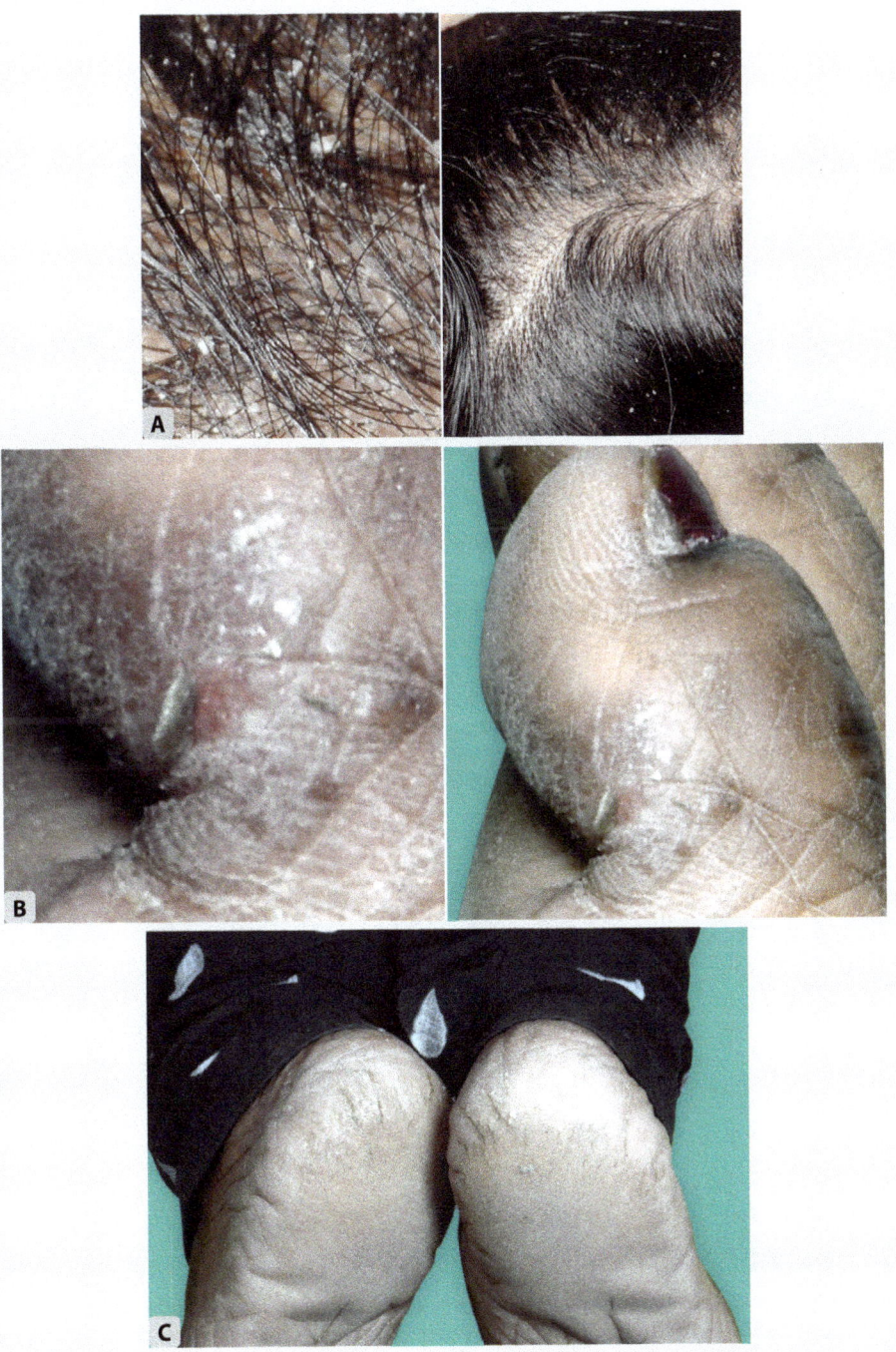

PATIENT 9: A 33-year-old housewife—7 years history of recurrent dandruff. (A) Scalp—visible desquamation; (B) Outer aspect of little toe—grouped vesicular eruption; and (C) Heels—hyperkeratosis (HK) and fissuring.

Patient 10

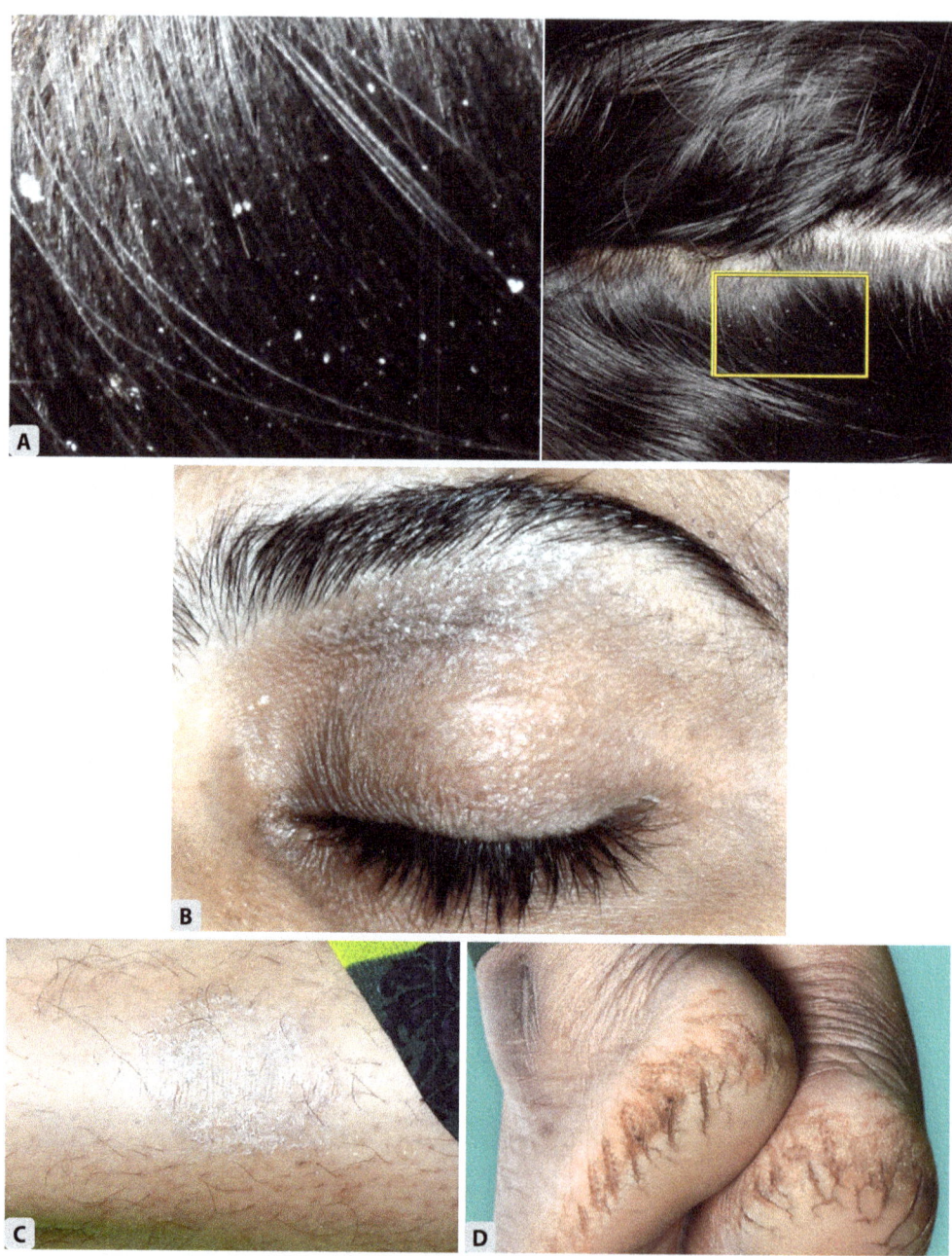

PATIENT 10: A 40-year-old housewife—2 years history of recurrent dandruff. (A) Scalp—visible desquamation (yellow box); (B) A thin plaque of psoriasis on her (left) upper eyelid; (C) A similar lesion on (right) shin; and (D) Heels—hyperkeratosis (HK) and fissuring.

Patient 11

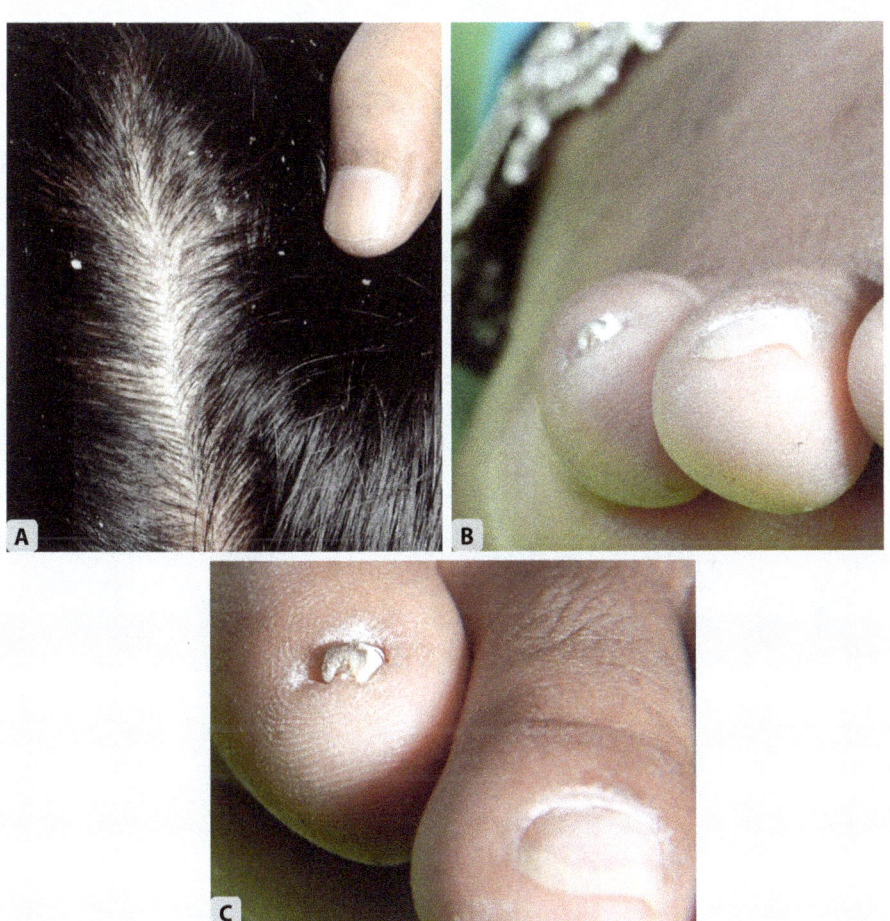

PATIENT 11: A 21-year-old housewife—3 months history of dandruff (A) Scalp—visible desquamation; (B) (Right) fourth toenail—angulation; and (C) (Right) little toenail (LTN)—tent-like elevation/pincer nail.

Patient 12A

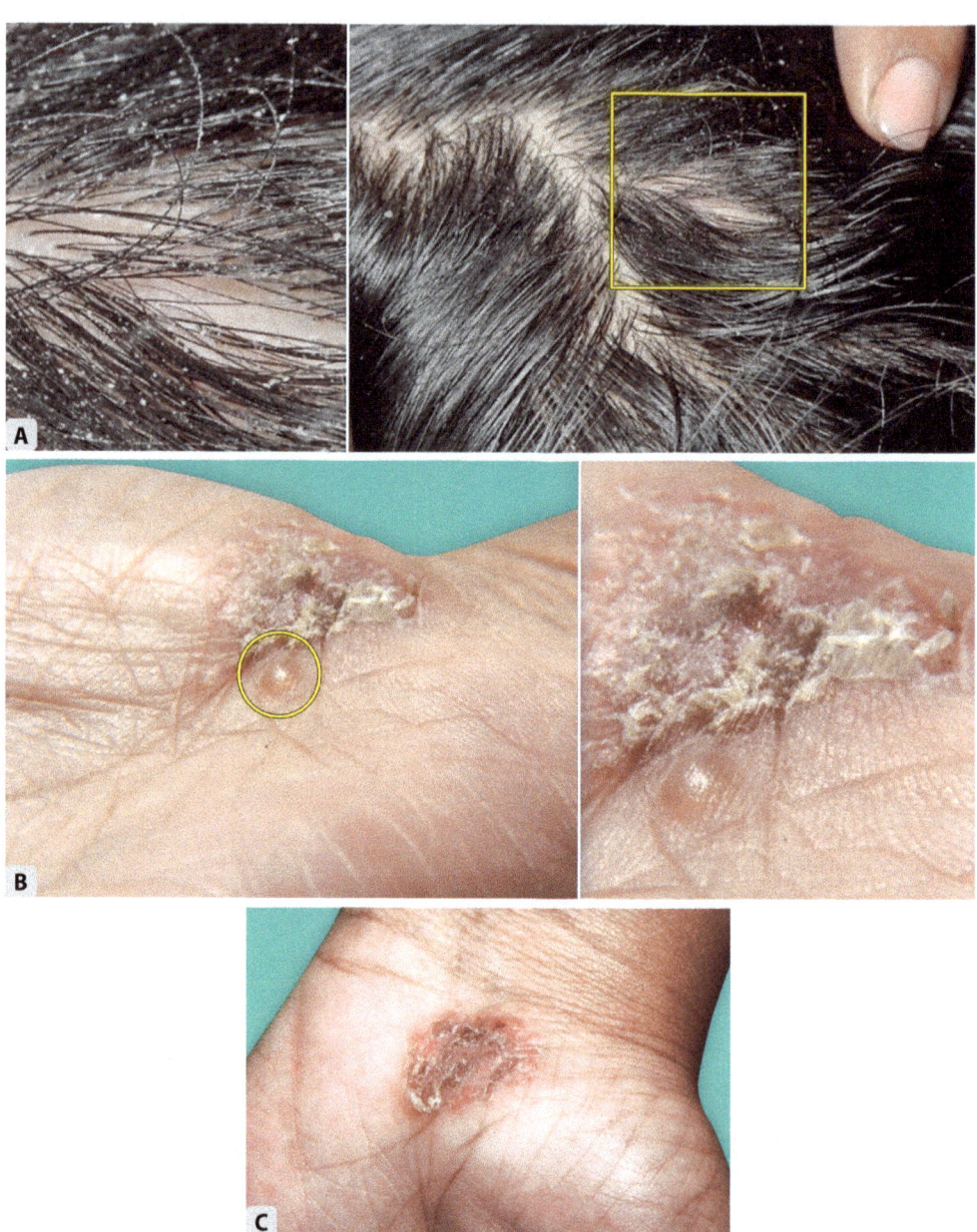

PATIENT 12A: A 23-year-old working woman—1 year history of scaling of scalp and recurrent vesicular eruption of palms and soles from the age of 5 years (18 years duration). (A) Occiput—visible desquamation (yellow box); (B) A seemingly eczematous plaque—in 5 o'clock position—an intact vesicle may be noted on (right) palm (yellow circle); and (C) Similar lesion in (left) palm as in "B".

Patient 12B

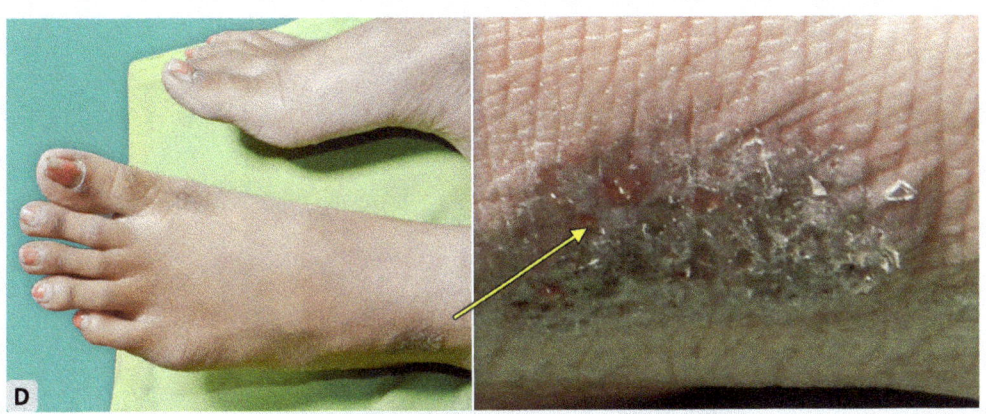

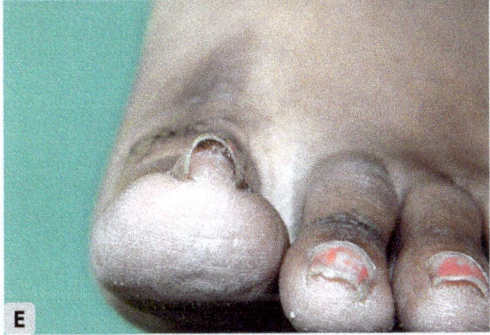

PATIENT 12B: A 23-year-old working woman—1 year history of scaling of scalp and recurrent vesicular eruption of palms and soles from the age of 5 years (18 years duration). (D) An excoriated psoriatic plaque—dorsum (left) foot (yellow arrow); and (E) (Left) great toenail (GTN)—pincer nail.

Patient 13

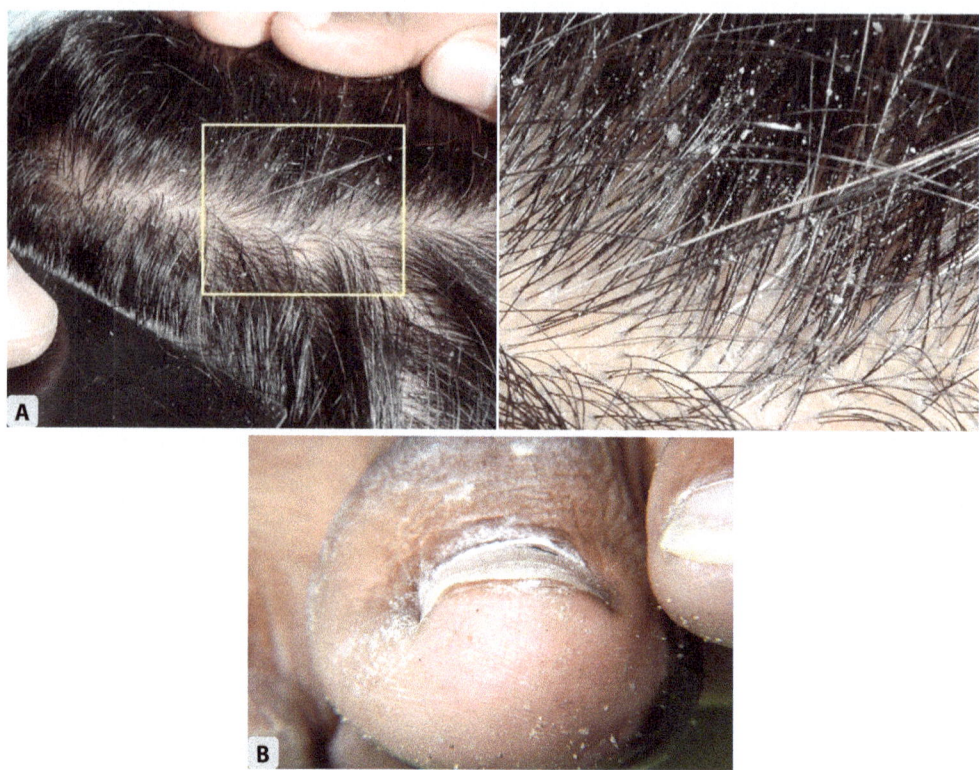

PATIENT 13: A 20-year-old engineering student—5 years history of recurrent episodes of dandruff. (A) Scalp—visible desquamation (yellow box); and (B) (Right) great toenail (GTN)—typical angulation.

Patient 14

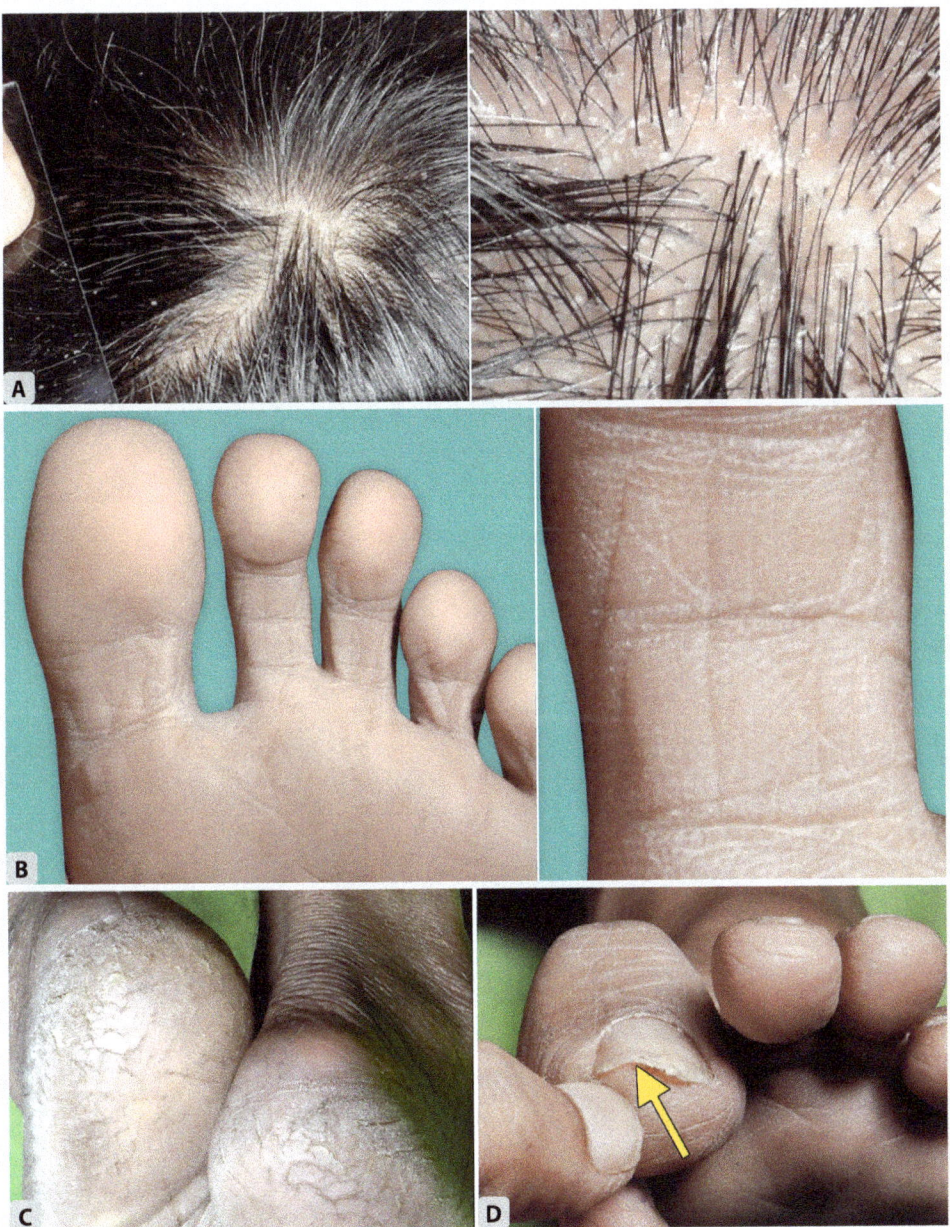

PATIENT 14: A 40-year-old male patient—12 years history of recurrent to persistent dandruff. (A) On stroking the occiput—remarkable desquamation elicited and follicular psoriasis demonstrated; (B) Under toes of (left) foot—mild HK; (C) Heels—HK and fissuring; and (D) (Left) GTN—typical angulation (yellow arrow).
(GTN: great toenail; HK: hyperkeratosis)

II. Dandruff in Children
(No. of Patients Depicted—8)

Patient 1

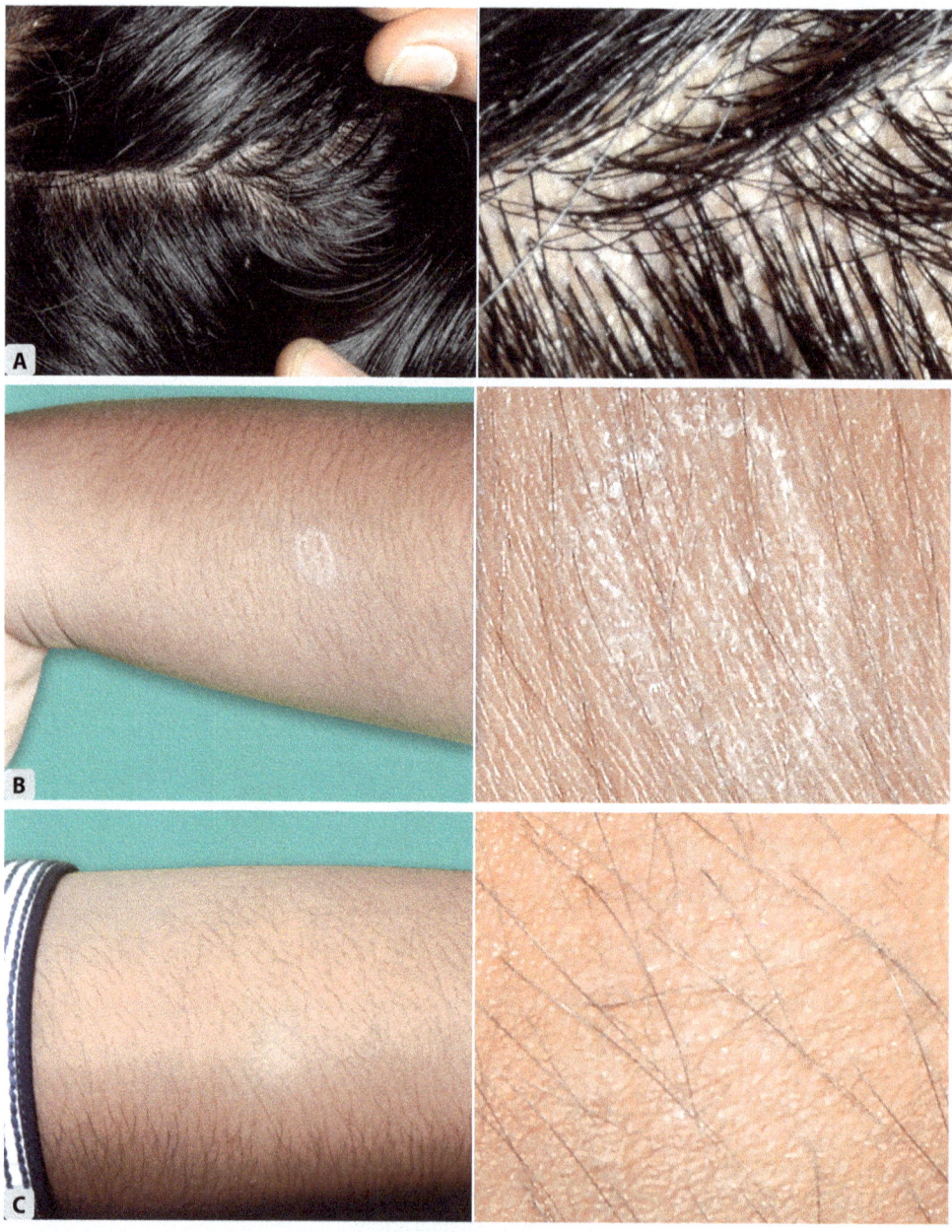

PATIENT 1: A 13-year-old female—2 months history of scaling scalp—brought by both her parents who are known psoriatics. (A) Scalp—visible desquamation; and (B and C) Both the forearms—very thin plaques with silvery white scales suggesting photosensitive psoriasis.

Patient 2

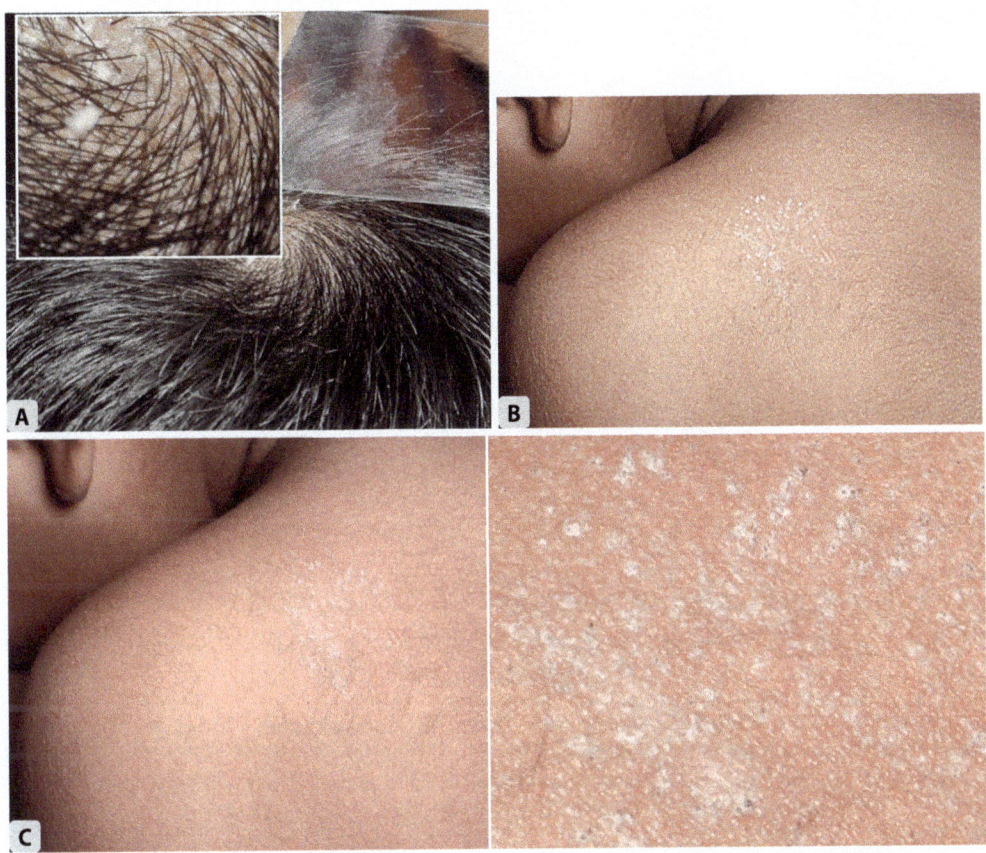

PATIENT 2: A 7-year-old boy—brought by his parents—2 days history of itching and scaling of scalp. (A) Apparently normal occiput—on stroking—turned scaly; (B) Grouped tiny papules mimicking lichen nitidus (LN); and (C) On stroking, LN-like lesions—display silvery white scales.

Patient 3

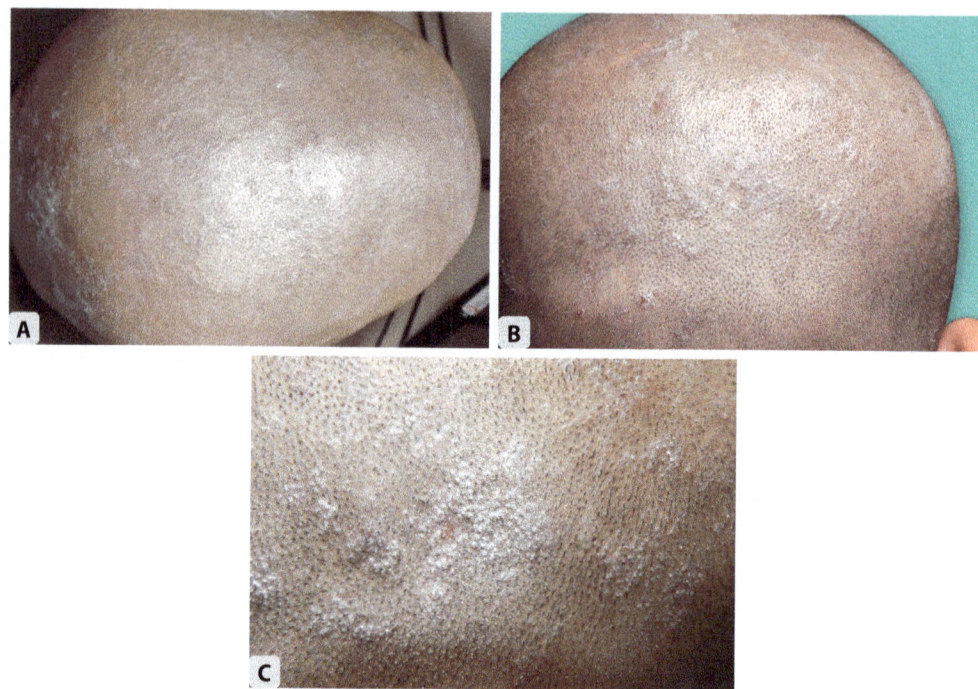

PATIENT 3: A 6-year-old boy—brought by his parents—tonsured head—6 months history of dandruff—scalp displayed fleshy, grouped, and papular eruption. (A) On stroking—fleshy papules turned scaly; (B) Occipital scalp—similar picture; and (C) (Left) parietal scalp—discrete, grouped, and coalescent papular eruption covered with typical silvery white scales.

Patient 4

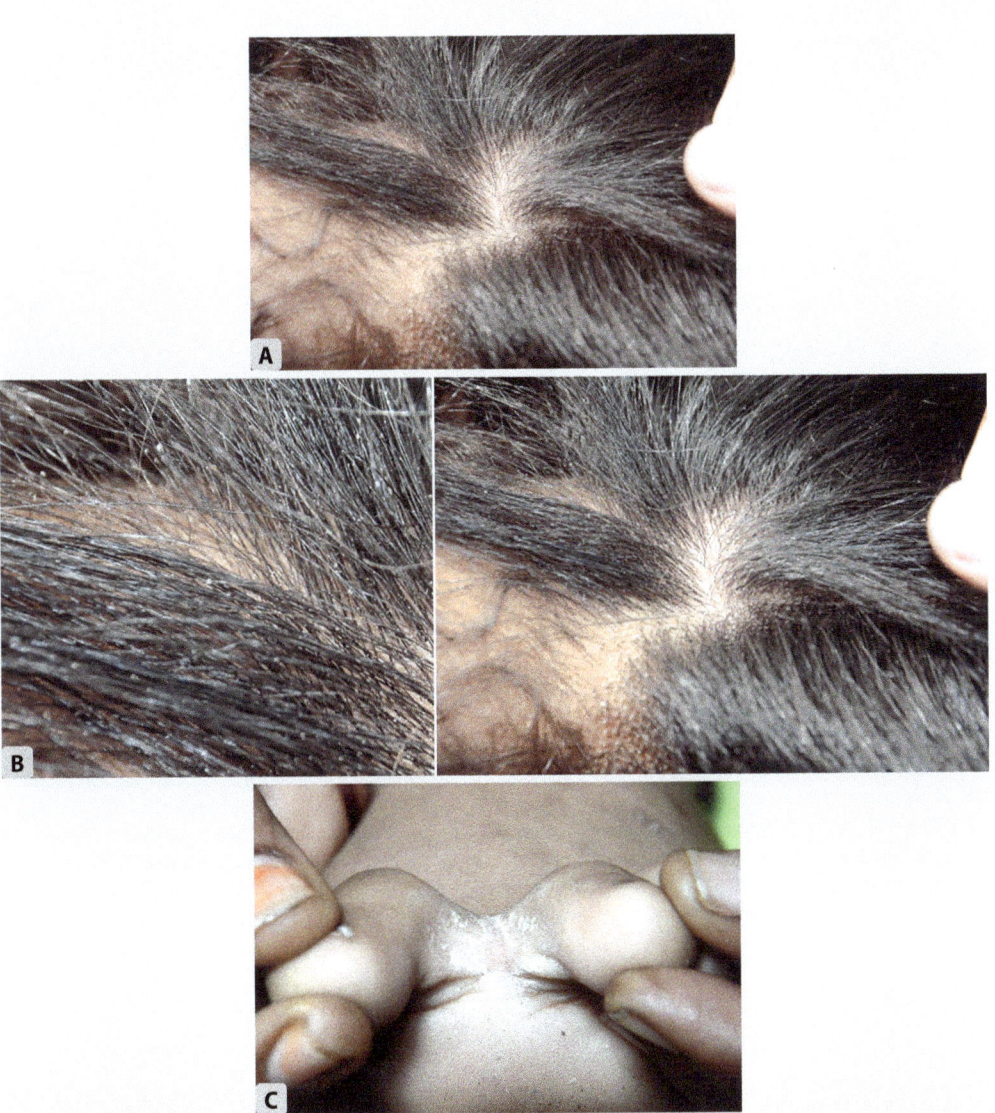

PATIENT 4: An 11-year-old female—brought by her mother—9 months history of dandruff. (A) Scalp—before stroking—minimal visible desquamation; (B) After stroking—profuse scaling elicited; and (C) (Left) foot first toe web—on stroking—turns scaly; no maceration—hence, candidal intertrigo may be ruled out.

Looking beyond the lesion is mandatory.

Patient 5

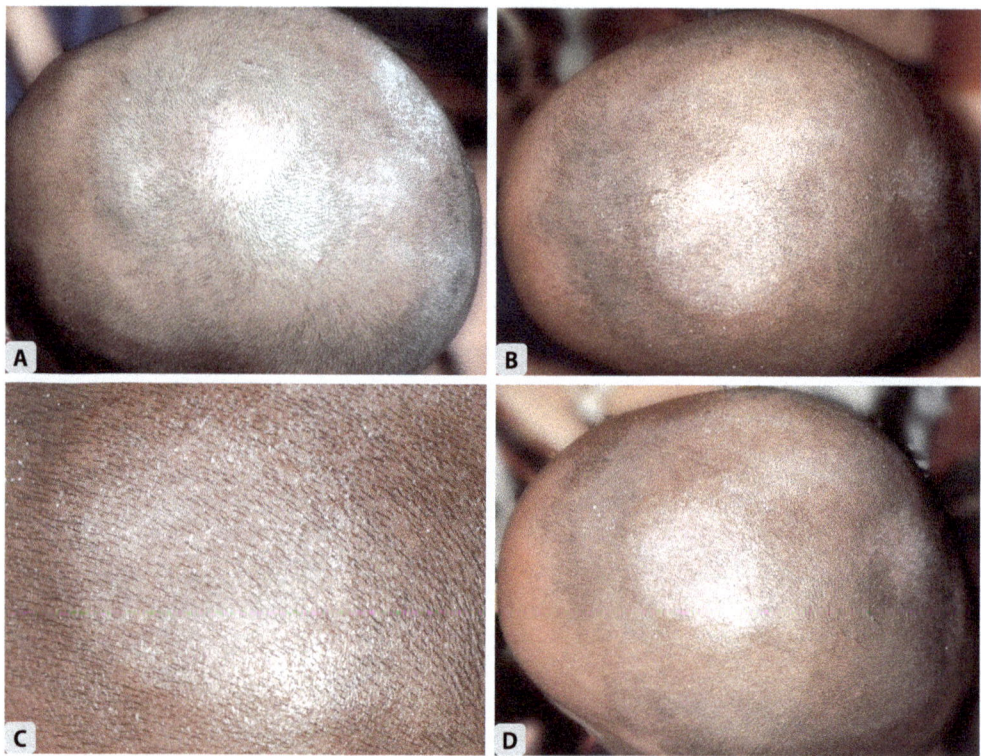

PATIENT 5: A 9-month-old male baby—brought by his paternal grandmother—condition of scaling scalp; she was instructed to bring her grandson with tonsured head; after 5 days, the child's father brought the child. (A) The scalp—multiple barely raised scaly patches of varying sizes all over; (B) On stroking, silvery white scale elicited; and (C and D) Close-up view of (B).

Patient 6

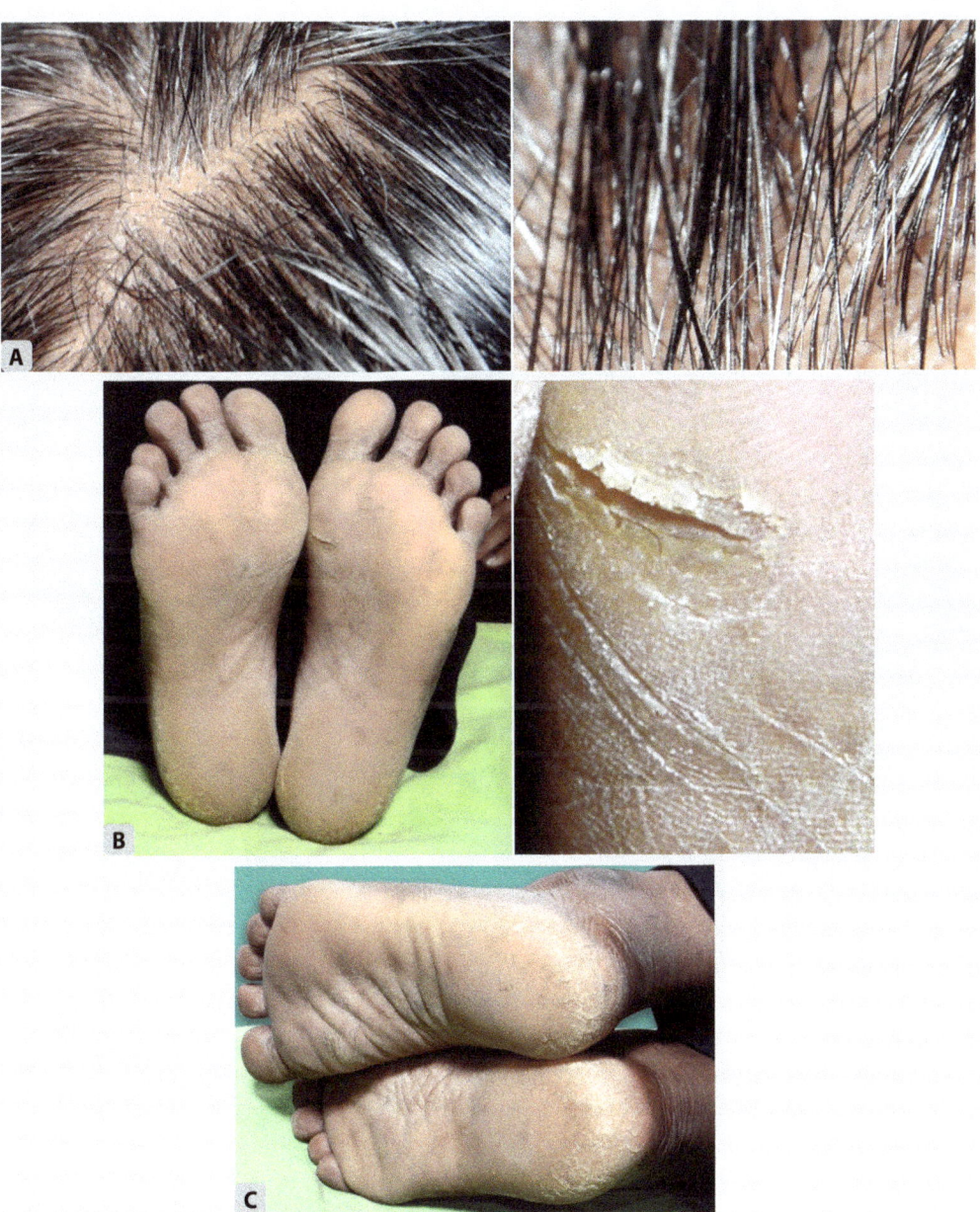

PATIENT 6: A 34-year-old male, father of patient 6. (A) Scalp—visible desquamation; (B) Plantar psoriasis involving insteps under toes—hyperkeratosis (HK); and (C) Heels—HK and fissuring.

Patient 7

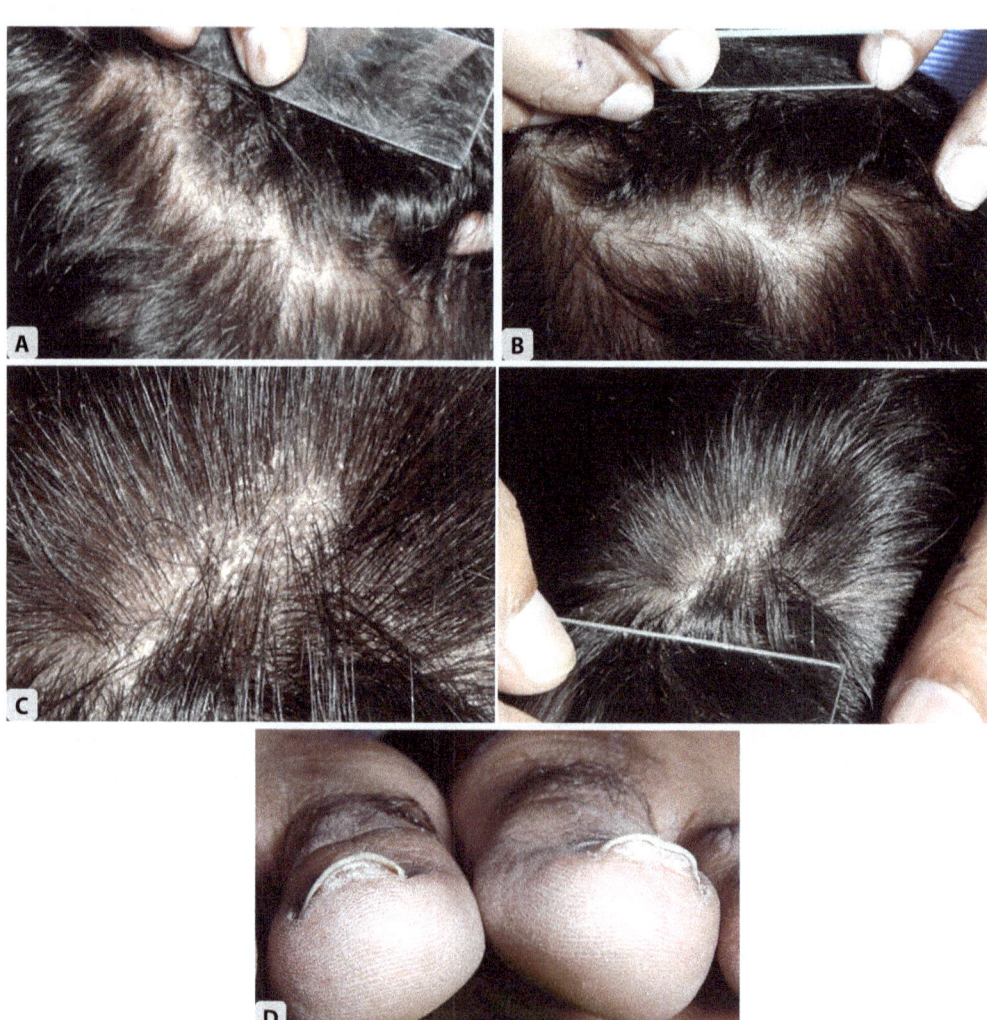

PATIENT 7: A 3-year-old male child—4 months history of dandruff. (A and B) On stroking the vertex—minimal desquamation; (C) On stroking the occiput—heavy desquamation; and (D) The child's father—both the great toenails (GTNs)—overcurvature with angulation.

Patient 8A

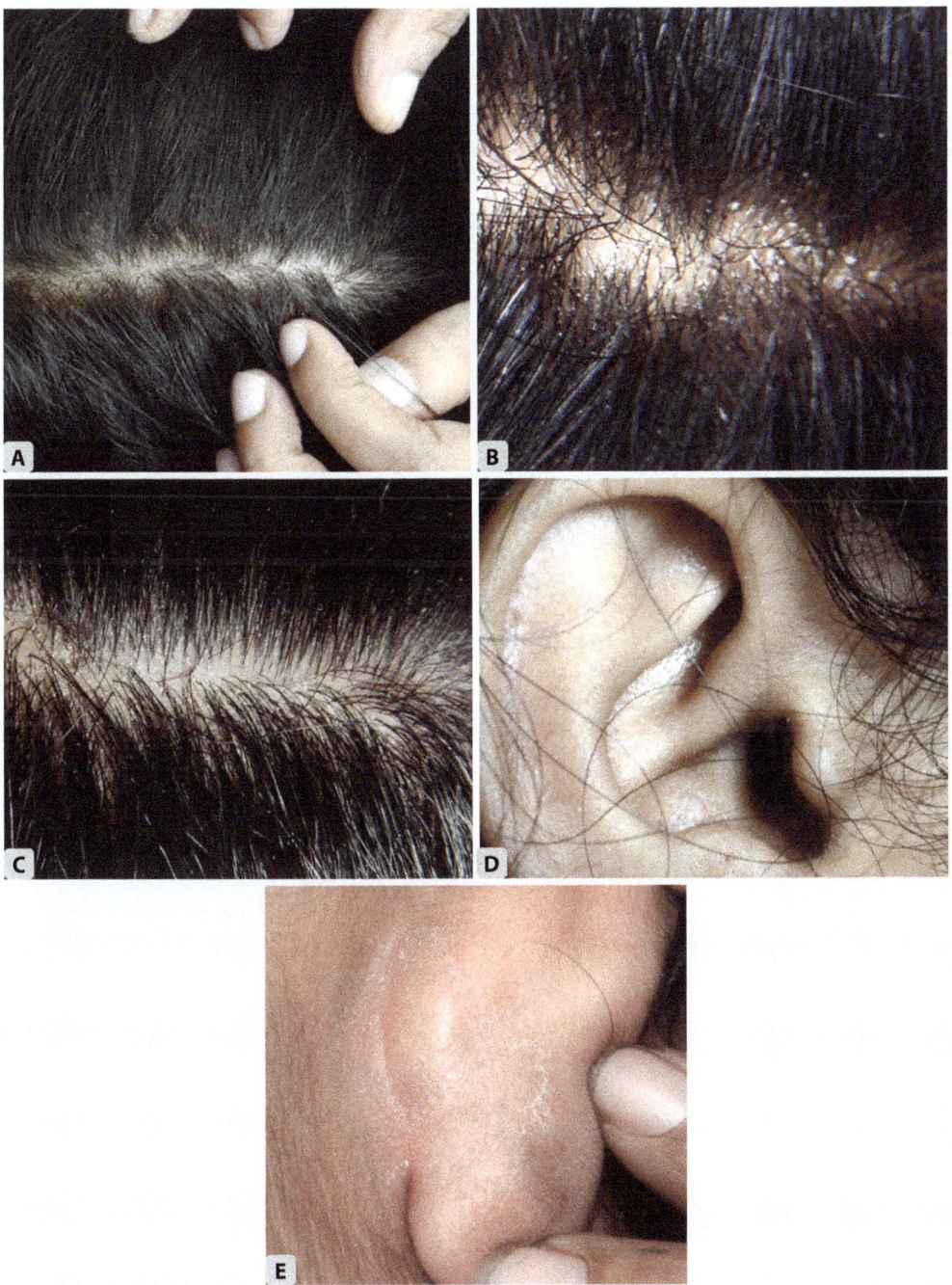

PATIENT 8A: An 11-year-old female—a student with 5 years history of dandruff (i.e., onset—at the age of 6 years). (A) Apparently normal scalp; (B) At the occiput end of hair parting—follicular psoriasis with visible desquamation—on stroking; (C) Entire length of hair parting turns scaly; (D) Interior of (right) external earlobe—silvery white scaly patches; and (E) (Right) retroauricular region—scaly erythema.

Patient 8B

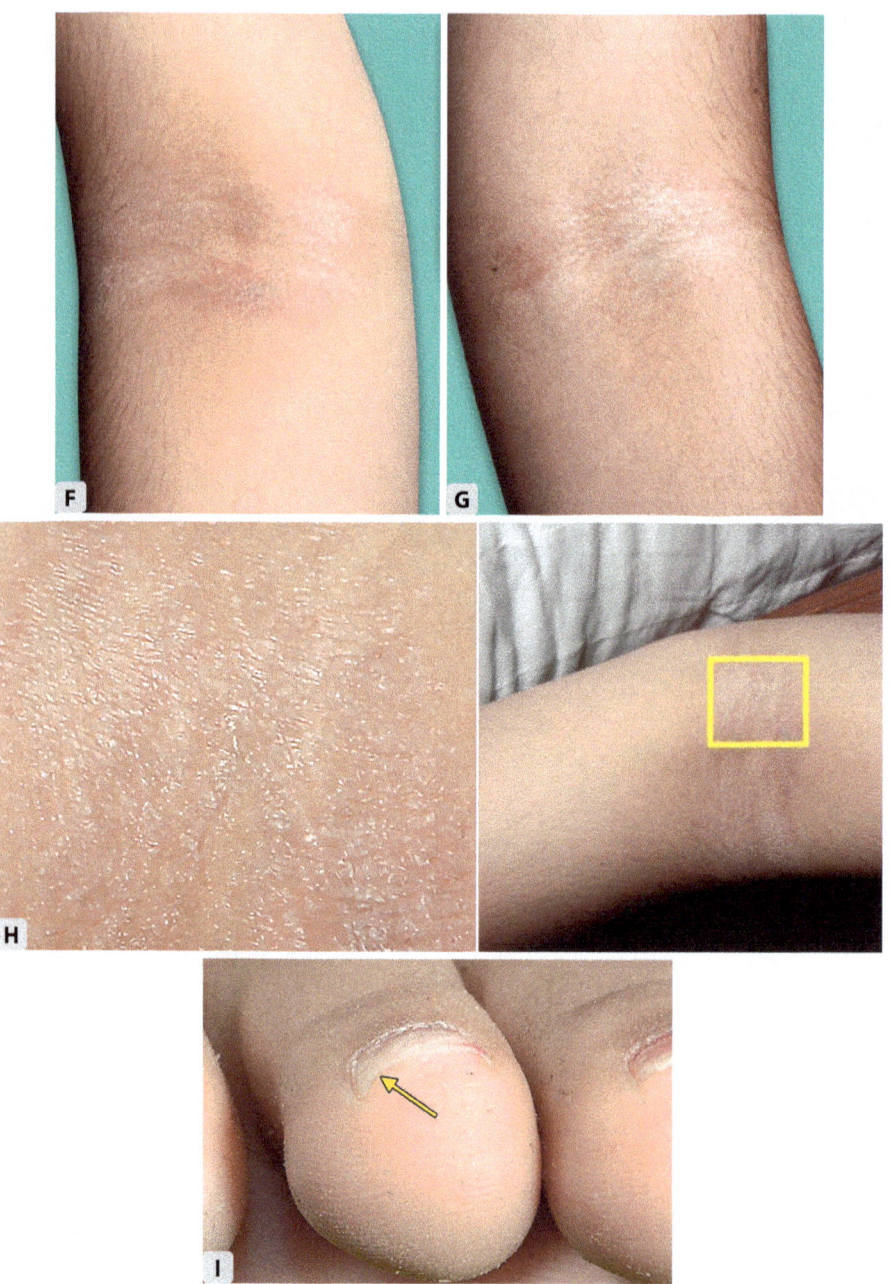

PATIENT 8B: (F and G) Both the antecubital fossa (ACF)—dermatitis; (H) (Left) ACF—scaly papular character of the dermatitis may be appreciated (yellow box); and (I) Middle toe of (right) foot—subtle angulation of nail plate (yellow arrow).
Additional information: History of a scaly patch on occipital scalp at the age of 5 months; no history of cradle cap.

Color Atlas of Dandruff

III. Subclinical Psoriasis Capitis
(No. of Patients Depicted—17)

Patient 1

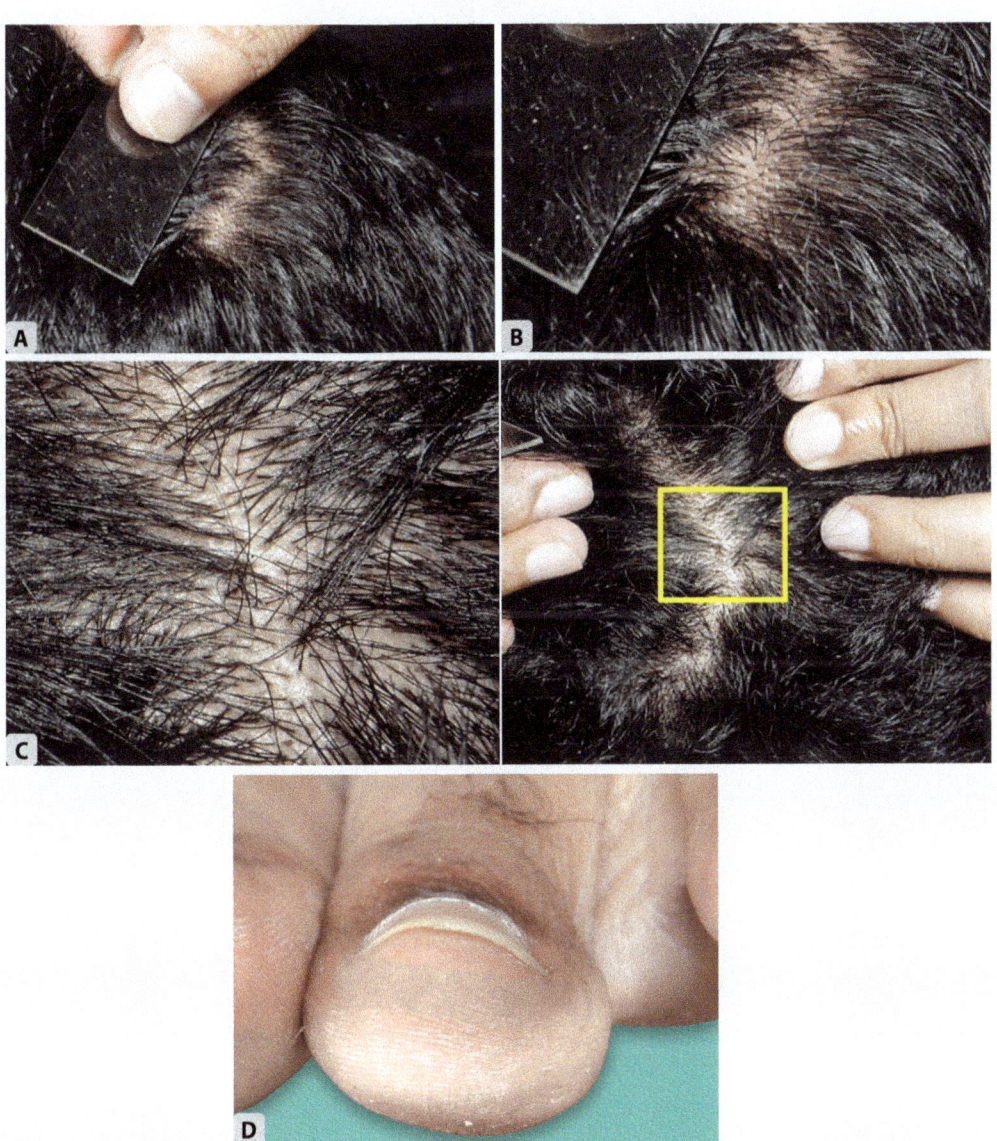

PATIENT 1: A 25-year-old male—5 years history of itching and scaling of scalp. (A) Apparently normal looking vertex; on stroking minimal desquamation; (B) On further stroking, a little more scaling obtained; (C) On further stroking—scalp displays silvery white scaling; and (D) (Left) great toenail (GTN)—increased curvature and angulation.

Patient 2

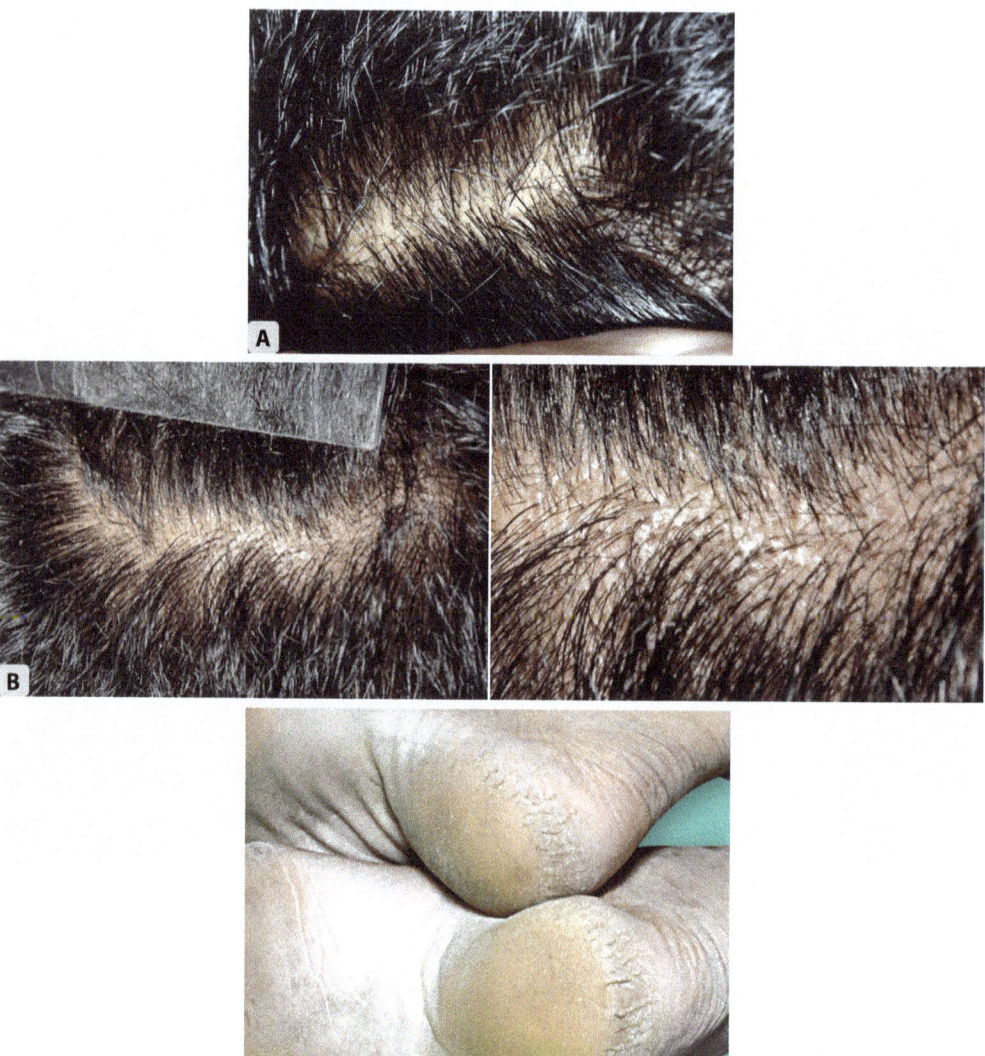

PATIENT 2: A 22-year-old two-wheeler mechanic—2 years history of dandruff. (A) Scalp—apparently normal; (B) Scalp—on stroking—significant silvery white scaling; and (C) Heels—hyperkeratosis (HK) and fissuring.

Patient 3

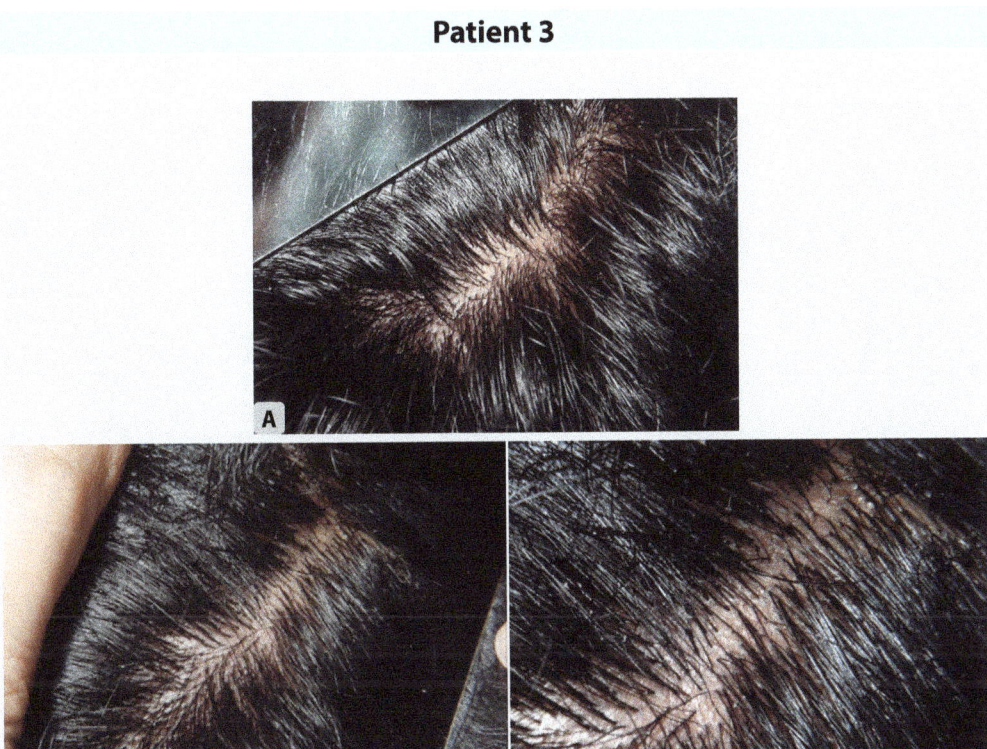

PATIENT 3: A 30-year-old male—a fruit vendor—2 years history of episodic dandruff. (A) Apparently normal scalp; and (B) On stroking—significant desquamation.

Patient 4

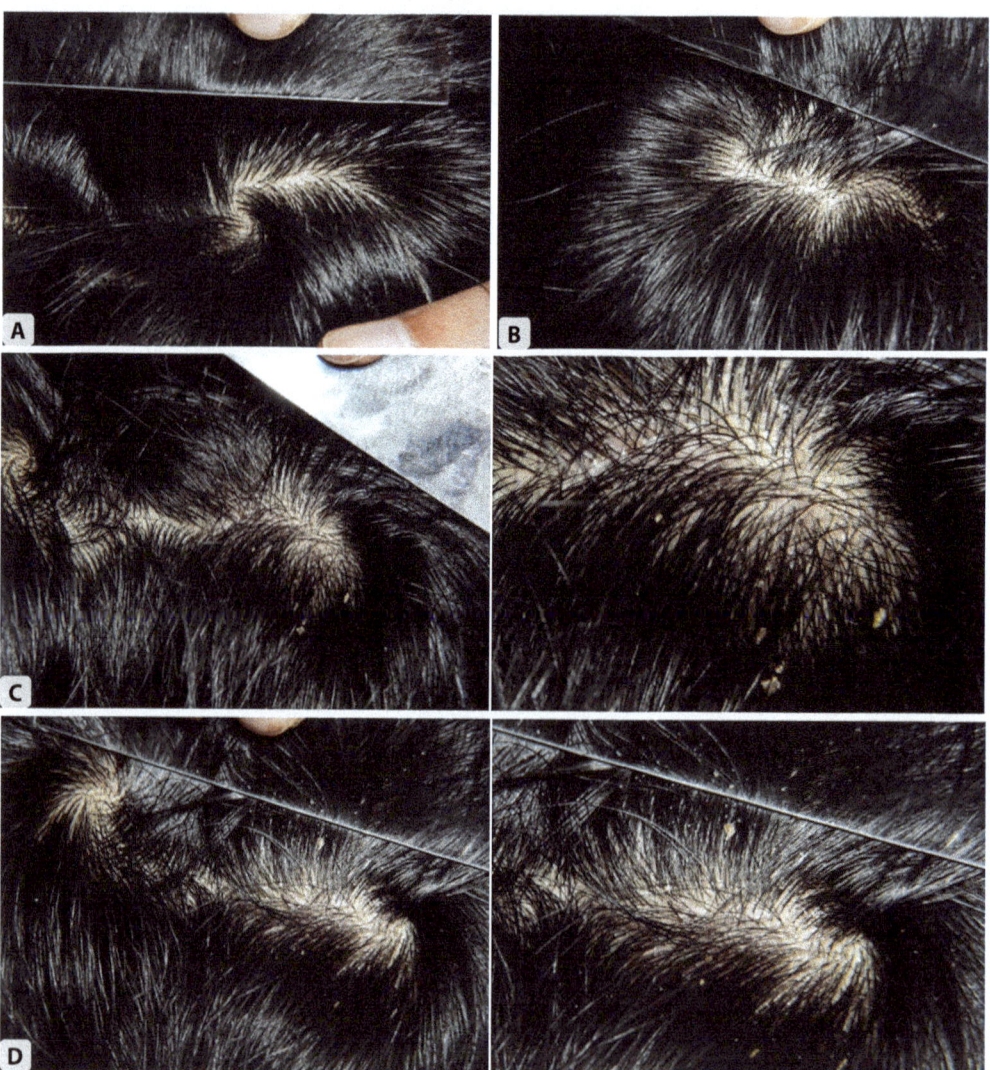

PATIENT 4: A 3-year-old female child—3 weeks history of itching and scaling of scalp (brought by her father). (A) A relatively apparently normal scalp; (B) On stroking—minimal desquamation; and (C and D) On further stroking, many more scales got displaced.

Further information: Child's mother develops fissuring of soles every winter since her marriage.

Patient 5

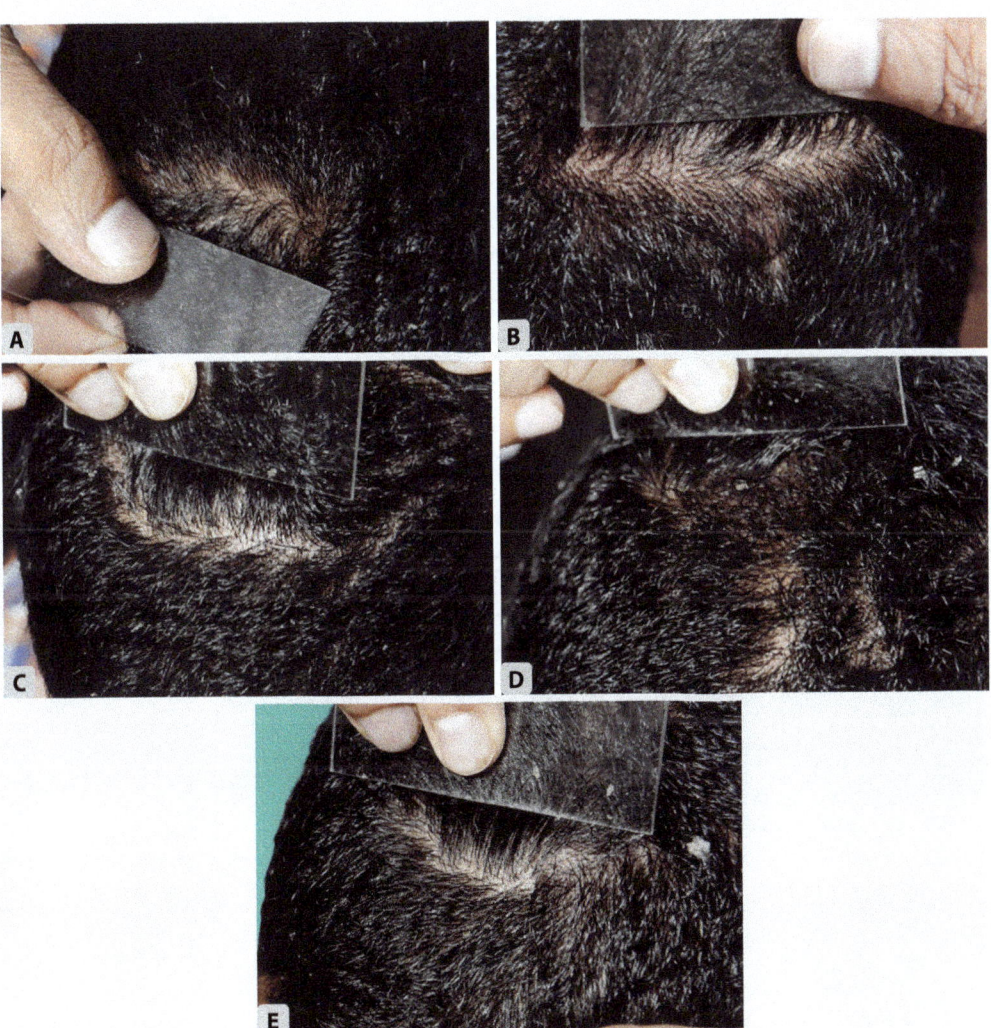

PATIENT 5: A 19-year-old engineering student—2 years history of scaling scalp associated with severe itching. (A and B) No visible desquamation; (C and D) On stroking, visible desquamation elicited; and (E) Relatively larger squames may be noted.

Patient 6

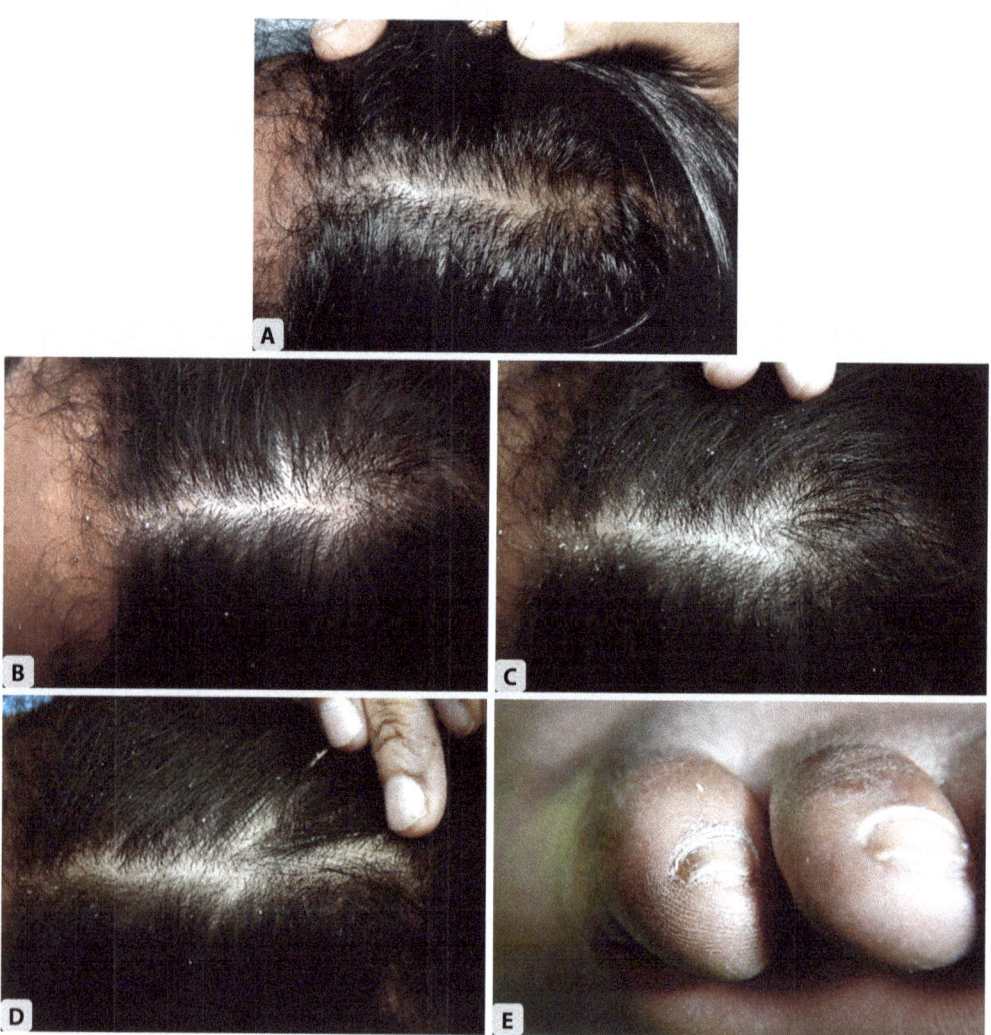

PATIENT 6: A 22-year-old female—a housewife—4–5 months history of scaling scalp. (A) Hair parting—no visible desquamation; (B to D) Significant visible desquamation on stroking; and (E) (Right) little toenail (LTN)—typical angulation.

Color Atlas of Dandruff

Patient 7A

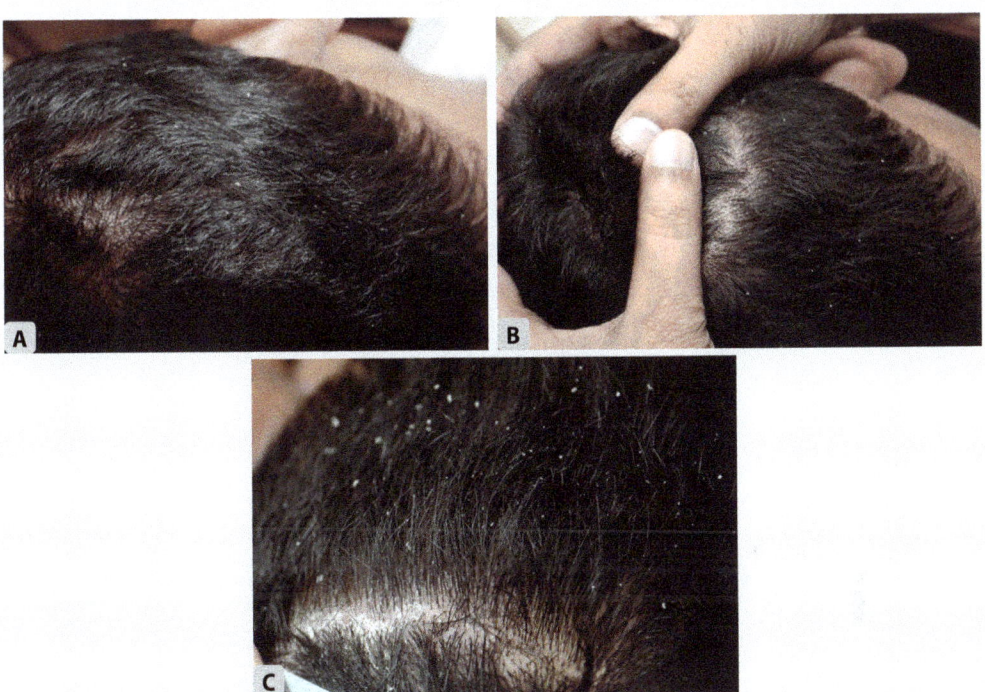

PATIENT 7A: A 24-year-old male—an employed engineer—1 year history of occasional itching associated with dandruff. (A) Minimal desquamation on scalp hair; (B) On stroking, minimal desquamation noted; and (C) Repeated strokes elicited remarkable number of squames.

Patient 7B (father of patient 7A)

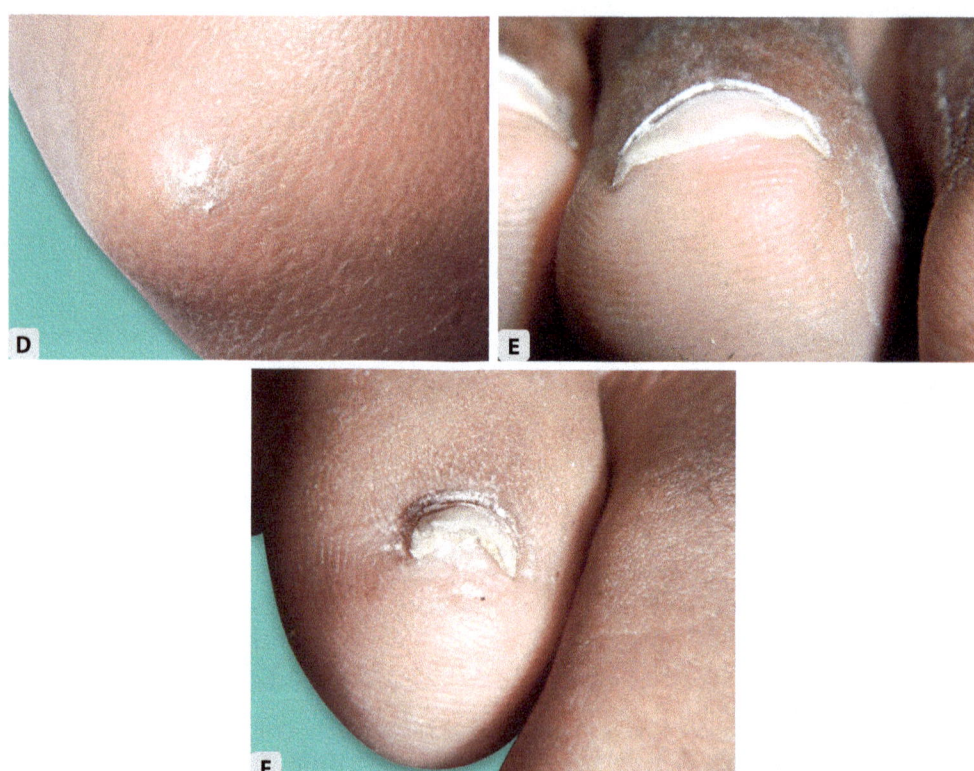

PATIENT 7B: (D) (Right) elbow—a thin plaque covered with silvery white scale; (E) Middle toe of (right) foot—angulation (on both sides); and (F) (Right) LTN—overcurvature and SUHK.

(LTN: little toenail; SUHK: subungual hyperkeratosis)

Thus, clues picked up from her father prove that the father is also a psoriatic.

Patient 8

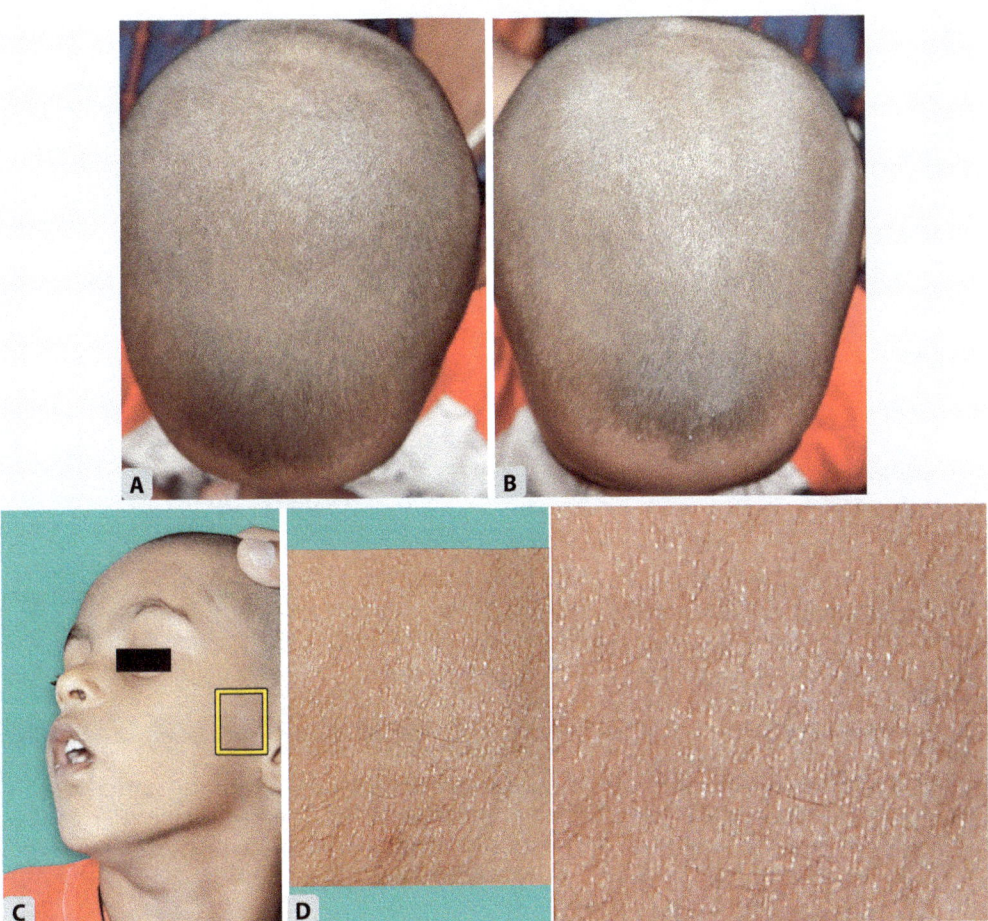

PATIENT 8: A 5-year-old male child with apparently normal scalp—brought by his father—8 months history of dandruff. (A) After a single stroke—multiple scaly patches become visible; (B) On further stroking—patches become more conspicuous; (C) Left side of face—pityriasis alba-like lesions (yellow box); and (D) Scaly papular character of pityriasis alba lesion may be noted.

Patient 9

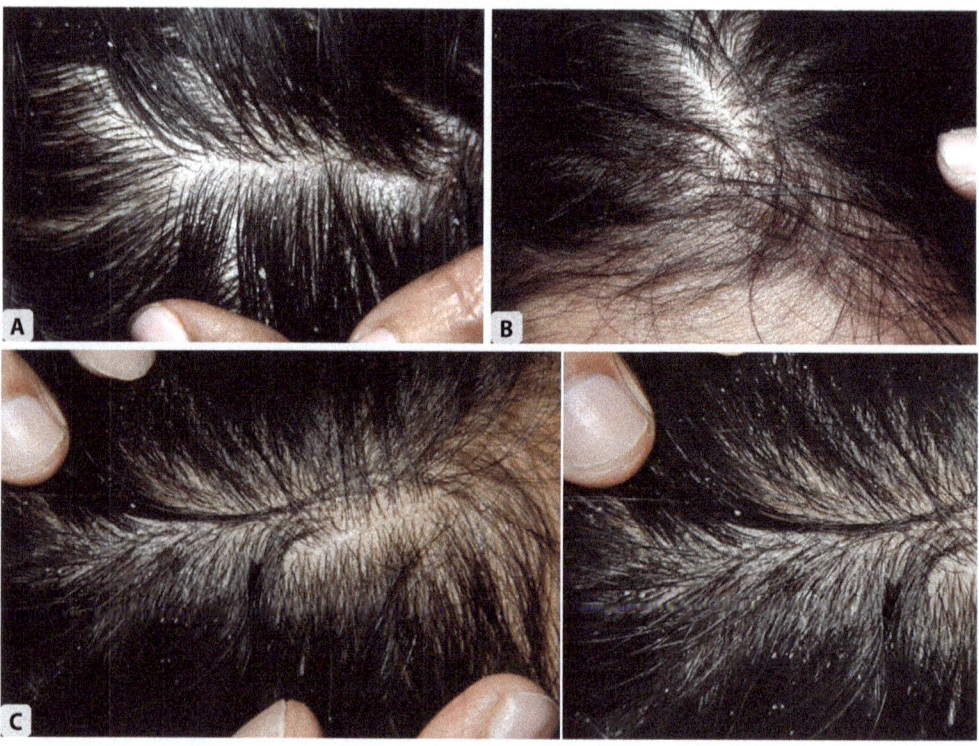

PATIENT 9: An 18-year-old female—an engineering student—1 year history of scaling scalp. (A) Multiple scaly plaques with heavy visible desquamation; (B) The frontal end of the hair parting—free of scales; and (C) On stroking, the frontal end of the hair parting—turns scaly with visible desquamation.

Patient 10

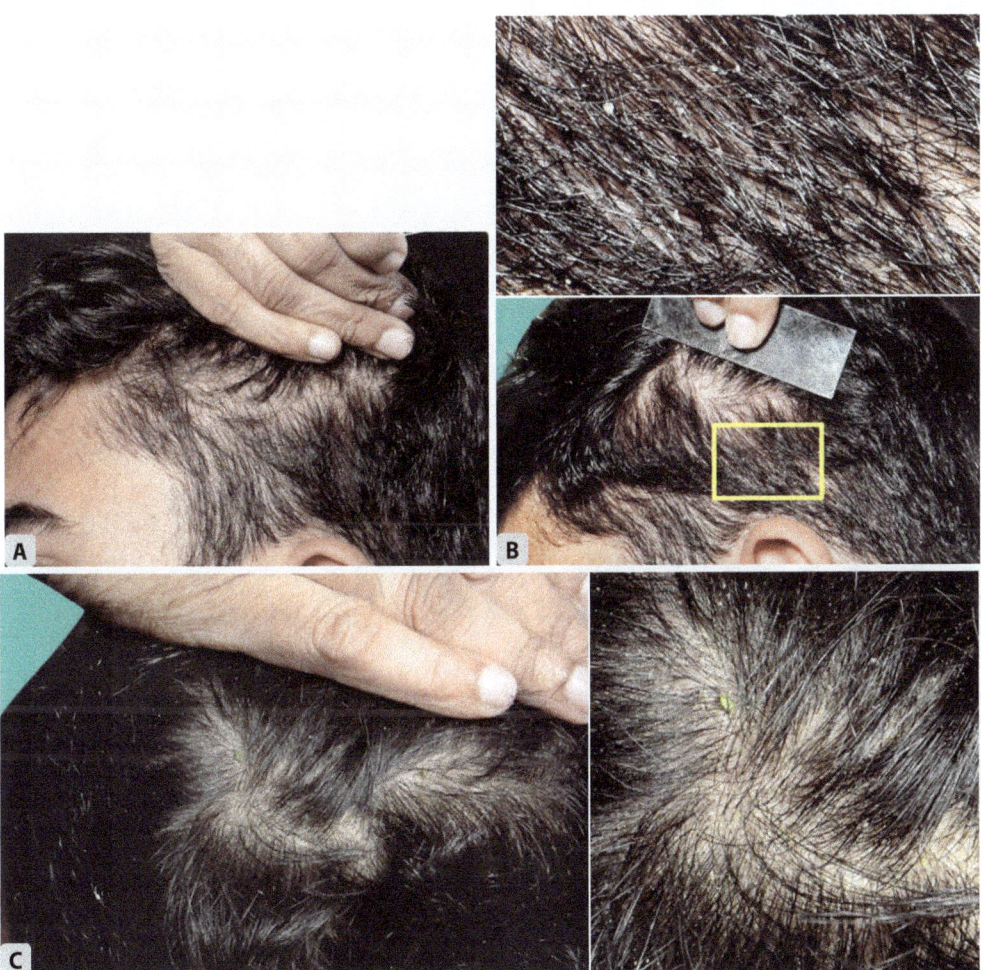

PATIENT 10: A 19-year-old male—a college drop-out—1 year history of dandruff. (A) Entire scalp—normal—no visible desquamation; (B) On stroking—parietal scalp—turns scaly with visible desquamation (yellow box); and (C) On stroking the occiput—significant scaling elicited.

Patient 11

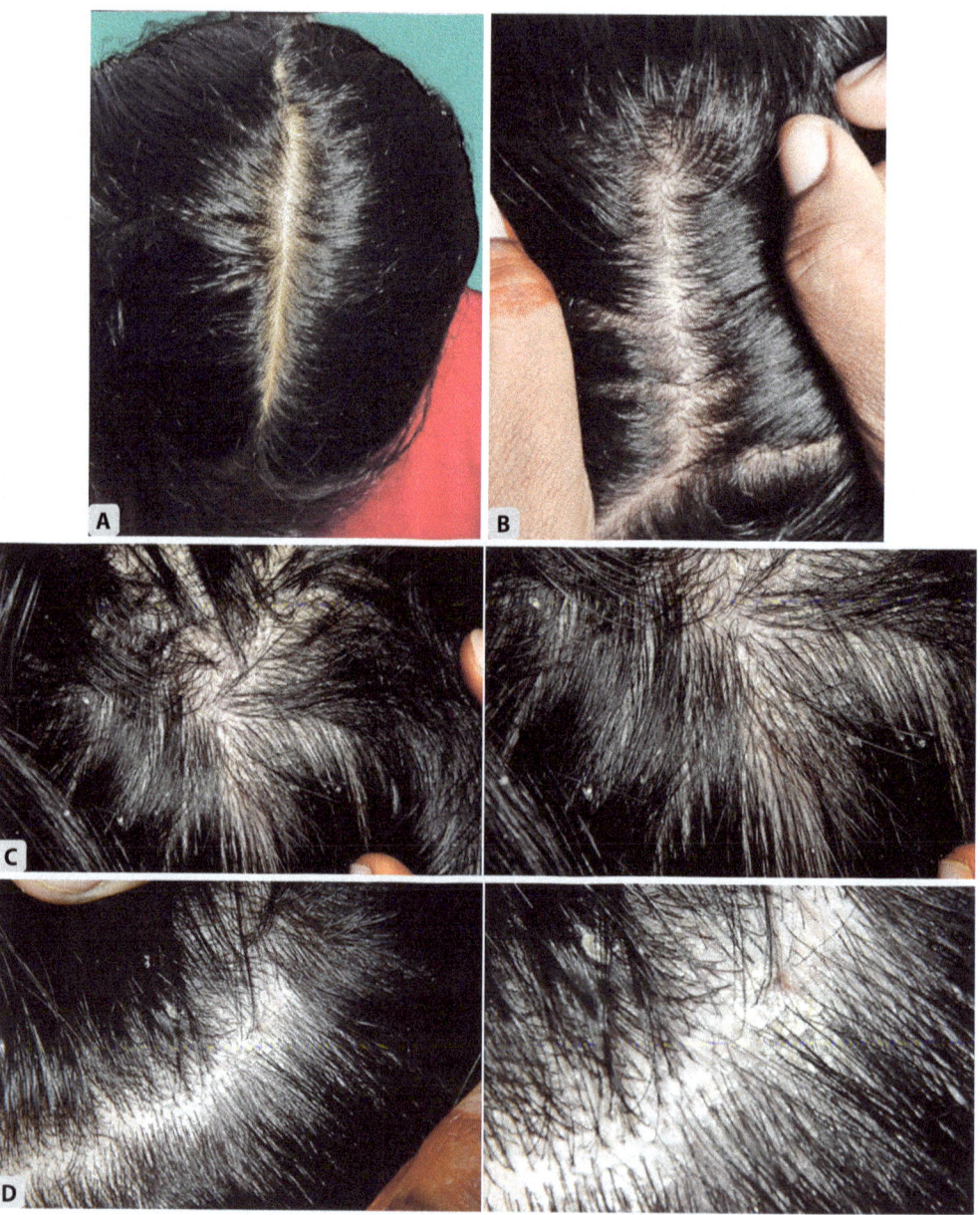

PATIENT 11: An 8-year-old female child—brought by her mother—2 months history of dandruff. (A and B) Entire scalp normal with no visible desquamation; (C) On stroking—occiput turns scaly; and (D) On stroking—hair parting over vertex also turns scaly.

Patient 12A

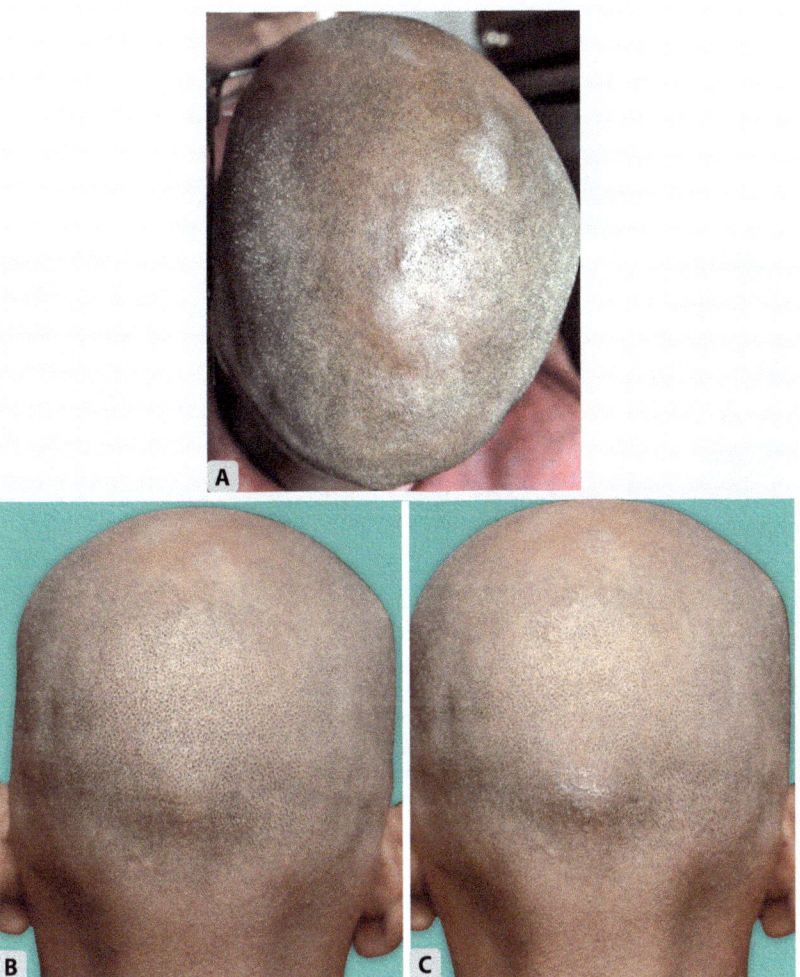

PATIENT 12A: A 58-year-old male—a clerk at a college—2 years history of dandruff—becomes worse in winter. (A) Tonsured scalp—multiple scaly patches; (B) Normal looking occipital scalp; and (C) On stroking, a typical psoriatic plaque manifests.

Patient 12B

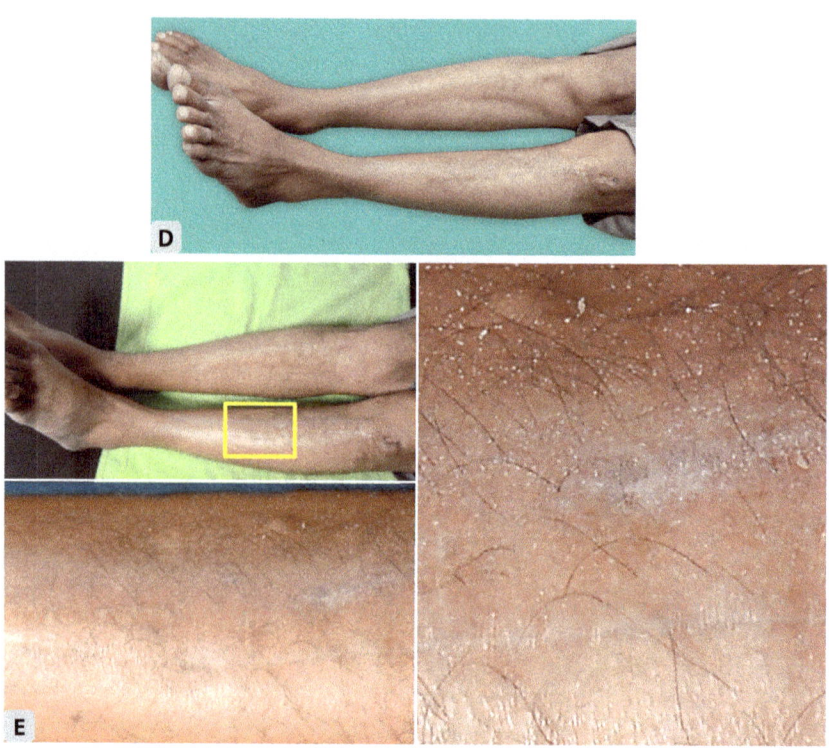

PATIENT 12B: (D) Skin over both lower legs—normal; and (E) On stroking the (left) lower leg—skin turns scaly with visible desquamation (yellow box).

Patient 13A

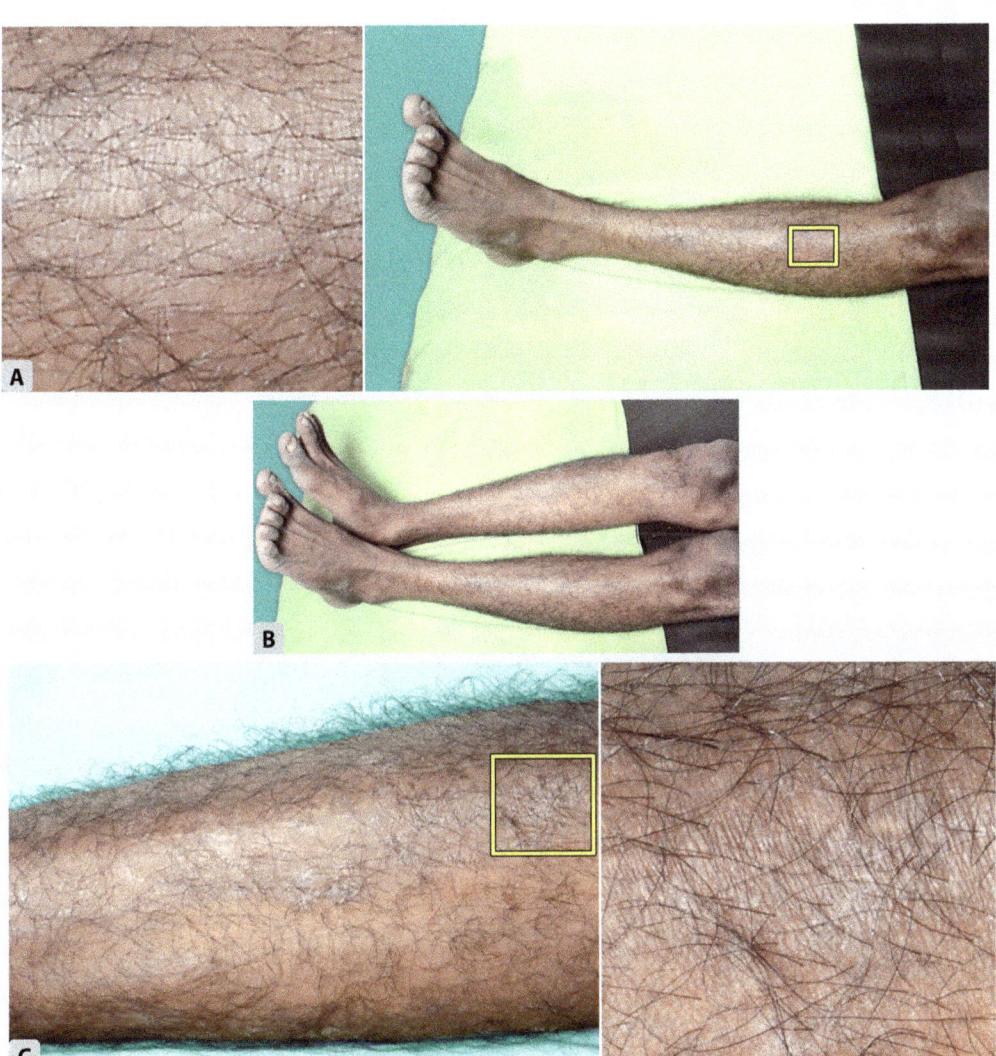

PATIENT 13A: A 42-year-old automobile mechanic—6 months history of itching all along both lower legs—more on (right) lower leg. (A) (Left) leg apparently normal except for mild dryness (yellow box); (B) On stroking—scaly patches appear; and (C) Silvery white scaly patch on (right) lower leg may be noted (yellow box).

*B and C suggest that there exists psoriasis in subclinical form.

Patient 13B

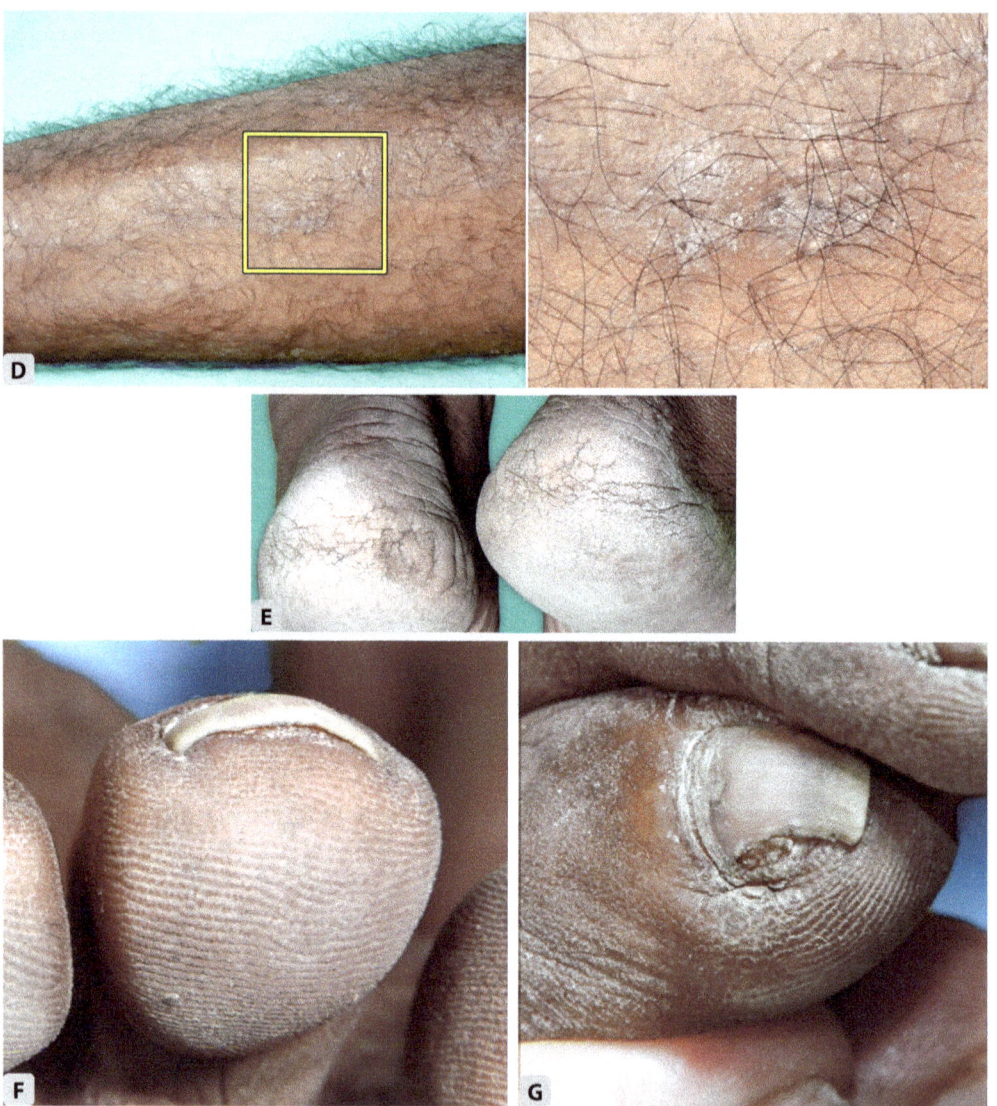

PATIENT 13B: (D) (Right) lower shin—similar lesion as in (C); (E) Heels—HK and fissuring; (F) (Right) second toe—angulation; and (G) (Right) LTN split and part of it lost.
(HK: hyperkeratosis; LTN: little toenail)

Angulation and LTN split are pathognomonic for psoriasis anywhere on body in any form—as per my clinical experience (APMCE).

Patient 14

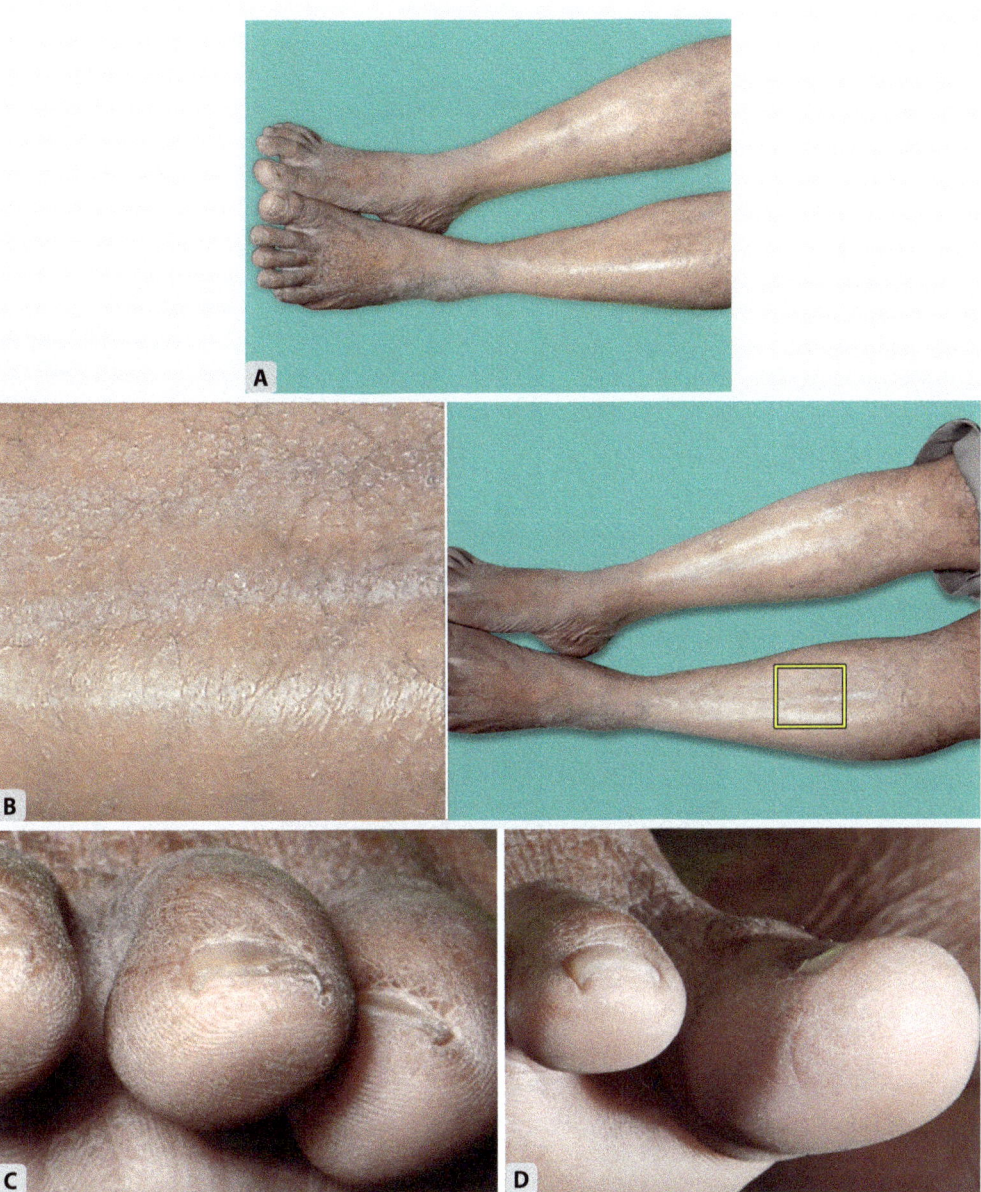

PATIENT 14: A 63-year-old male—an agriculturist—2 months history of itching of both lower legs. (A) Both the lower legs—seemingly normal; (B) On stroking the shins—skin turns silvery white; and (C and D) Fourth toenail (TN) of (left) foot and second TN of (right) foot—angulation.

Patient 15A

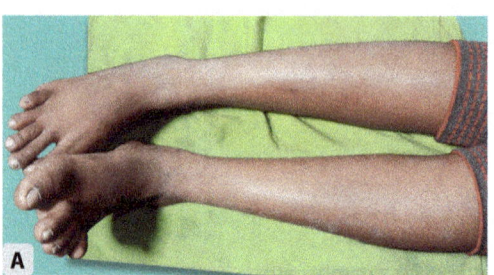

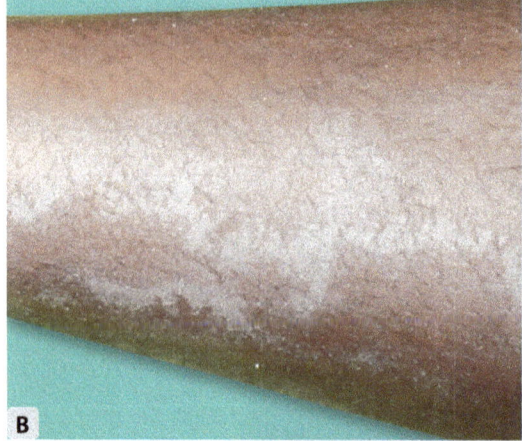

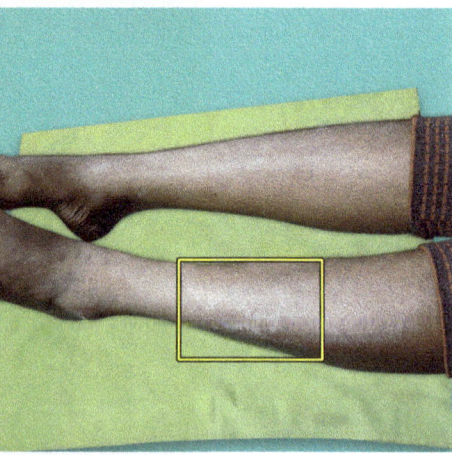

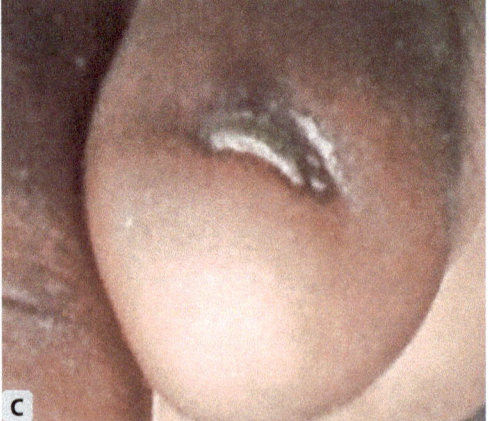

PATIENT 15A: A 16-year-old male student—1 month history of itching of both lower legs. (A) On stroking—both the lower legs—(which were seemingly normal)—turned scaly; (B) Skin over (left) lower leg turns scaly (silvery white nature of the scales may be noted) (yellow box); and (C) (Left) little toenail (LTN)—displays subtle angulation.

Patient 15B

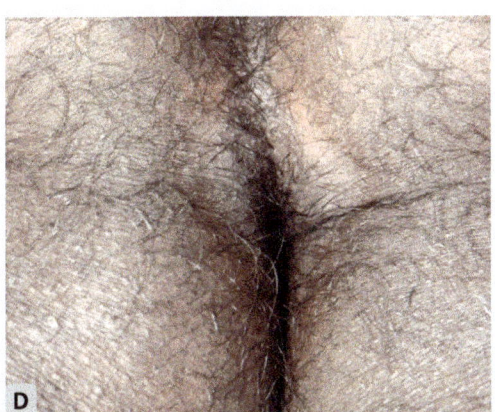

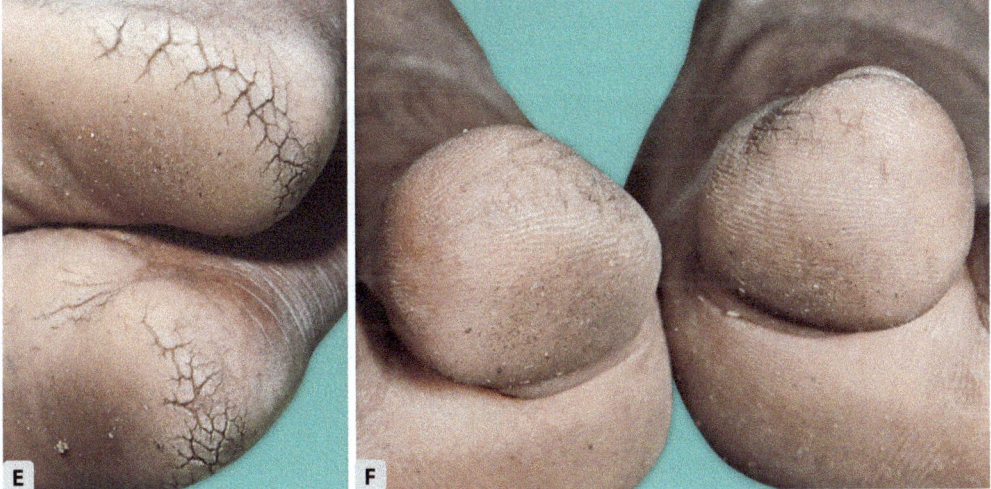

PATIENT 15B: A 40-year-old male—father of patient 15(A)—an agriculturist provides clues for psoriasis. (D) Natal cleft—erythema, scaling maceration; (E) Both heels—hyperkeratosis (HK) and fissuring; and (F) Pads of both great toes (GTs)—cracking.
Dryness, fissuring, and cracking suggest psoriatic diathesis (because of absence of granular layer which results in impaired barrier function).

Patient 16

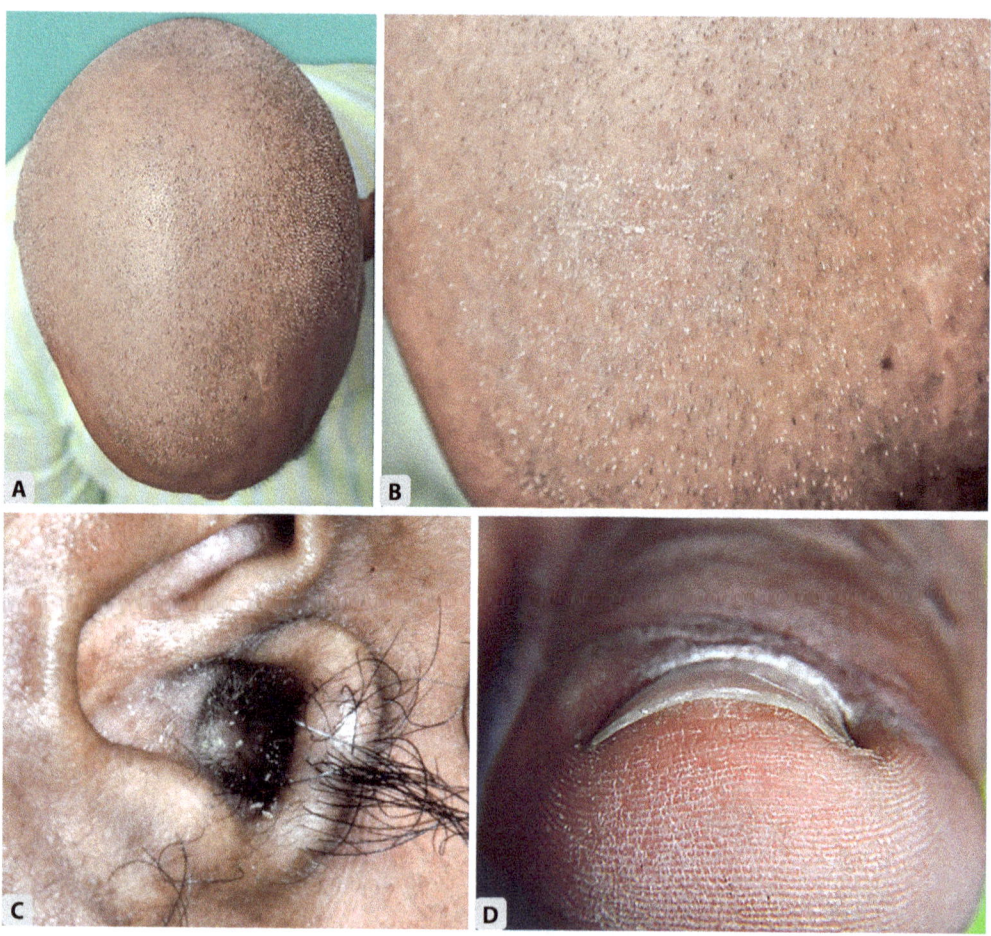

PATIENT 16: A 42-year-old cloth merchant—6 years history of dandruff. (A) Tonsured head—appears normal (nonscaly); (B) On stroking—skin over frontal scalp—turns scaly; (C) Concha and EAC—erythematous scaly patches and scales on hair; and (D) (Right) GTN—arch-like elevation.
(EAC: external auditory canal; GTN: great toenail)

Patient 17

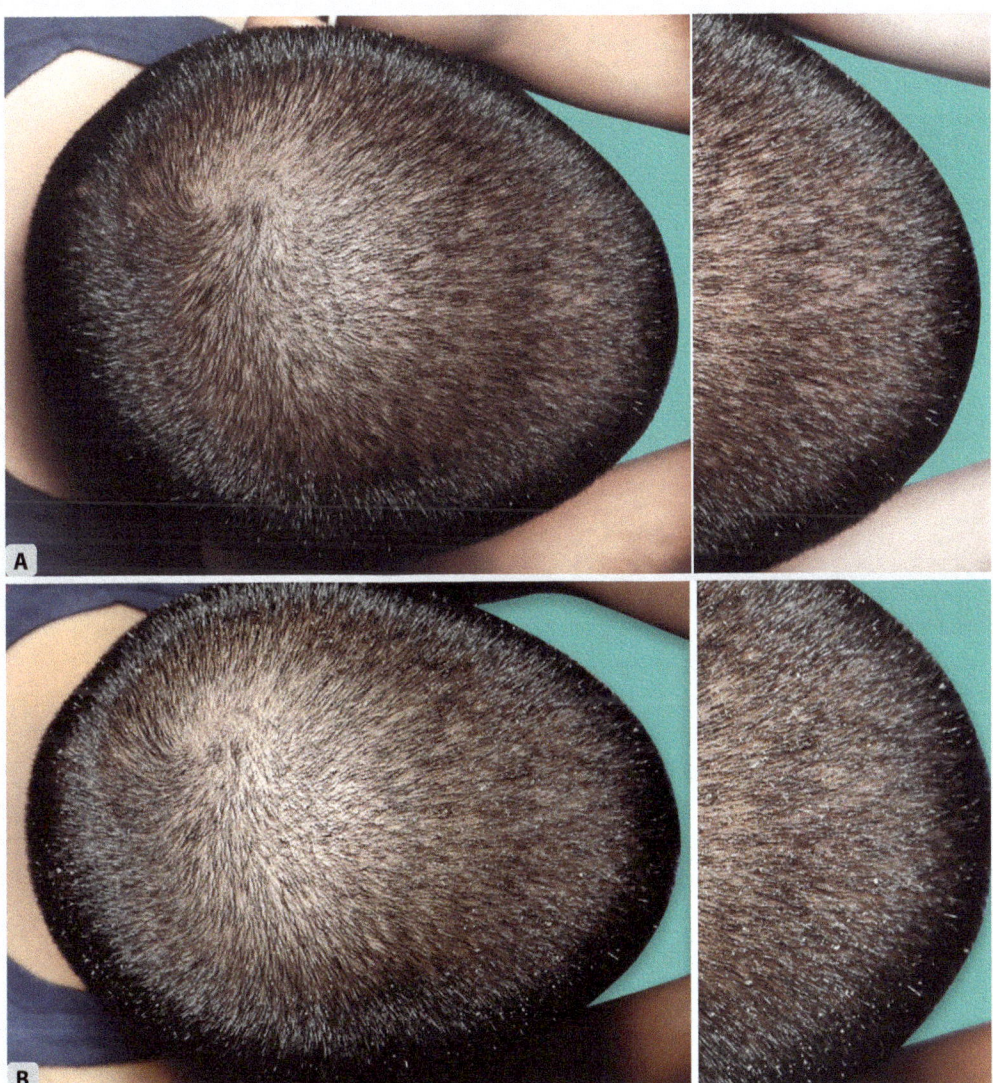

PATIENT 17: A 21-year-old male—an unemployed graduate—4 months history of dandruff—2 weeks history of tonsuration. (A) Apparently normal scalp (free of scaling); and (B) Stroking elicits significant visible desquamation.

Additional information: History of groin itch.

IV. Sebopsoriasis Masquerading as Seborrheic Dermatitis
(No. of Patients Depicted—28)

Patient 1

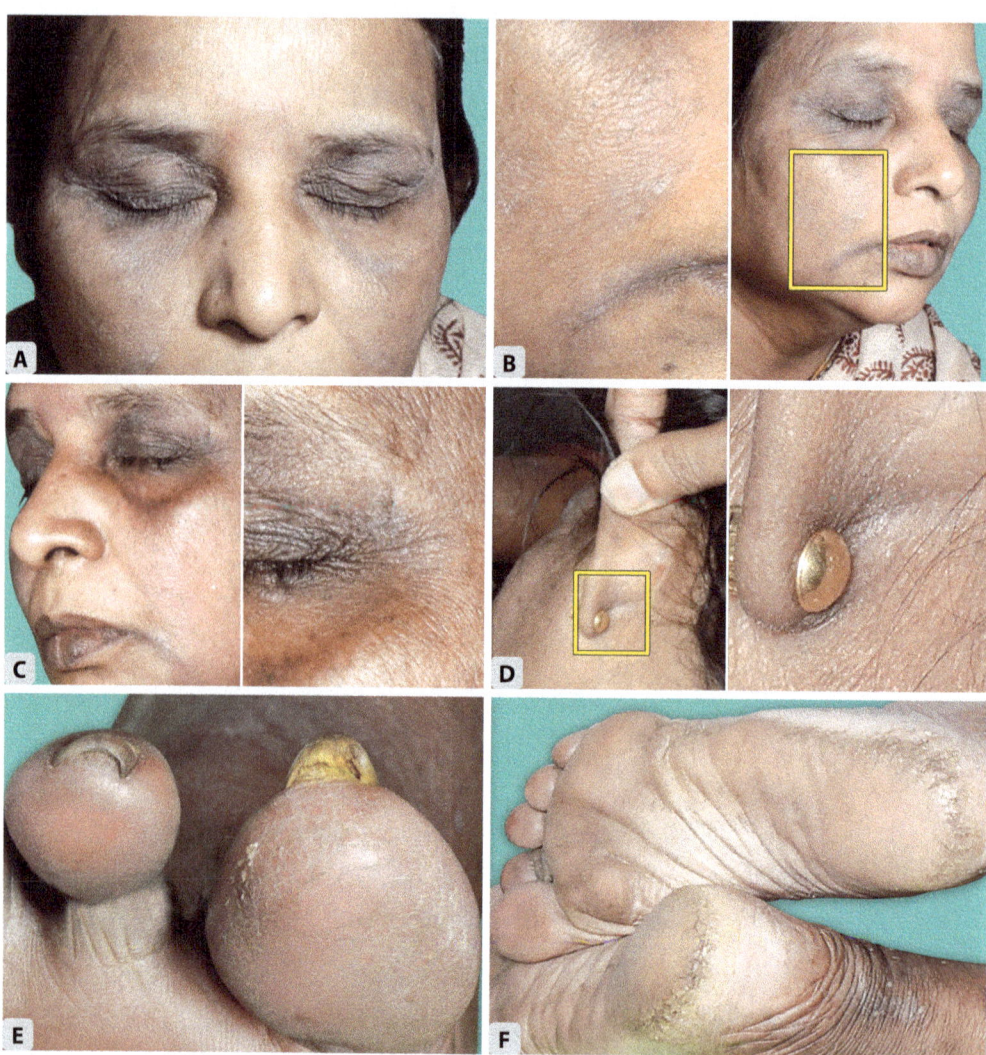

PATIENT 1: A 62-year-old female—a ruralite—3 weeks history of itching of face. (A) Scaly dermatitis involving seborrheic sites; (B) Psoriatic character of the scale may be noted (yellow box); (C) Erythema and dry (not greasy scaling) scaling of the eyelid and outer canthus; (D) Retroauricular erythema and dry scaling (yellow box); (E) Sides of (right) toepad—HK—scaling with minimal cracking; overcurvature of (right) GTN; and (F) Heels—HK and fissuring.

(GTN: great toenail; HK: hyperkeratosis)

Patient 2

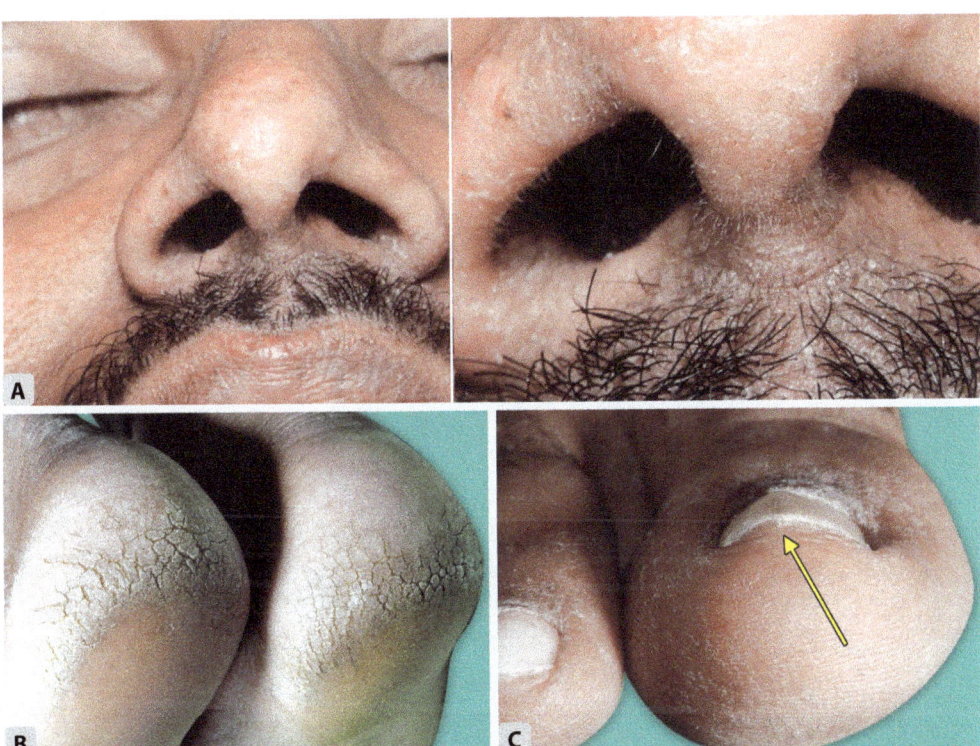

PATIENT 2: A 32-year-old male—an agriculturist—1 month history of itching and scaling of nostril rims and moustache area. (A) Erythema and scaling of nostril rims and upper lip; (B) Heels—HK and fissuring; and (C) (Right) GTN—angulation (yellow arrow).
(GTN: great toenail; HK: hyperkeratosis)

Patient 3A

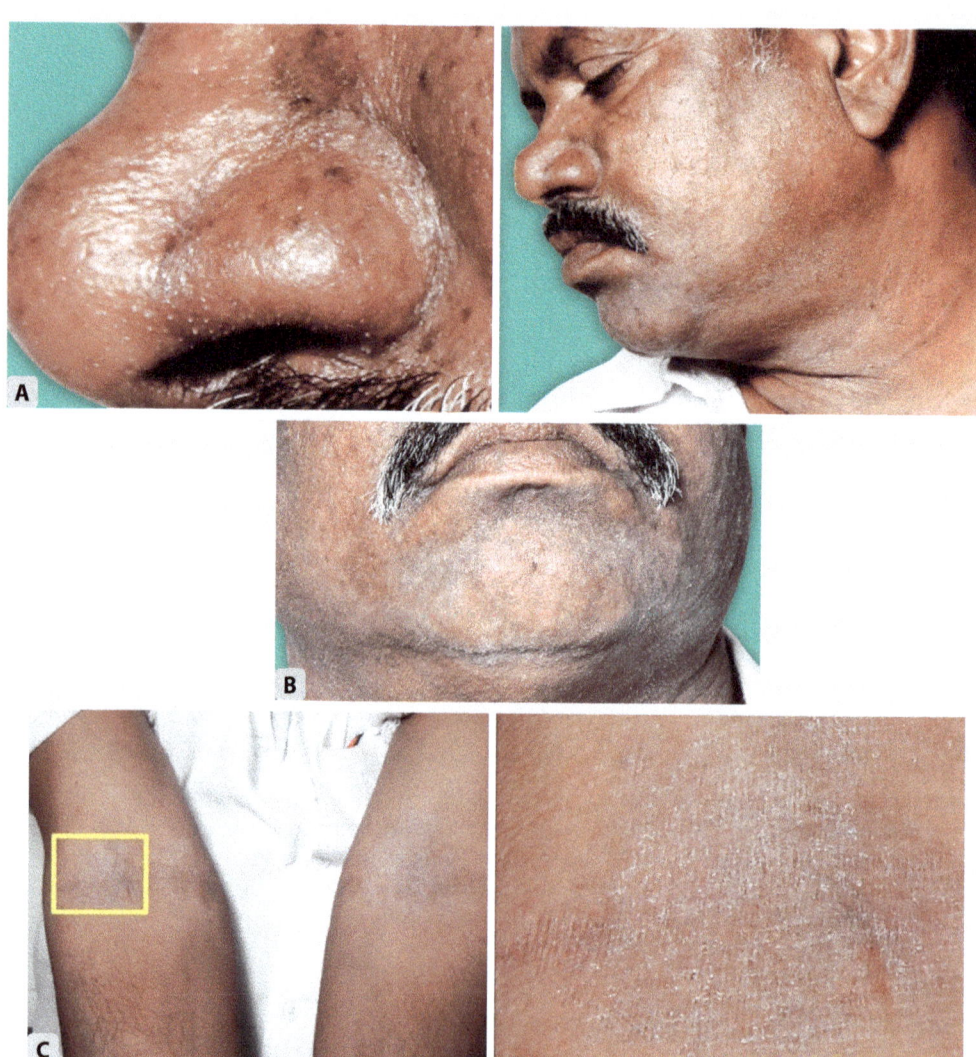

PATIENT 3A: A 45-year-old male—an agriculturist—6 months history of itching and scaling of beard region and scalp. (A) Beard region—submental region, adjacent neck, (L) retronasal fold—scaly patches (yellow box); (left) retronasal fold—scaling; (B) Irregularly coalescent scaly patches; and (C) Both the ACF—scaly papular eruption against the back drop of dry scaly skin (yellow box).

Patient 3B

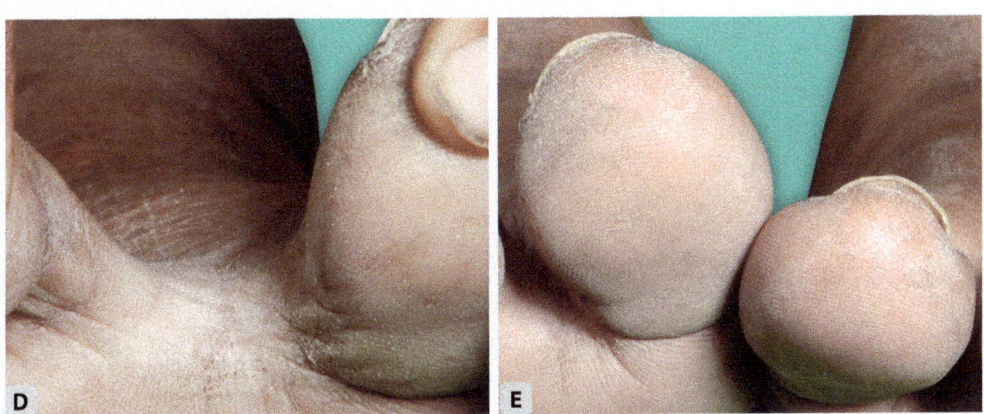

PATIENT 3B: (D) First (right) toe web—HK and scaling. Lateral aspect of (right) great toe (GT) similar findings; and (E) Both the GTNs—arch shaped (overcurved). Pulps of both the GTs—scaly.
(GTNs: great toenails; HK: hyperkeratosis)

Patient 4A

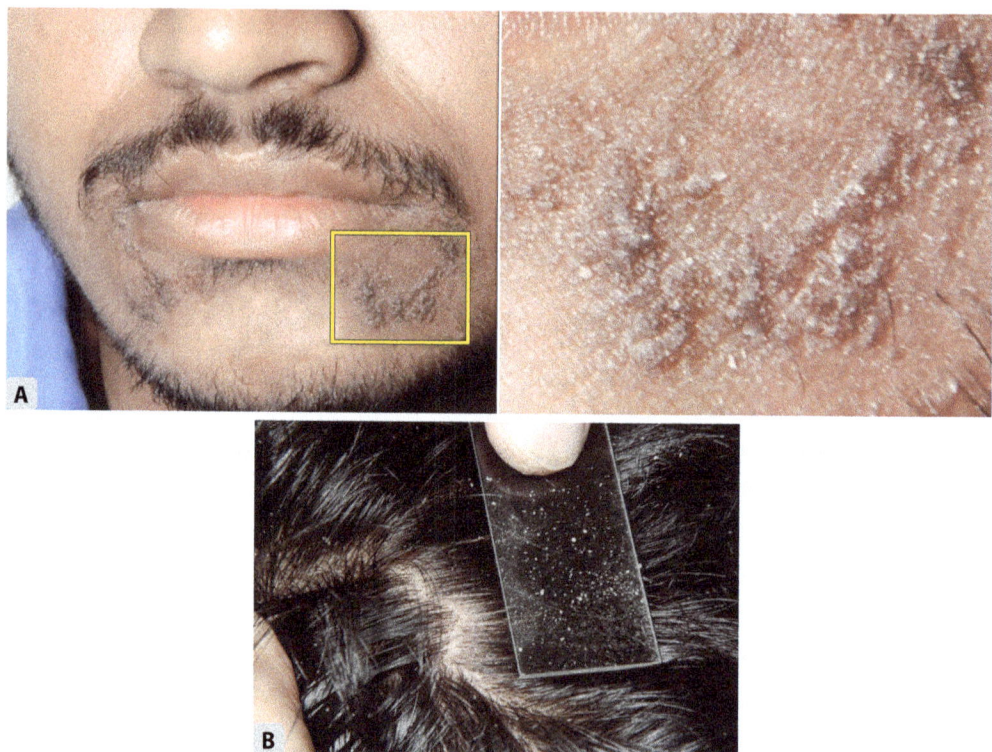

PATIENT 4A: A 16-year-old male—a student—3 days history of sudden onset of asymptomatic eruption below (left) half of lower lip. (A) Dirty brown, irregularly, coalescent papules (yellow box); and (B) Vertex—visible desquamation.

Patient 4B

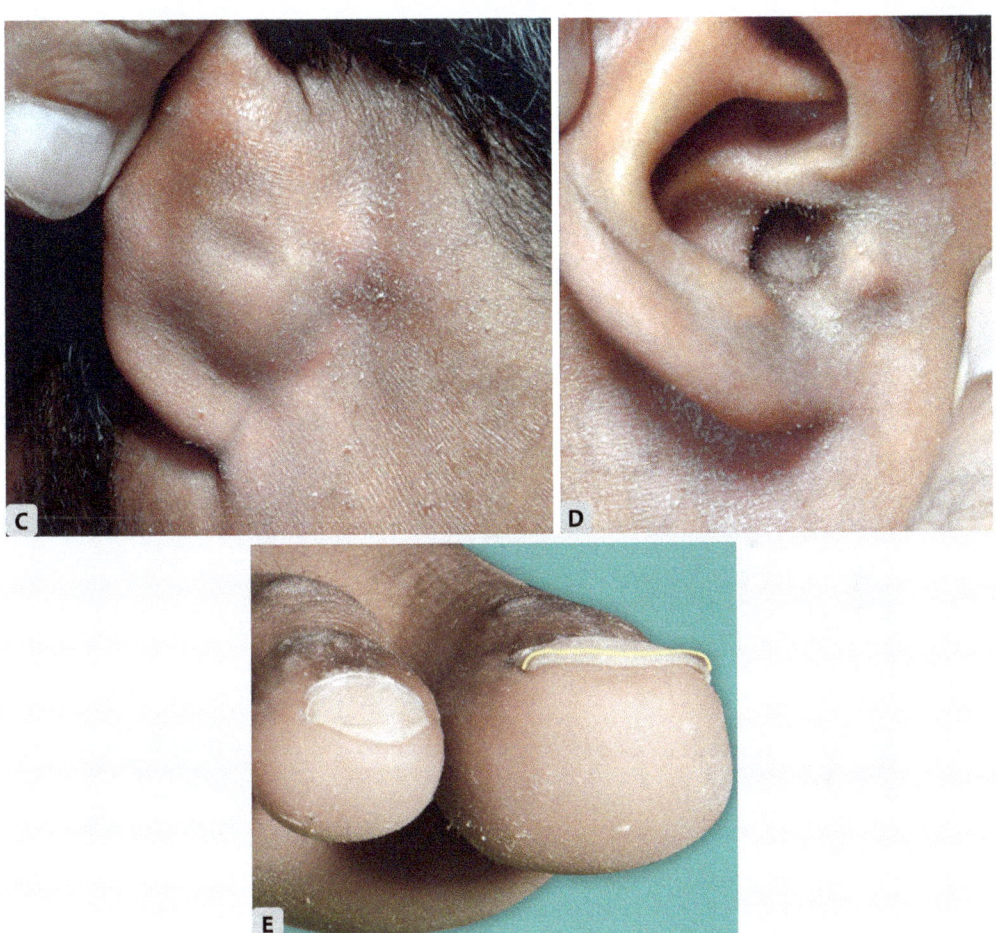

PATIENT 4B: (C) (Left) retroauricular area—mild erythema and nongreasy scales; (D) (Right) auditory canal and periauricular area—erythematous patches with powdery scales; and (E) (Right) great toenail (GTN)—subtle asbestos sheet-shaped nail plate.

Thus, this is a case of sebopsoriasis; the morphology of the lesions below lower lip is atypical/misleading.

Patient 5

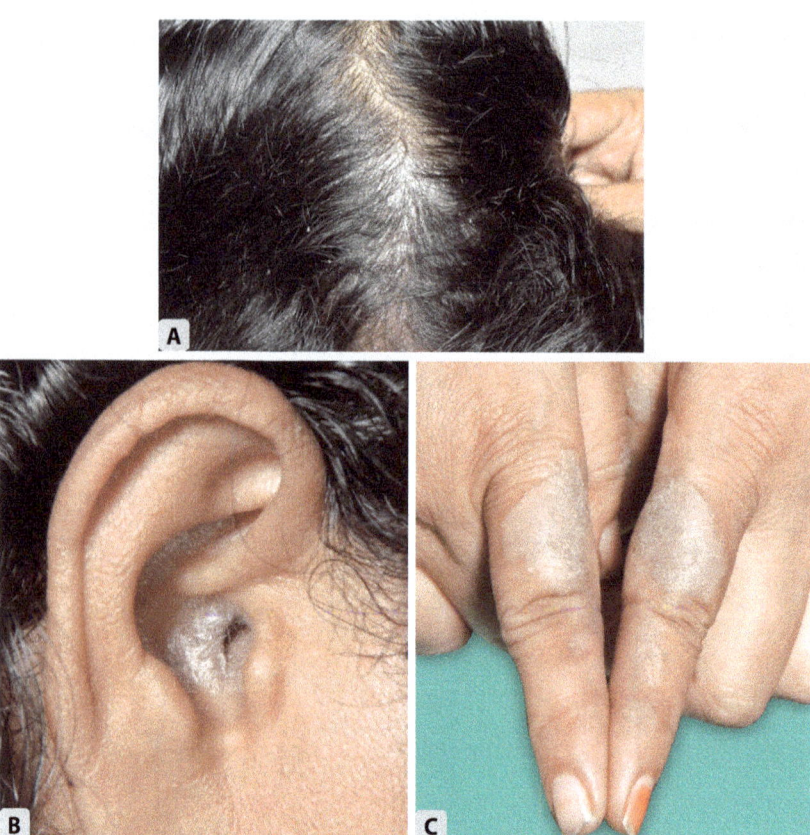

PATIENT 5: A 40-year-old housewife—1 year history of dandruff. (A) Occipital scalp—silvery white scaly plaque; (B) Interior of (right) external earlobe—typical psoriatic lesions; and (C) Both index fingers—barely raised, slightly erythematous scaly plaques (history of applying some topical medicament now and then).

Patient 6A

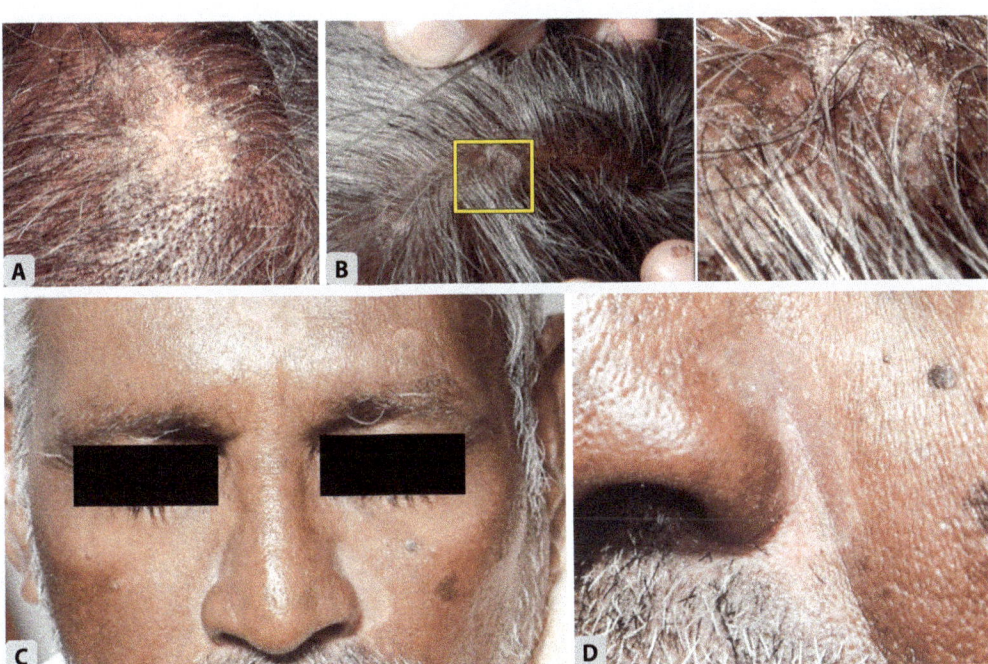

PATIENT 6A: A 68-year-old male—an agriculturist—2 years history of itchy and scaly patches on scalp and elsewhere (lesions typically found in seborrheic distribution). (A) Occiput—a large erythematous scaly patch; (B) Vertex—a scaly plaque—silvery white character of the scale may be noted (yellow box); (C) Nasolabial folds—erythematous scaly patches extending into moustache area; and (D) Similar lesion as in (C).

Patient 6B

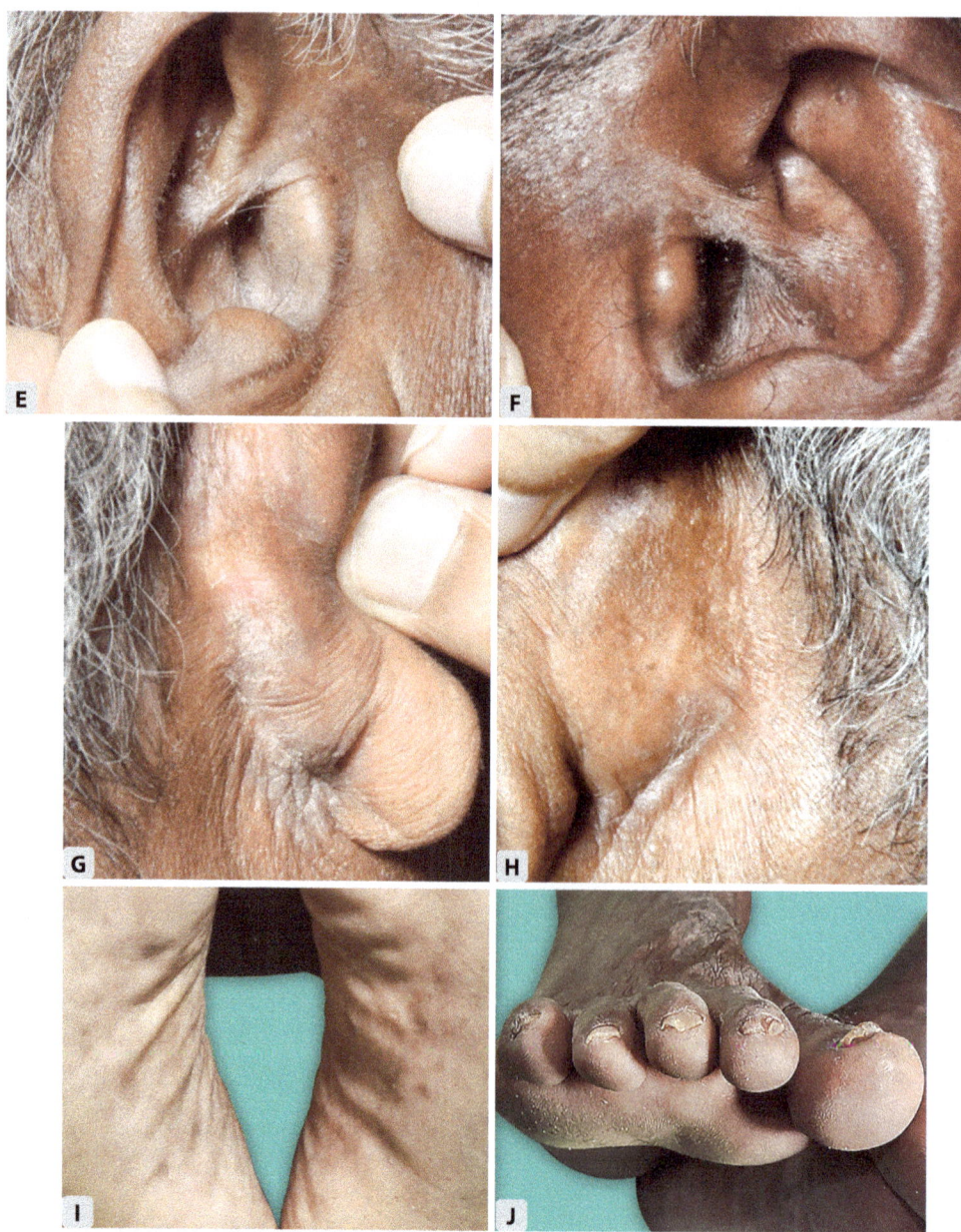

PATIENT 6B: (E and F) Both the external auditory canals—erythematous scaly patches; (G) (Right) retroauricular area—erythematous scaly plaques; lower down a little hypertrophic lesion may be noted; (H) Similar lesion as in (G); (I) Insteps—plantar psoriasis in evolution; and (J) All the nail plates of (right) foot distorted.

Hypertrophic lesions in psoriasis are well-known, but not described in respect of seborrheic dermatitis (SD). Phospholipid is described to contribute to softness of nail plate; perhaps, in psoriasis, phospholipids in nail plates increased making the nail plates more softer; therefore, it may be assumed that trauma may mold the soft nail plate into different shapes.

Patient 7

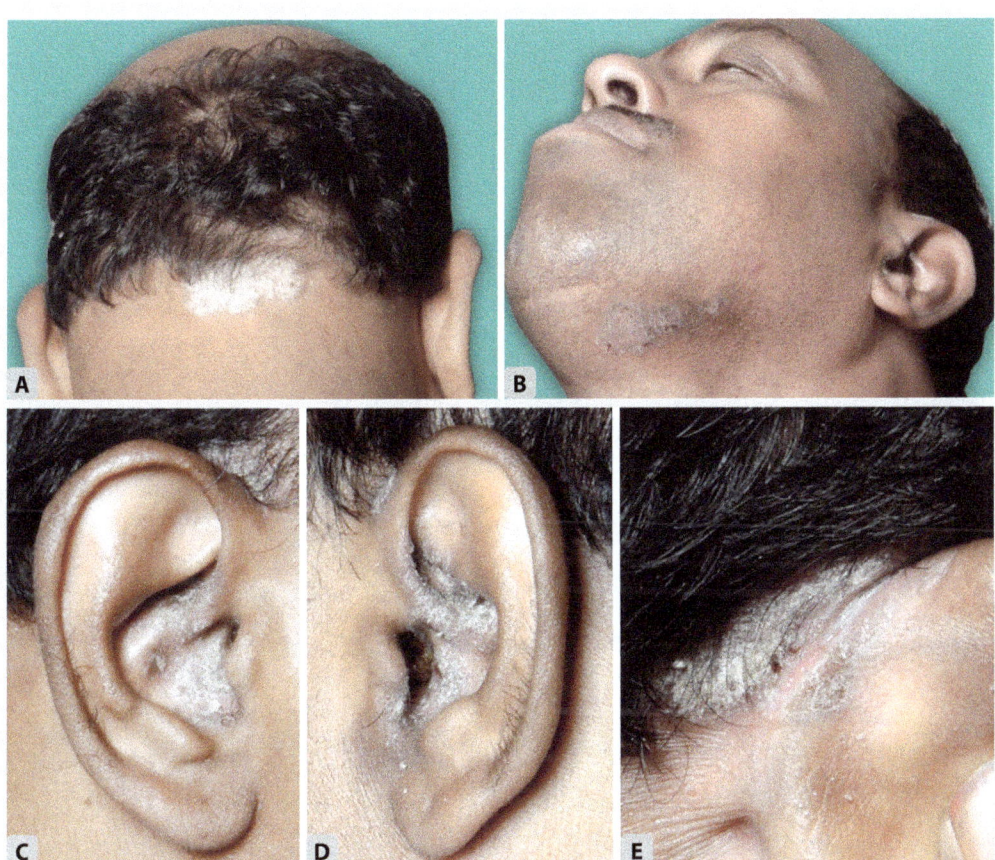

PATIENT 7: A 49-year-old male—a businessman—1.5 years of itchy lesions in neck and earlobes with a past history of dandruff. (A) Nape of neck—typical psoriatic plaque; (B) (Left) submental region—psoriatic plaque; (C and D) Earlobes—psoriatic lesions; and (E) (Right) retroauricular area—psoriatic plaque with fissure.

Patient 8A

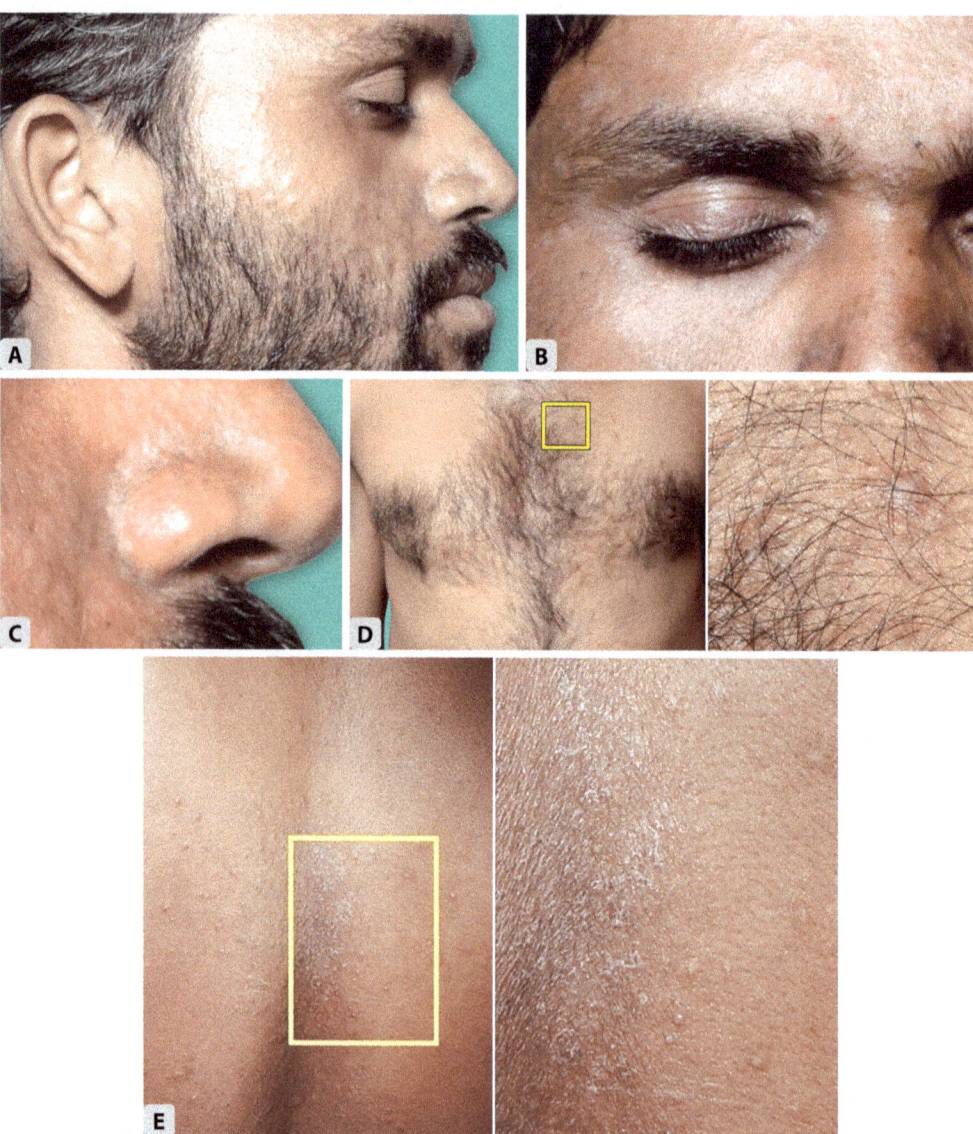

PATIENT 8A: A 28-year-old male—a mason—8 months history of itchy eruption involving face, chest, and back. (A) (Right) side of face—multiple flesh-colored follicular and interfollicular papular eruption; (B) Forehead and glabella—similar lesions as in (A); (C) (Right) retro ala groove—mild erythema and scaling; (D) IM skin—similar lesions as in (A) (yellow box); and (E) Midline of the back—scaly papular eruption (yellow box).

Patient 8B

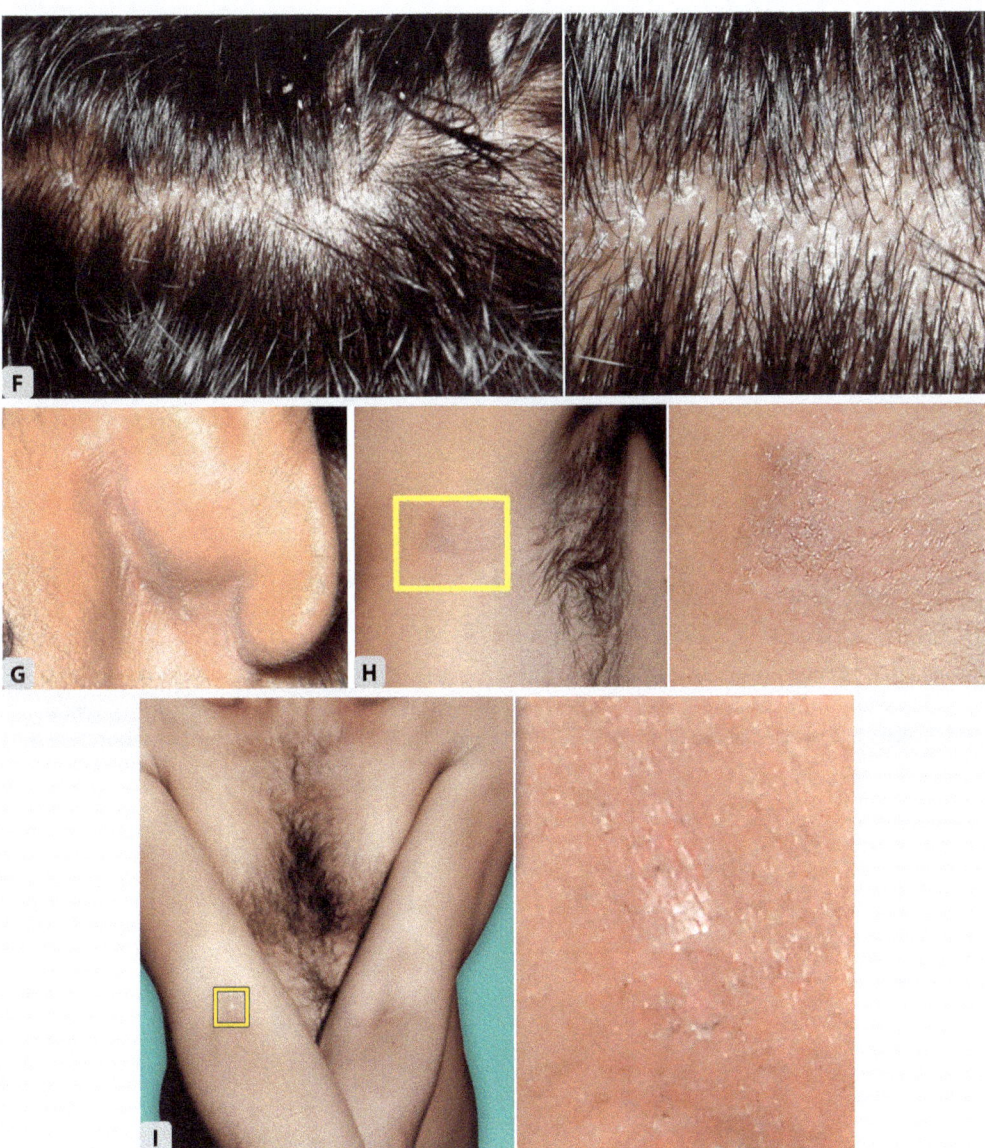

PATIENT 8B: (F) Scalp—multiple follicular silvery white scaly papules; (G) (Right) retroauricular area—erythema, scaling, and fissuring; (H) (Right) axilla—erythematous plaque—composed of multiple, closely set scaly papules; and (I) (Right) ACF—psoriatic plaque in evolution.

Patient 9A

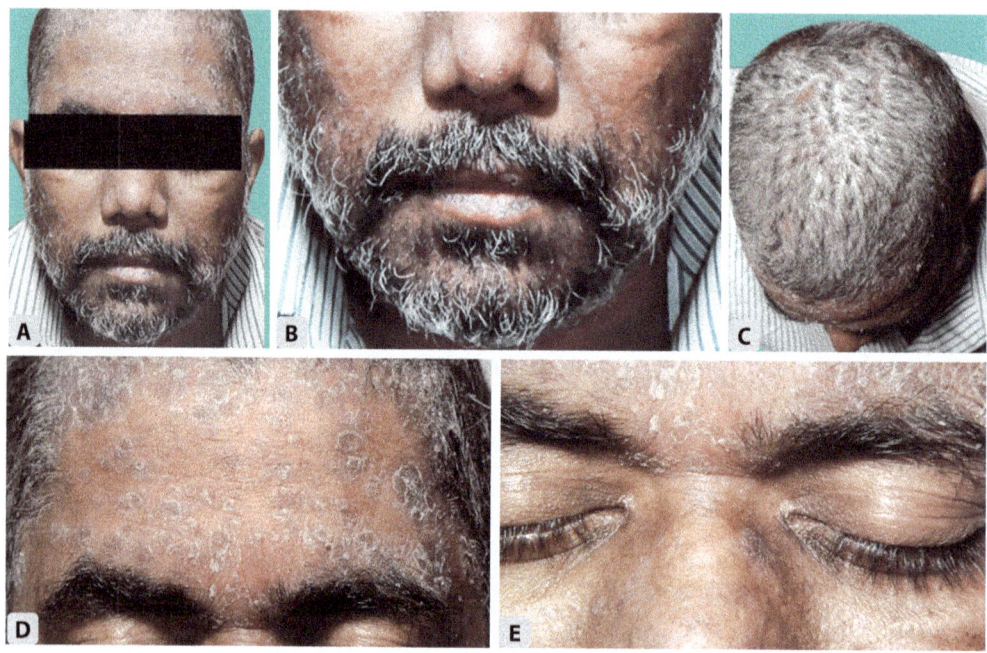

PATIENT 9A: A 47-year-old male—a bus driver—3 years history of itching, dandruff, and scaling of face and trunk. (A and B) Face—seborrheic dermatitis (SD)-like picture; (C) Scalp—pityriasis amiantacea-like picture; and (D and E) Close-up view of face—typical involvement of seborrheic sites.

Color Atlas of Dandruff

Patient 9B

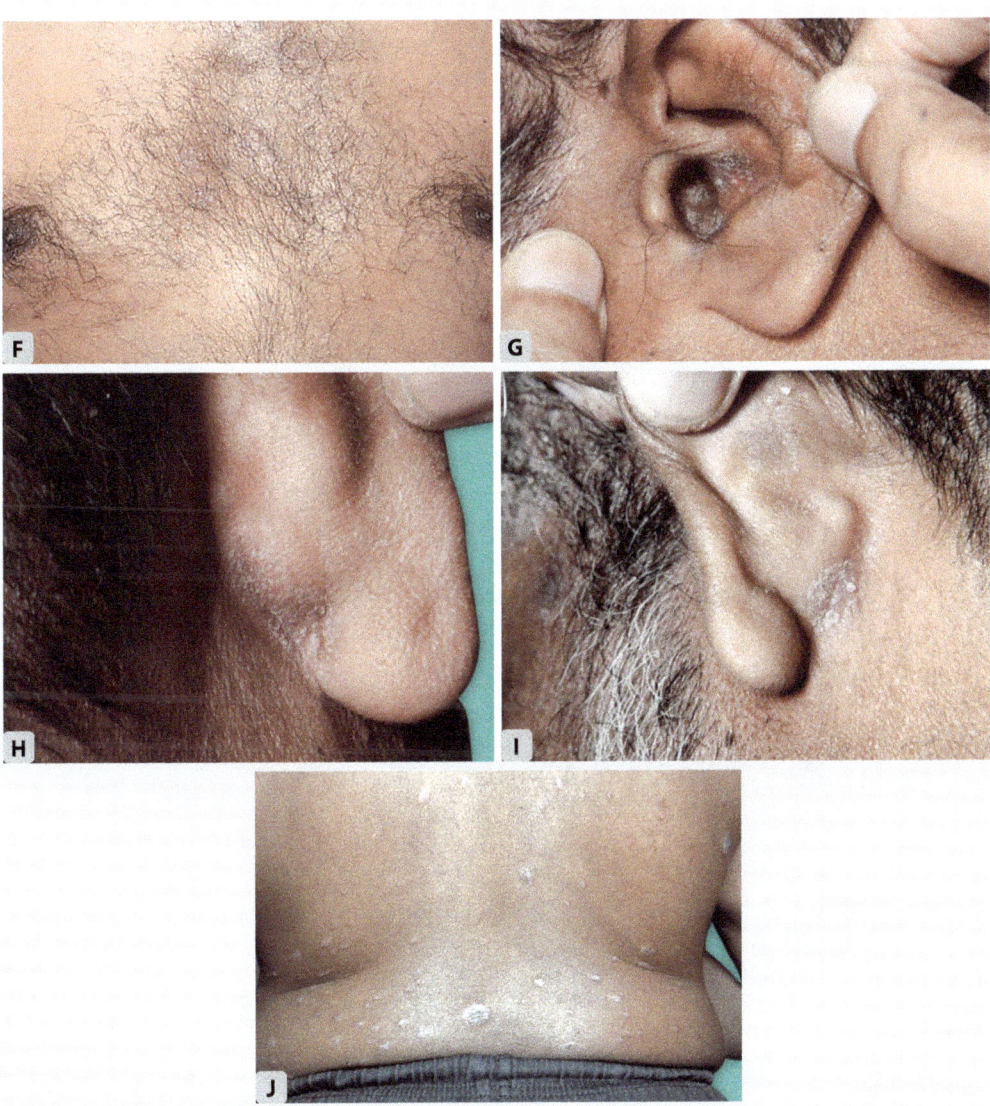

PATIENT 9B: (F) IM skin—very thin scaly plaques; (G) (Left) auditory canal—scaly plaques; (H and I) Both the retroauricular areas—similar lesions as in (G); and (J) Posterior trunk—plaque type psoriasis. *Sebopsoriasis (MA—SD) as a part of psoriasis vulgaris.*

Patient 10

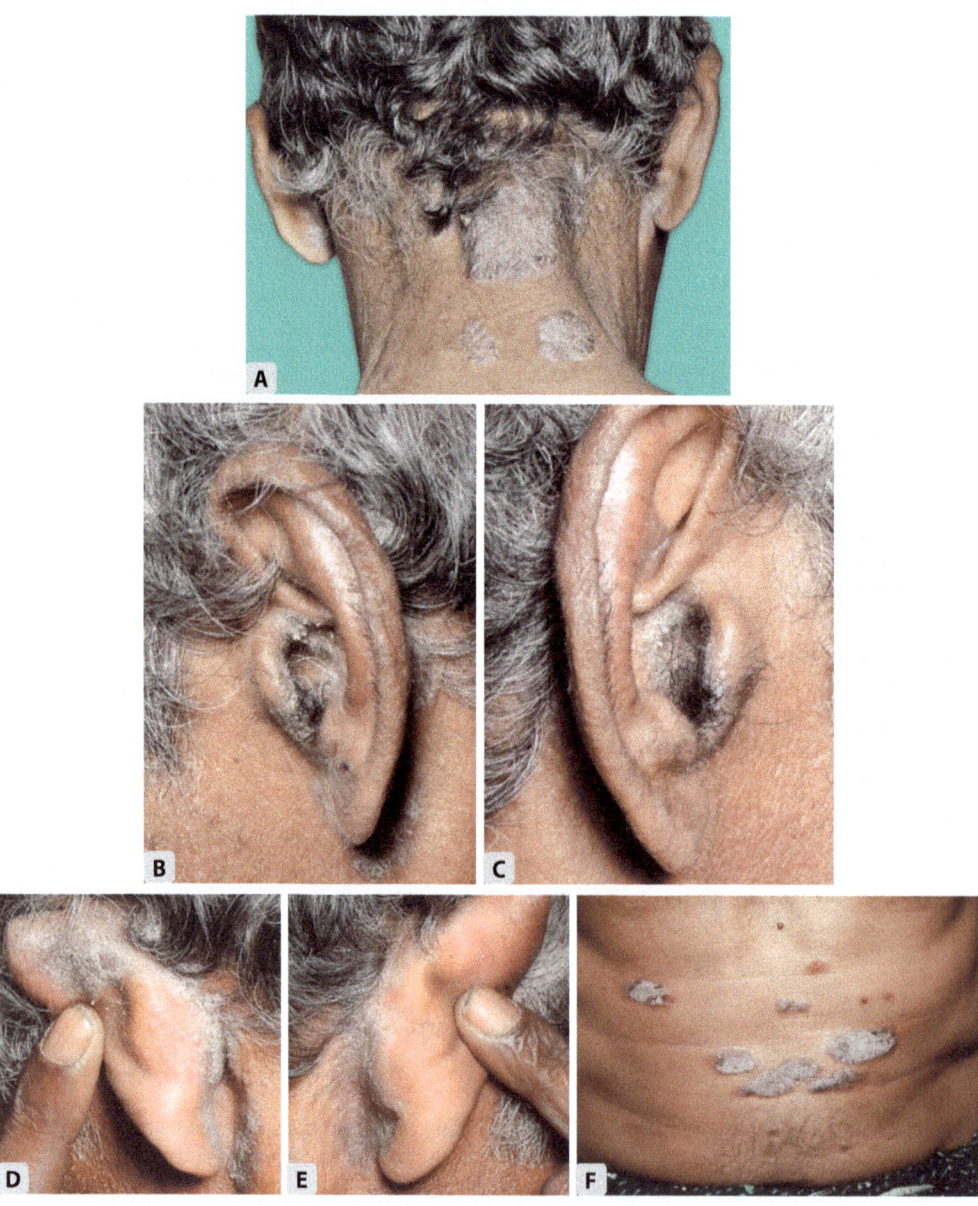

PATIENT 10: A 55-year-old male—an agriculturist—6 years history of itchy patches on face and body. (A) Nape of neck—scaly plaques of psoriasis; (B and C) Both the external auditory canals—scaly lesions; (D and E) Both the retroauricular areas—similar lesions as in B and C; and (F) Anterior trunk—chronic plaque psoriasis.

Sebopsoriasis is a component of chronic plaque psoriasis vulgaris.

Patient 11

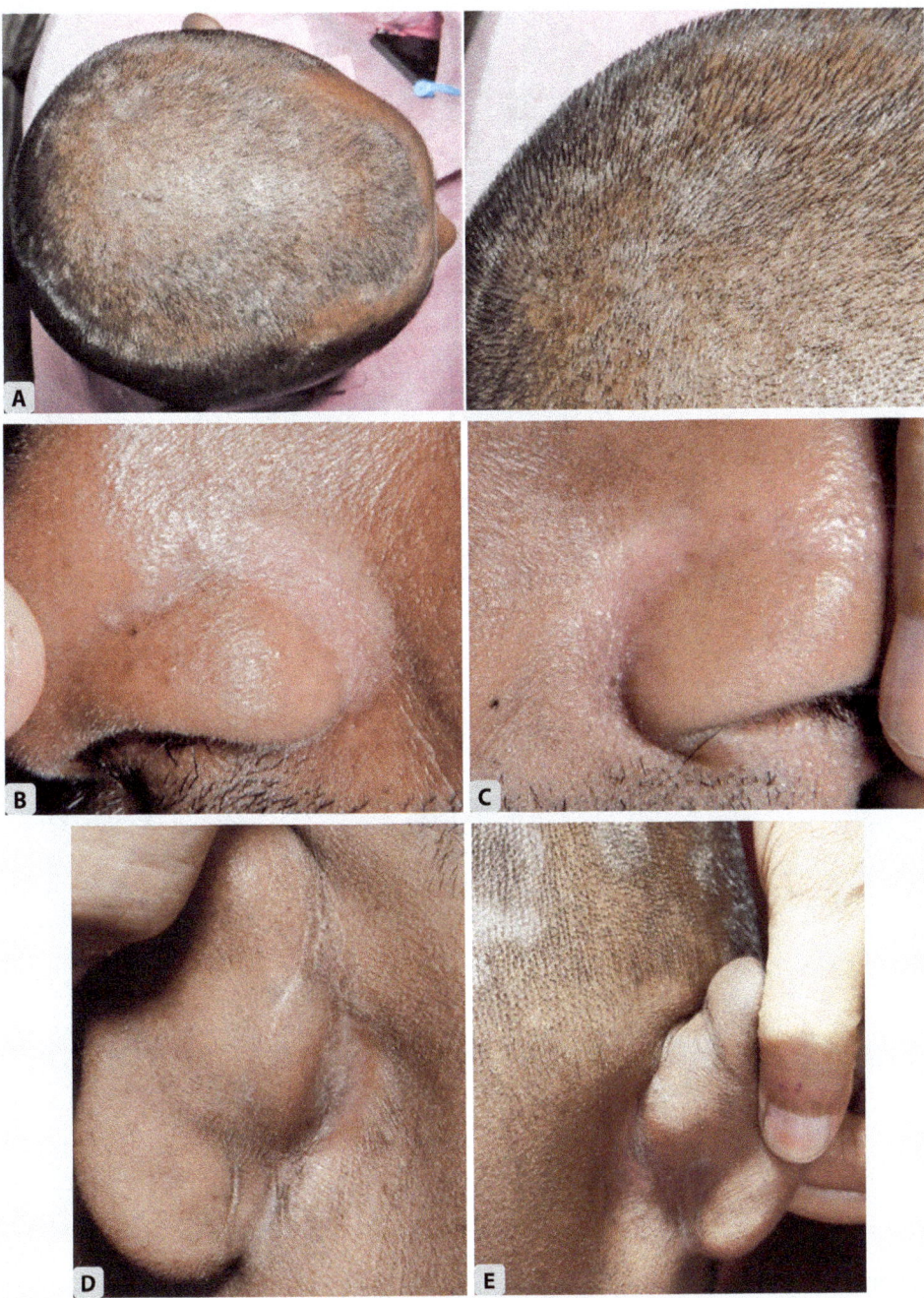

PATIENT 11: A 27-year-old male—a sales executive—2 years history of dandruff. (A) Scalp—discrete and coalescent scaly plaques; (B and C) Both the retro ala nasi—erythema and scaling; and (D and E) Both the retroauricular areas having erythema, scaling, and mild maceration.
This case of exclusive sebopsoriasis has the potential to be mistaken to seborrheic dermatitis (SD).

Patient 12A

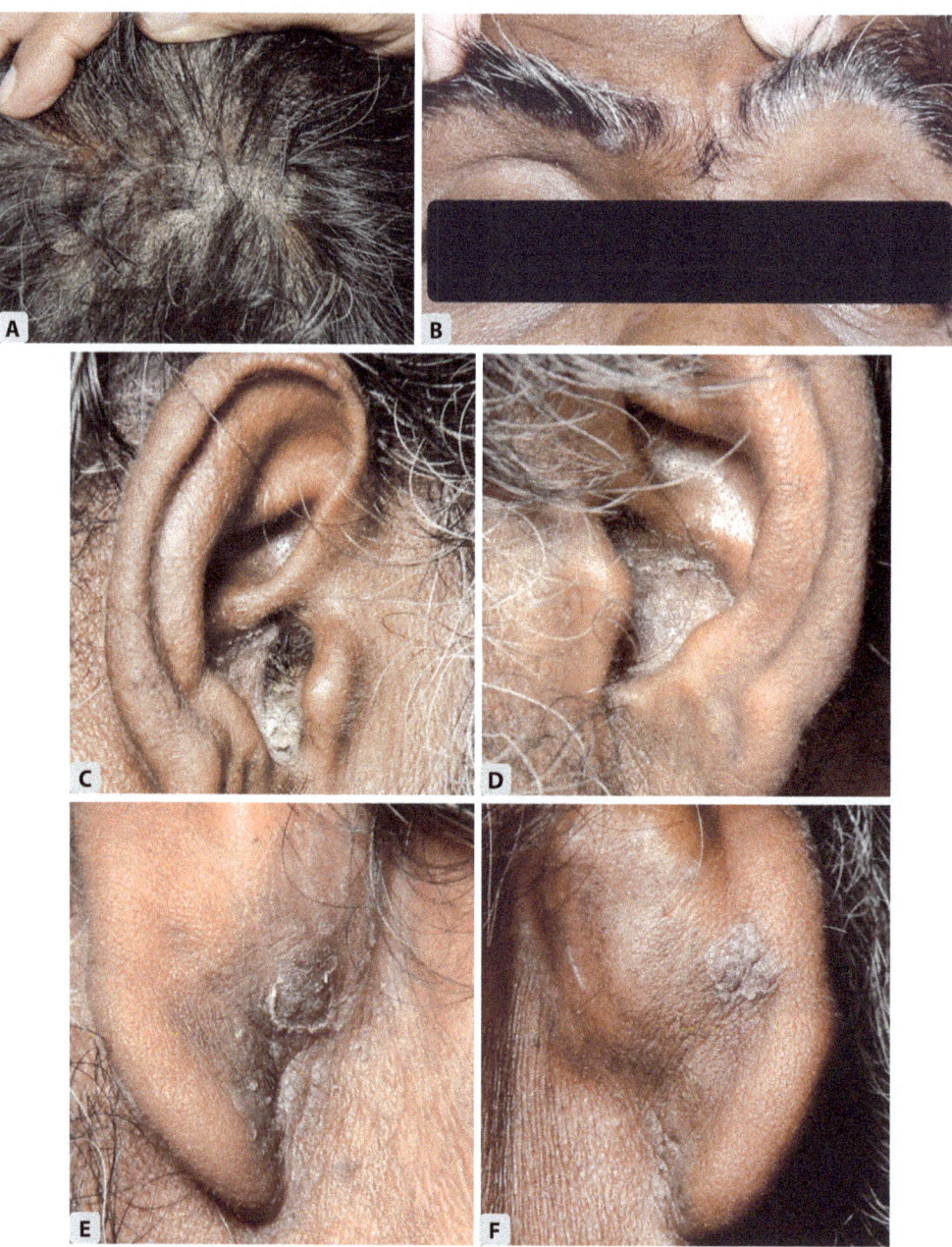

PATIENT 12A: A 50-year-old male—an agriculturist—3 years history of dandruff, itching, and scaling of eyebrows. (A) Occiput—coalescent scaly plaques; (B) Eyebrows—scaly; (C and D) Both the external auditory canals—scaly patches; and (E and F) Back of pinnae and retroauricular grooves—scaly plaques.

This presentation is likely to be mistaken to seborrheic dermatitis (SD).

Patient 12B

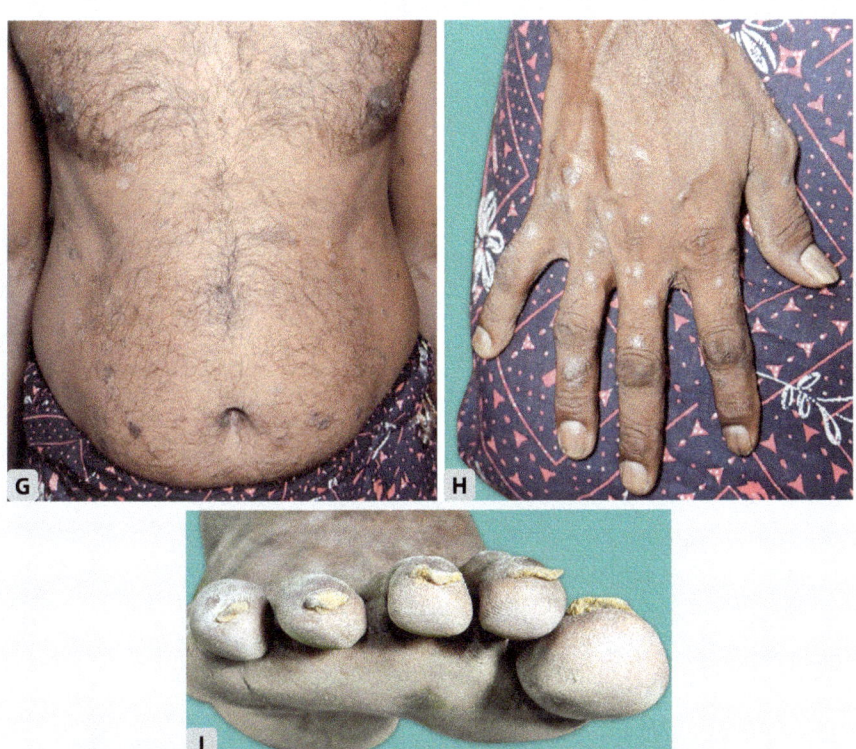

PATIENT 12B: (G and H) Anterior trunk and dorsum of (right) hand—scaly plaques of varying sizes; and (I) All the toenails (TNs) of (right) foot—deformed and (right) middle TN—asbestos sheet shaped. *Thus, it is a case of psoriasis vulgaris with a component of sebopsoriasis.*

Patient 13

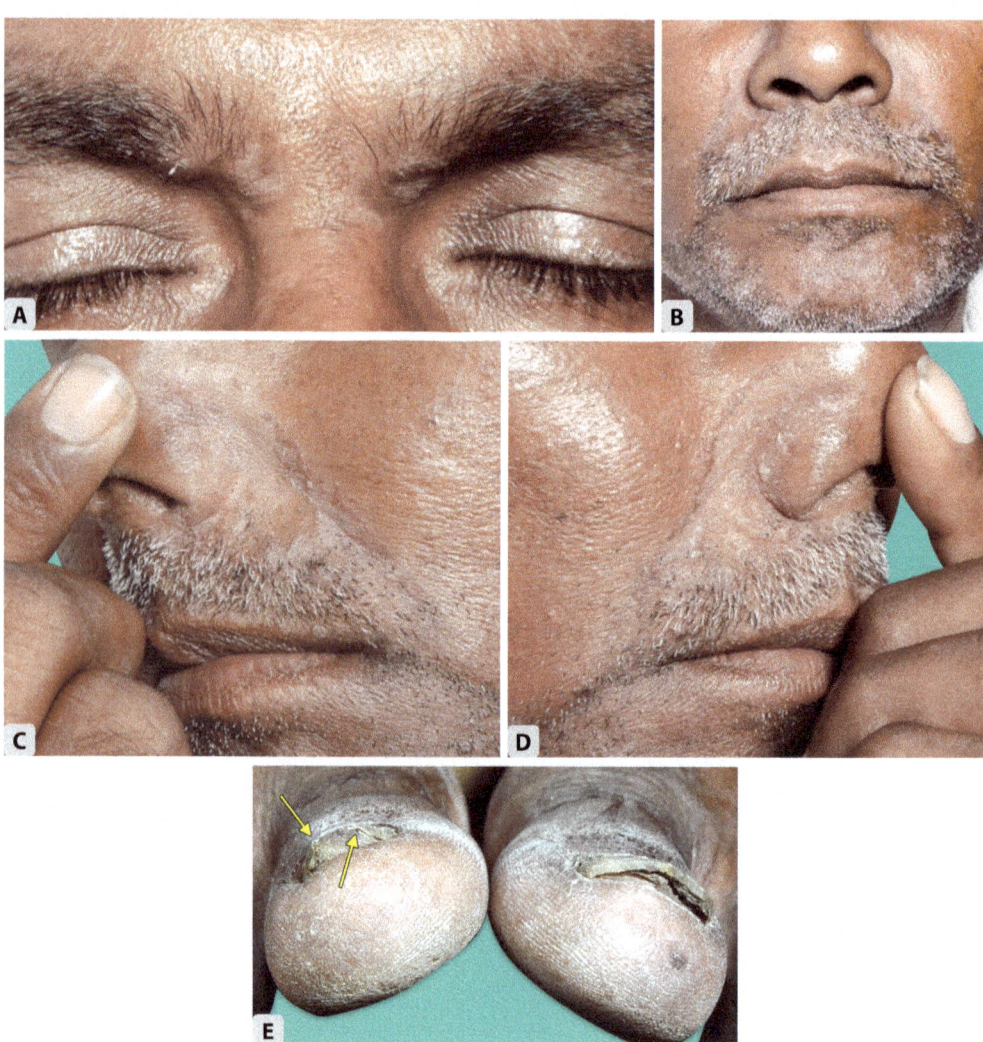

PATIENT 13: A 52-year-old male—an agriculturist—9 months history of itchy and scaly lesions on face. (A to D) Face—typical involvement of all the seborrheic sites of face characterized by erythema and scaling; and (E) Both the GTNs—SUHK; (right) GTN may be found angulated at two points suggested by yellow arrows.
(GTNs: great toenails; SUHK: subungual hyperkeratosis)
This case may be readily mistaken to seborrheic dermatitis (SD) of face; angulated (right) great toenail (GTN) tilts the balance in favor of psoriasis (i.e., sebopsoriasis).

Patient 14

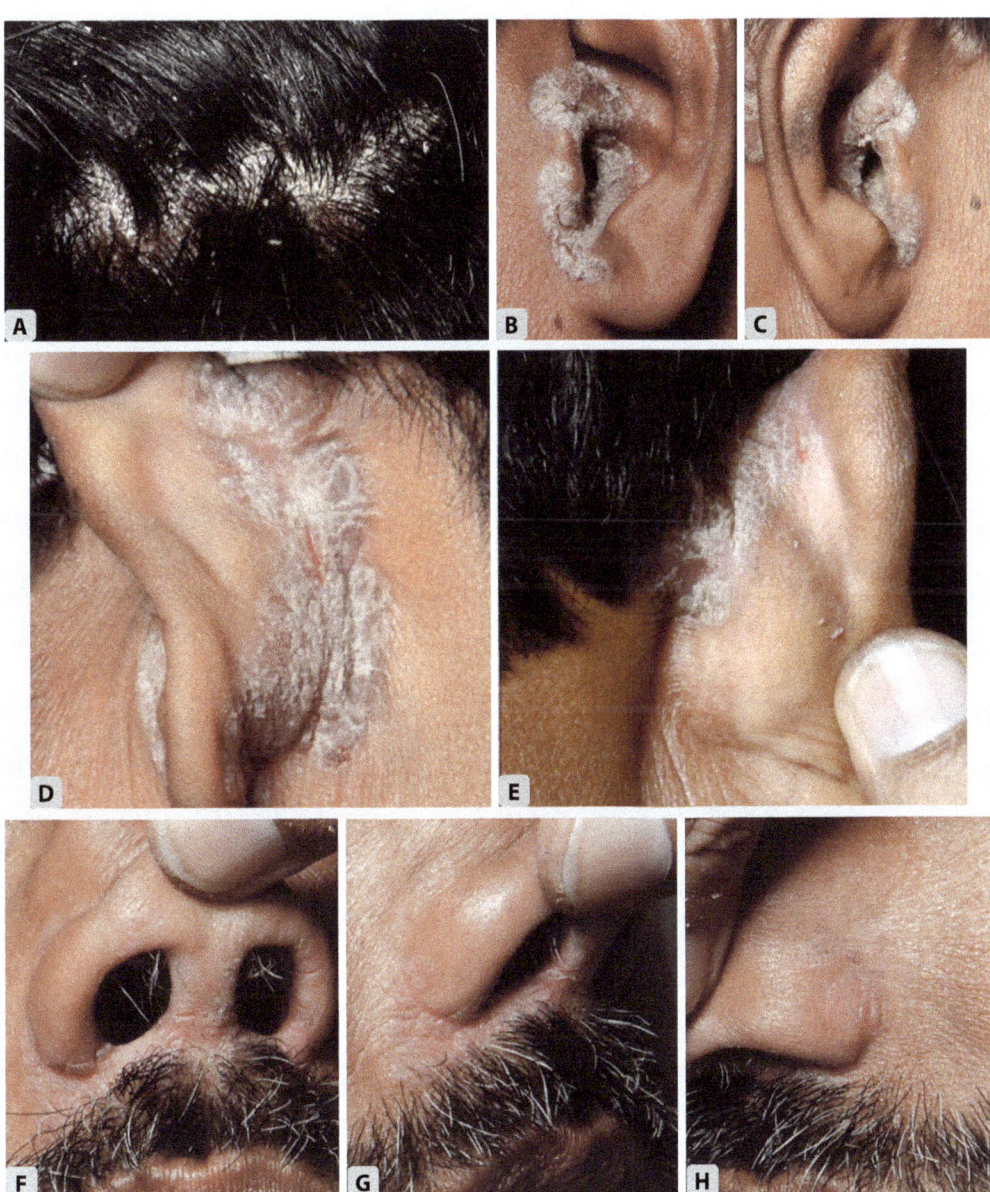

PATIENT 14: A 42-year-old male—a provisions merchant—10 years history of dandruff. (A) Scalp—scaly plaques; (B to E) External earlobes—scaly plaques; and (F to H) Rims of nostrils and nasolabial folds—erythema, scaling, and cracks.

This distribution of lesions may tempt an young dermatologist to diagnose the case as seborrheic dermatitis (SD), but the silvery white scale and morphology of lesions elsewhere tilt the balance in favor of sebopsoriasis.

Patient 15

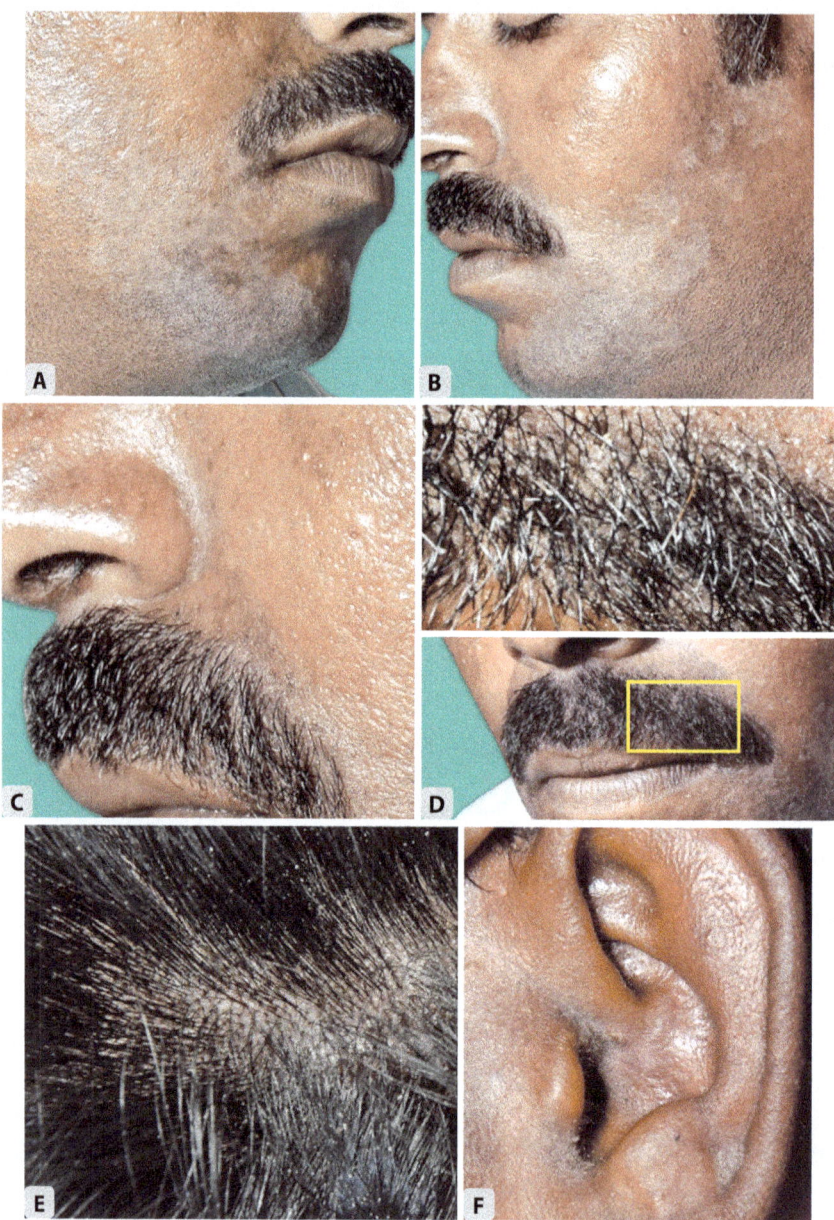

PATIENT 15: A 36-year-old male—a bearer in a way side hotel—1 year history of dandruff and 6 months history of itchy lesions on face; history of applying a TM to facial lesions. (A and B) Sides of face—pityriasis versicolor-like lesions; (C and D) (Left) side of face—patches extending into (left) end of moustache; upper lip—scales may be noted (yellow box); (E) Scalp—scaly plaques with silvery white scales; and (F) (Left) external earlobe—erythematous, scaly patches.

This case may be mistaken to either pityriasis versicolor or seborrheic dermatitis (SD). But on looking beyond the lesions, scalp displays silvery white scales which clinch the diagnosis of sebopsoriasis.

Color Atlas of Dandruff | 95

Patient 16A

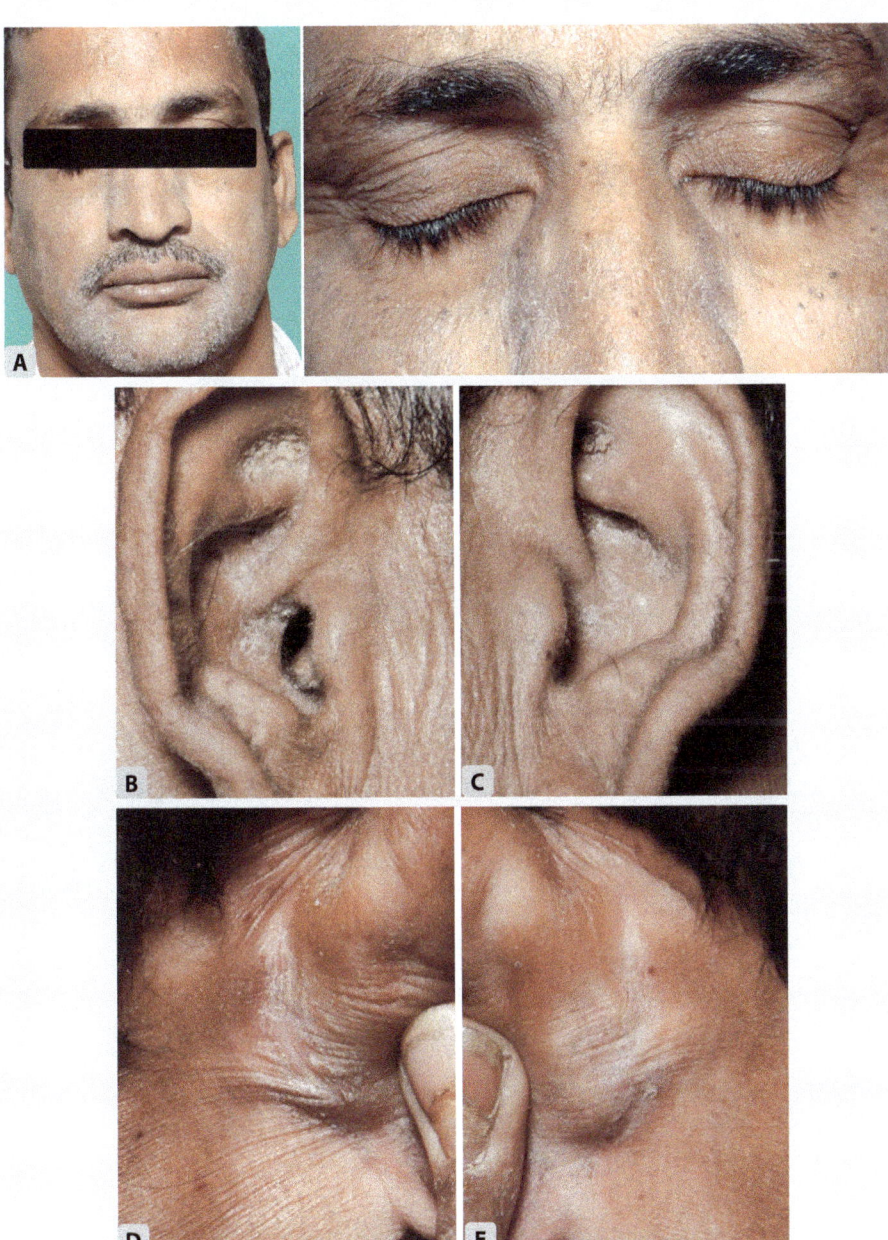

PATIENT 16A: A 55-year-old male—an agriculturist—5 months history of itching of face. (A) Face—diffuse, dry, and scaly dermatitis; (B and C) External earlobes—navicular fossae—nongreasy yellowish scales; external auditory meatus and elsewhere—erythematous scaly plaques; and (D and E) Both the retroauricular areas—erythema and scaling.

Face, in this agriculturist, at a glance, may offer a picture of ABCD; dry yellow scales may confuse the dermatologist and lead to a diagnosis of seborrheic dermatitis (SD) instead of sebopsoriasis.

Patient 16B

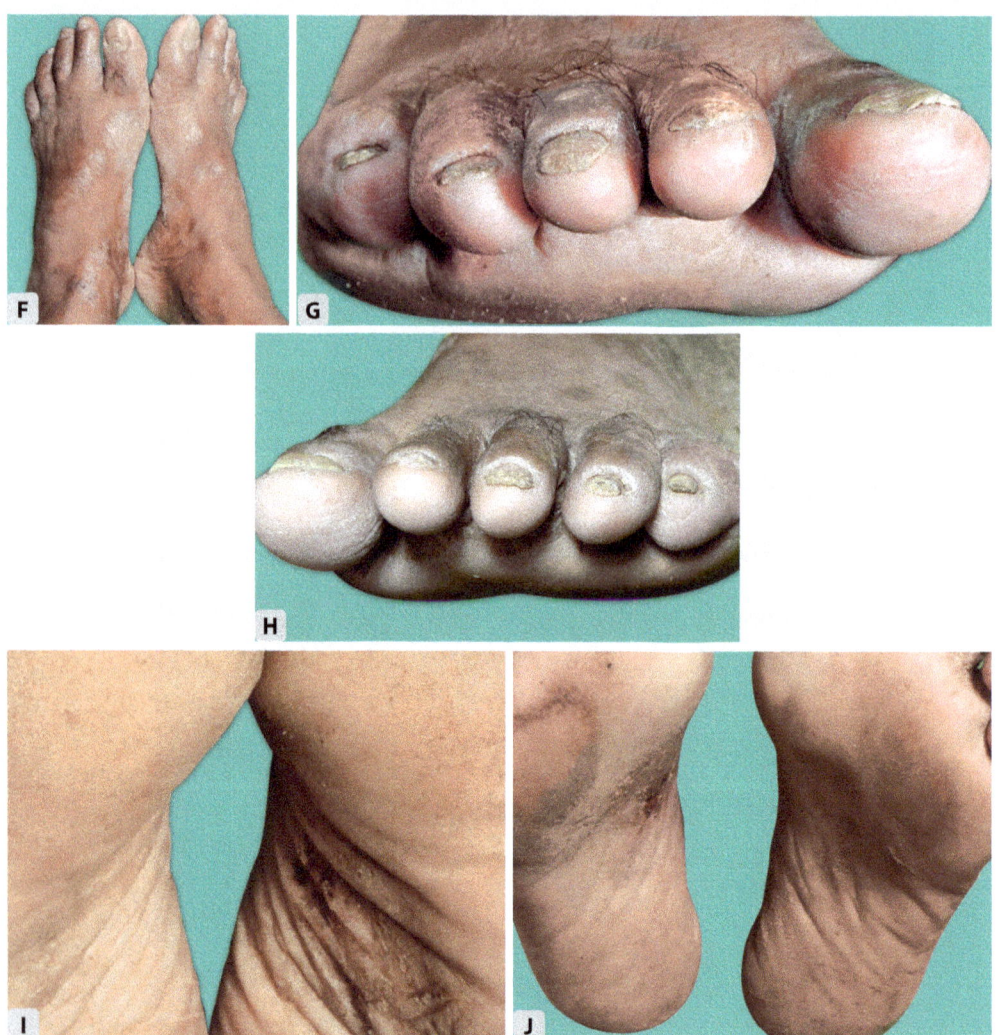

PATIENT 16B: (F) Dorsae of feet—multiple thin scaly plaques; (G and H) Almost all the toenails (TNs) are abnormal; and (I and J) Both the insteps—plantar psoriasis.

These photos provide clues to the diagnosis of psoriasis.

Patient 17

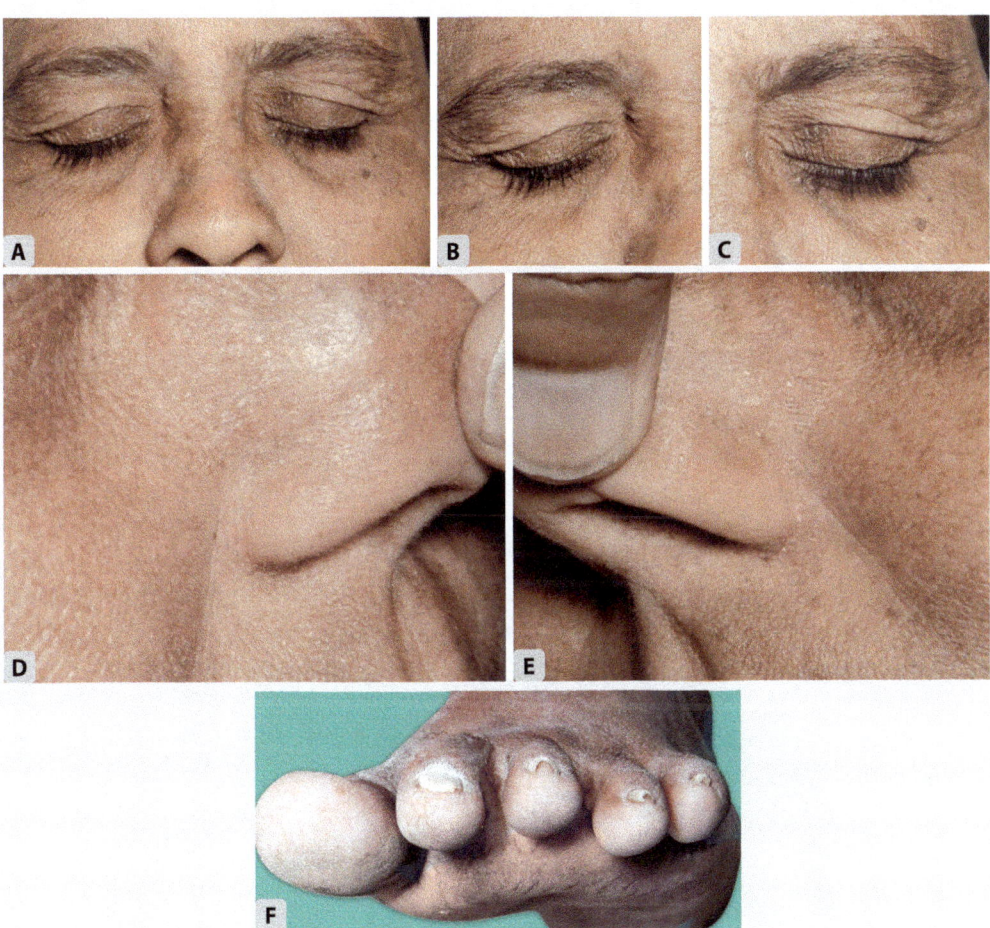

PATIENT 17: A 44-year-old female—a housewife—6 months history of itchy rash on her face. (A to C) Face—offers a picture of SD; (D and E) Nasolabial furrows—subtle erythema and scaling; and (F) Third, fourth, and fifth TNs of (left) foot—pincer nails.

(SD: seborrheic dermatitis; TNs: toenails)

The most common cause of pincer nails is psoriasis in this region—as per my clinical experience (APMCE).

Patient 18

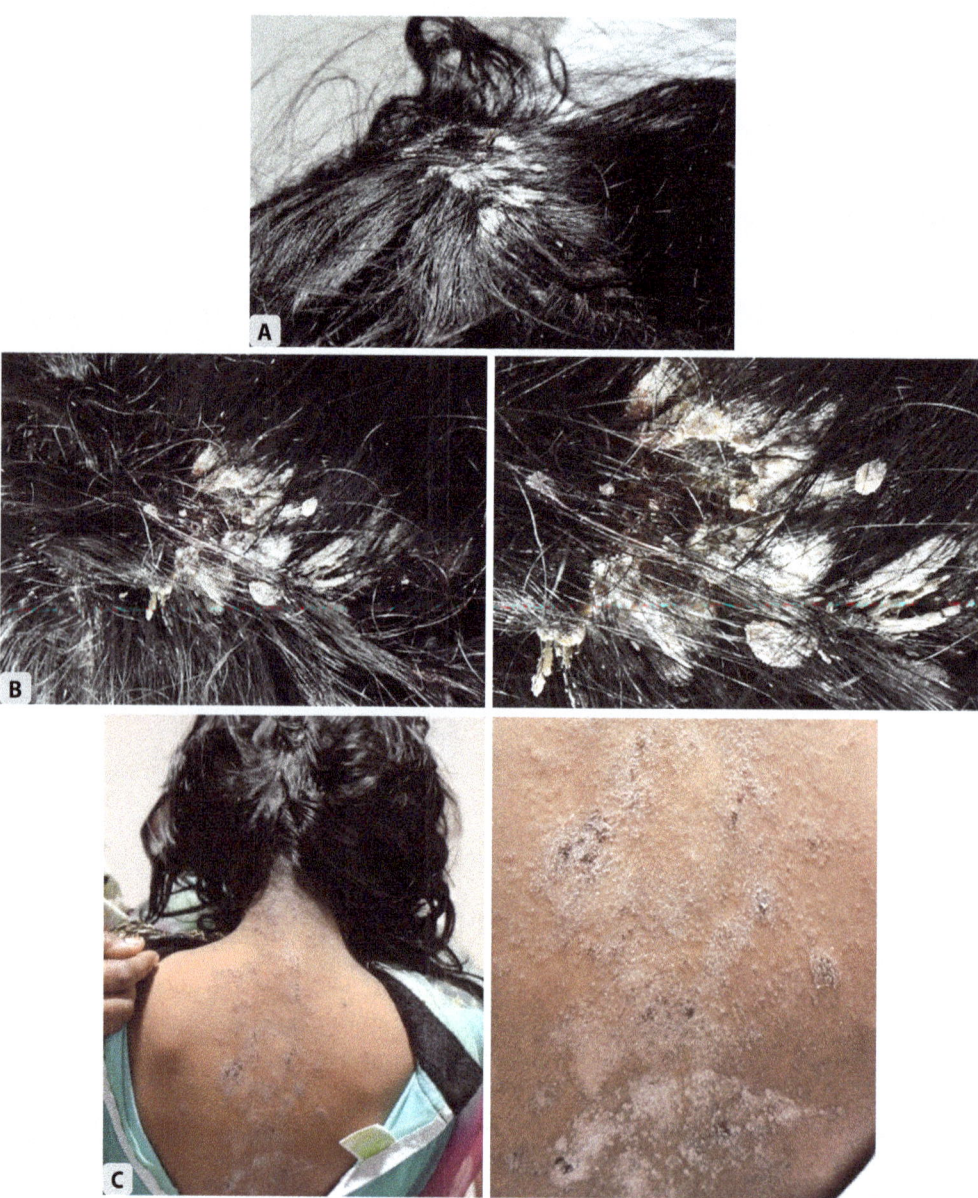

PATIENT 18: A 13-year-old female—an inmate of a school hostel—10 months history of itching and scaling of scalp and back (3 months). (A and B) Scalp—typical pityriasis amiantacea; and (C) Upper back—psoriatic plaques in evolution.
Involvement of interscapular skin may be mistaken to seborrheic dermatitis (SD) as the etiology of pityriasis amiantacea.

Patient 19A

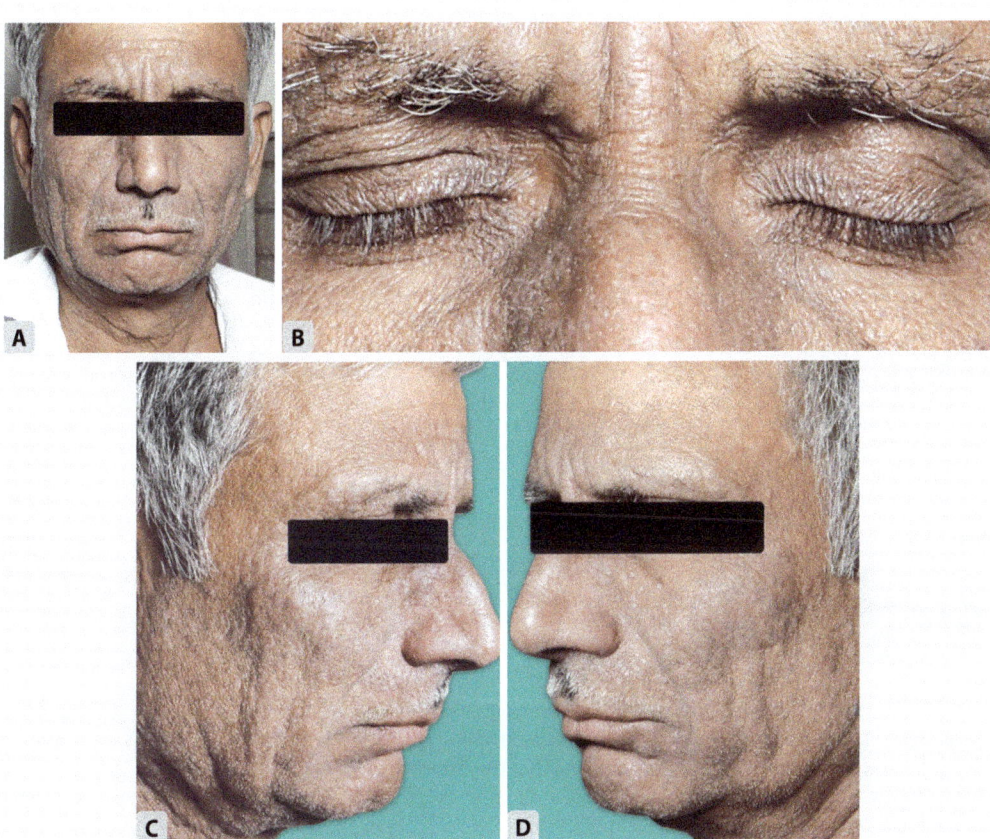

PATIENT 19A: A 50-year-old male—an agriculturist—2 years history of itching of face and scalp. (A to D) Face—diffuse, scaly dermatitis of face including eyelids with scanty papulation.
This facial dermatitis, too, may be mistaken to parthenium dermatitis in this agriculturist.

Patient 19B

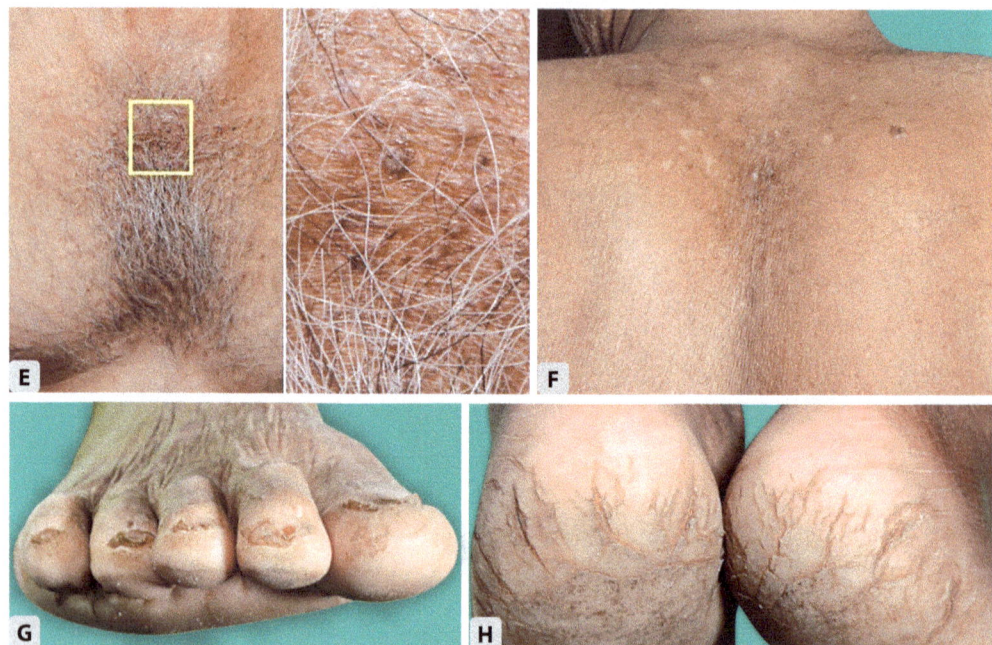

PATIENT 19B: (E) IM skin—follicular and interfollicular papules (yellow box); (F) Upper mid-back—amidst a population of flesh-colored papules, a solitary silvery white scaly papule may be noted; (G) (Right) foot—all the toenails (TNs) distorted; and (H) Soles—heavy fissuring.
The facial dermatitis and papules in the IM skin and upper midback may mislead to a diagnosis of seborrheic dermatitis (SD). The toenails and fissuring of soles provide clues to psoriasis.

Patient 20A

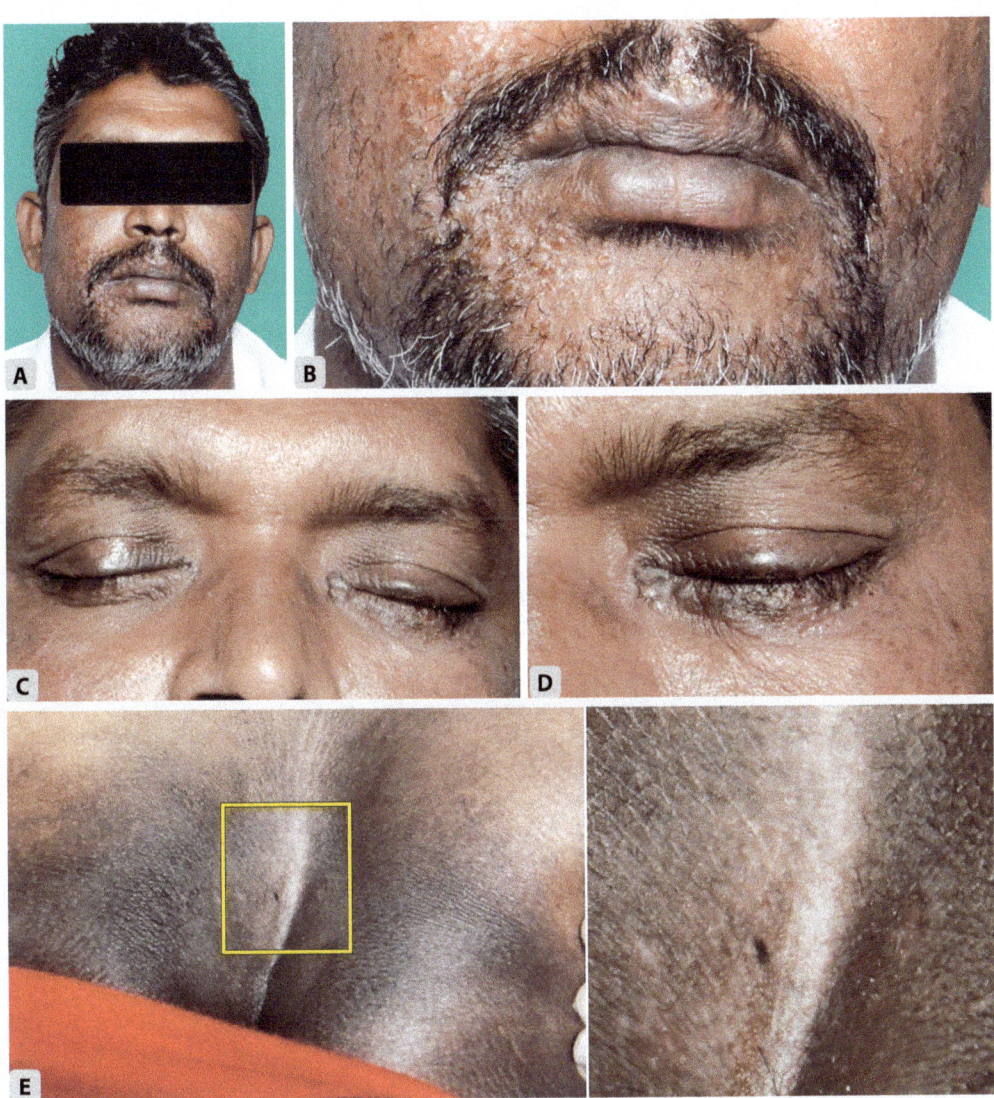

PATIENT 20A: A 40-year-old male—a painter—2 months history of itchy lesions on face. (A to D) Face—blepharitis; a perioral impetiginized, eczematous eruption; and (E) Upper natal cleft— mild erythema with subtle maceration (yellow box).
This case may be mistaken to seborrheic dermatitis (SD).

Patient 20B

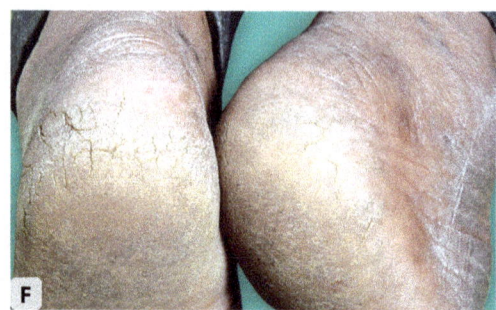

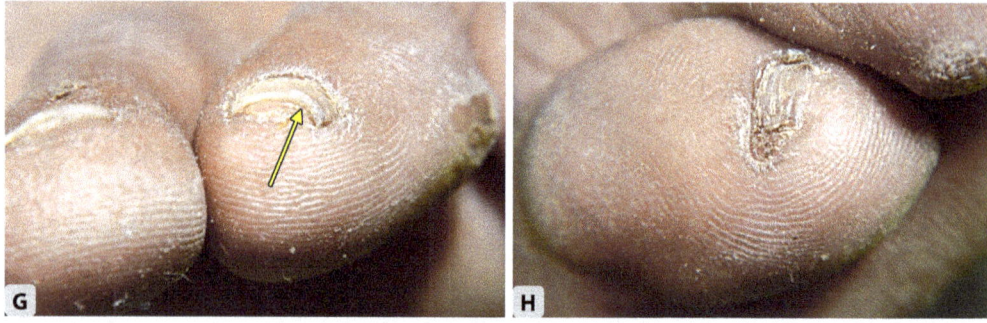

PATIENT 20B: (F) Hindfeet—HK and fissuring; (G) (Left) foot—fourth TN—angulation (yellow arrow); and (H) (Right) foot—(left) LTN—split.

(HK: hyperkeratosis; LTN: little toenail)

Little toenail (LTN) split is a pathognomonic nail sign for psoriasis in this region—as per my clinical experience (APMCE). Thus, this presentation proves to be a case of sebopsoriasis mimicking seborrheic dermatitis (SD).

Patient 21

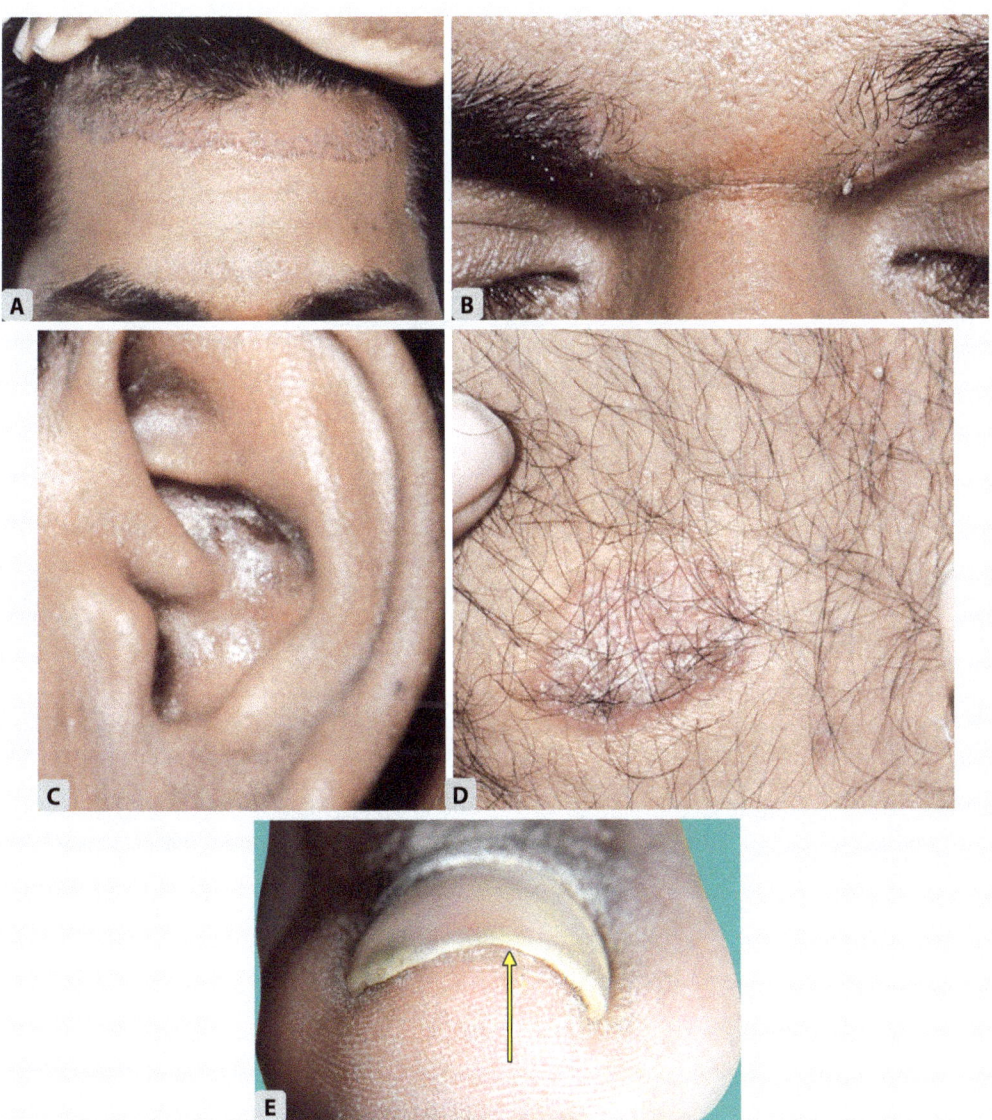

PATIENT 21: A 26-year-old male—an unemployed engineer—6 years history of scaling scalp and 2 months history of forehead patch. (A) Forehead—corona seborrheica-like plaque; (B) Medial eyebrows—scaly; (C) (Left) ear concha—thin erythematous scaly plaques; (D) IM skin—psoriatic plaques of varying sizes; and (E) (Left) great toenail (GTN)—subtle angulation (yellow arrow).

Patient 22

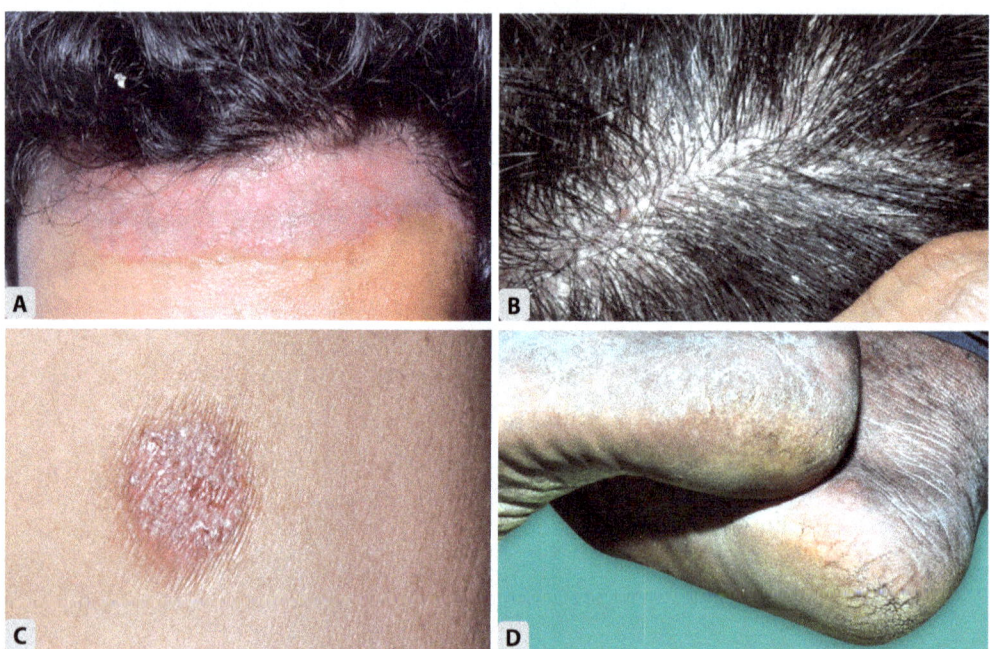

PATIENT 22: A 45-year-old male—a vegetable vendor—2 years history of dandruff and 3 months history of forehead eruption. (A) Forehead—corona seborrheica-like lesion; (B) Vertex—profuse silvery white scales; (C) (Right) outer arm—a discoid eczematous plaque-like psoriatic lesion; and (D) Foot borders—hyperkeratosis (HK) and fissuring.

Older editions of major textbooks used to describe extension of scaly plaque beyond the frontal hairline as a characteristic feature of seborrheic dermatitis (SD), but as per my clinical experience (APMCE) this extension is more a feature of psoriasis vulgaris.

Patient 23A

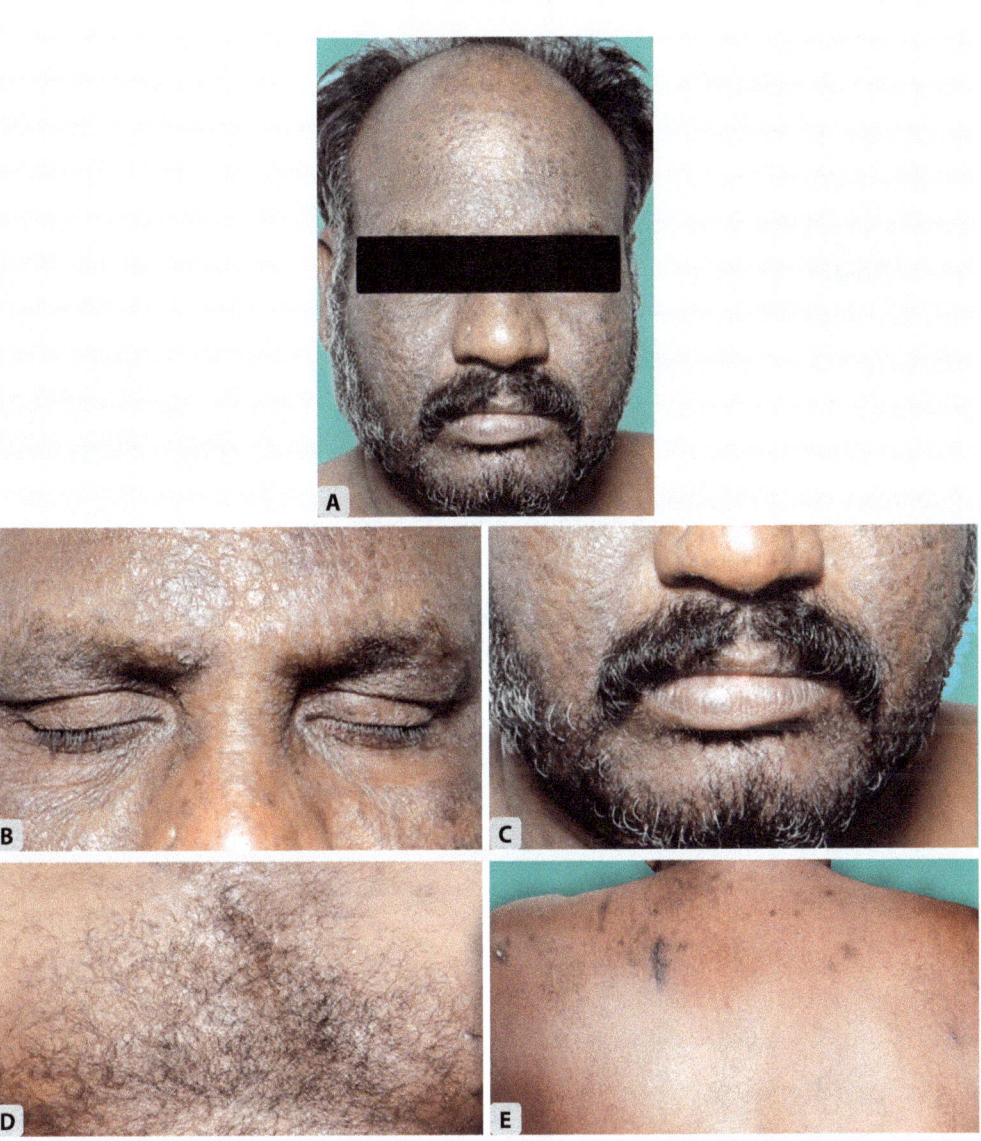

PATIENT 23A: *Continued*

Patient 23A

Continued

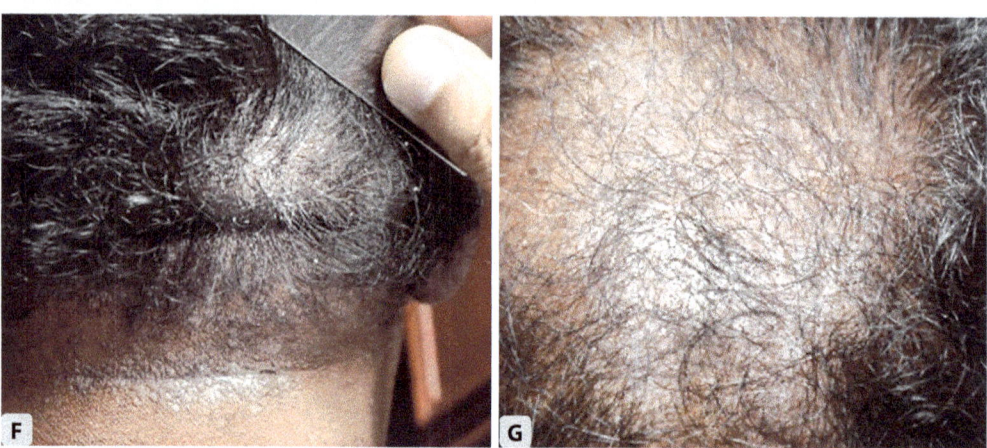

PATIENT 23A: A 55-year-old male—a mason—2 years history of itchy rash of face and chest. (A to C) Face—a dense, dusky red, discrete, and coalescent papular eruption; (D) IM skin—multiple faintly erythematous scaly patches; (E) Upper back—postinflammatory pigmentary changes; (F) Occipital scalp and nape of neck—multiple coalescent scaly papular eruption; and (G) Occiput—entire skin over occiput is scaly.

The seborrheic distribution of the lesions may result in wrong labeling of the case as seborrheic dermatitis (SD).

Patient 23B

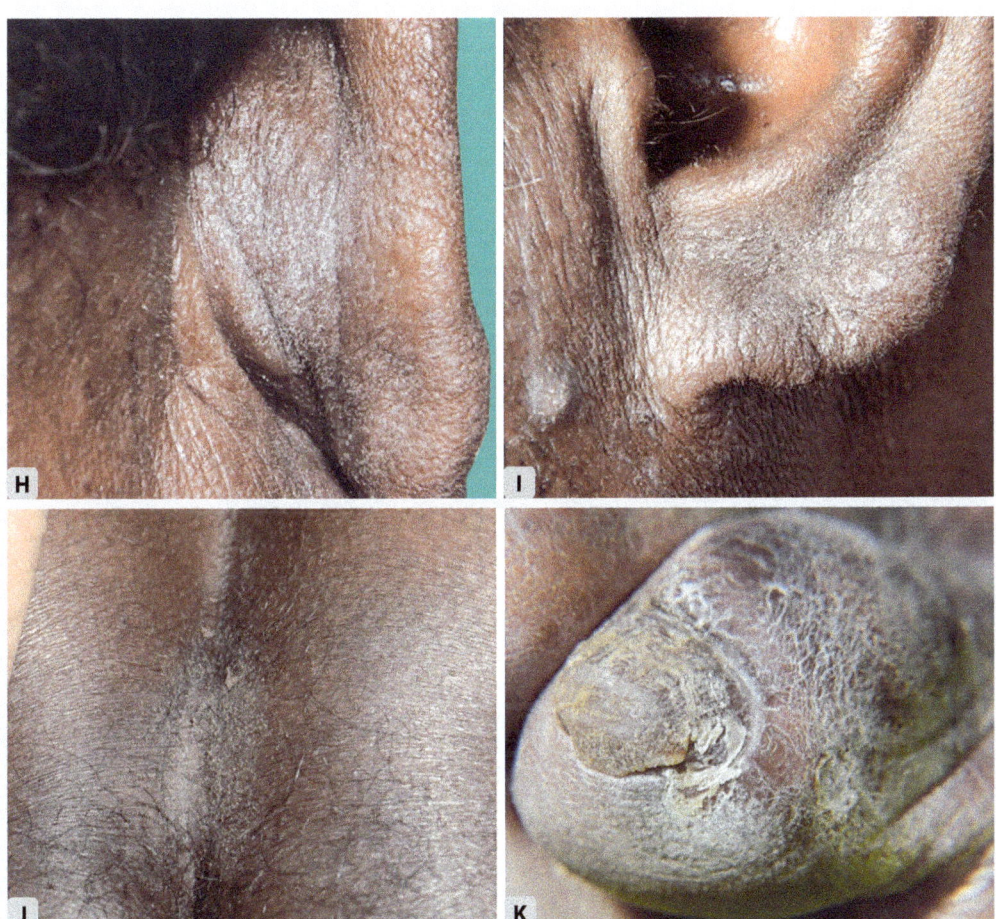

PATIENT 23B: (H) (Right) retroauricular area—diffusely scaly; (I) (Left) external ear lobule—diffusely scaly. A scaly plaque may be noted anterior to (left) ear lobule; (J) Upper natal cleft—mild erythema and scaling; and (K) (Left) little toenail (LTN)—split.

These clues help in diagnosing the case as psoriasis.

Patient 24

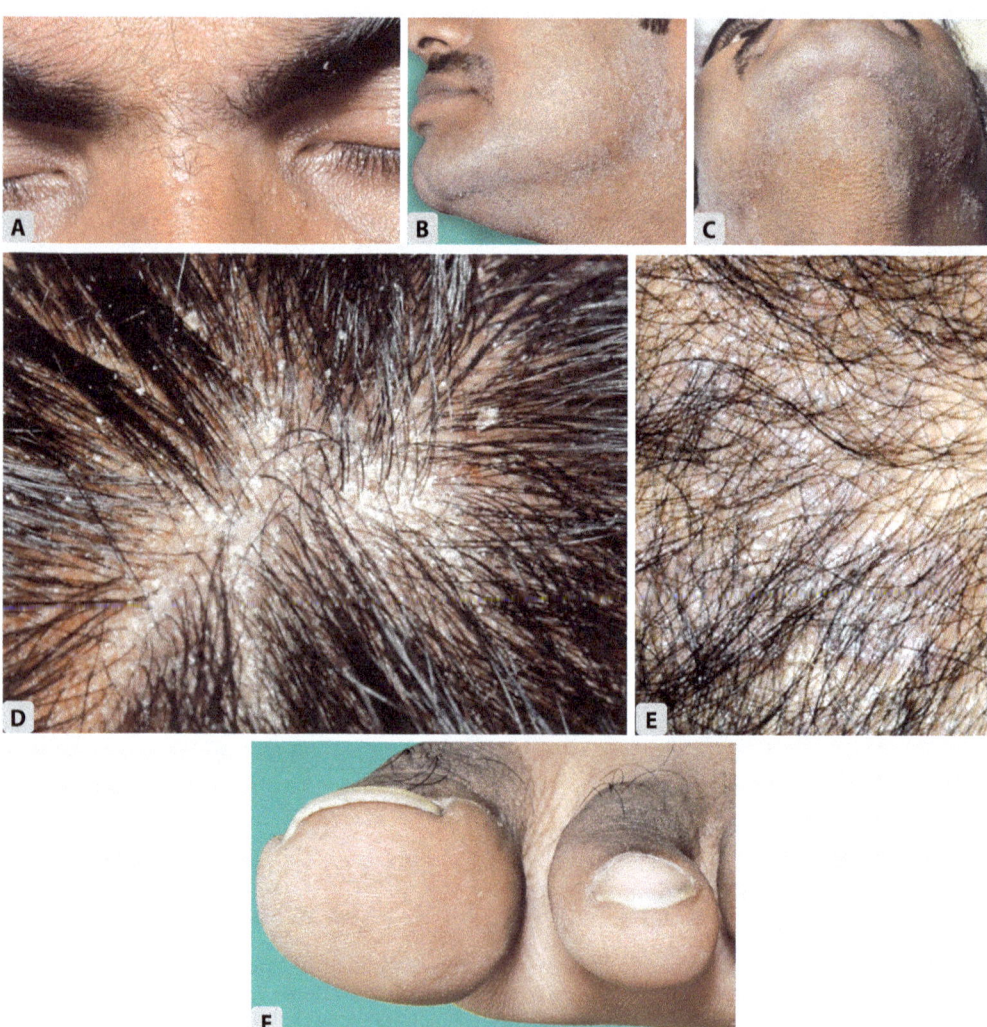

PATIENT 24: A 26-year-old male—a sales executive for a private company—2 years history of dandruff and 6 months history of itchy lesions on face and chest. (A) Glabella and medial eyebrows—scaly; (B and C) Sides of face and submandibular skin—multiple thin, coalescent, and scaly plaques; (D) Occiput—silvery white scales; (E) IM skin—a few erythematous scaly plaques; and (F) (Left) great toenail (GTN)—typical angulation.

The facial lesions may be mistaken to seborrheic dermatitis (SD).

Patient 25

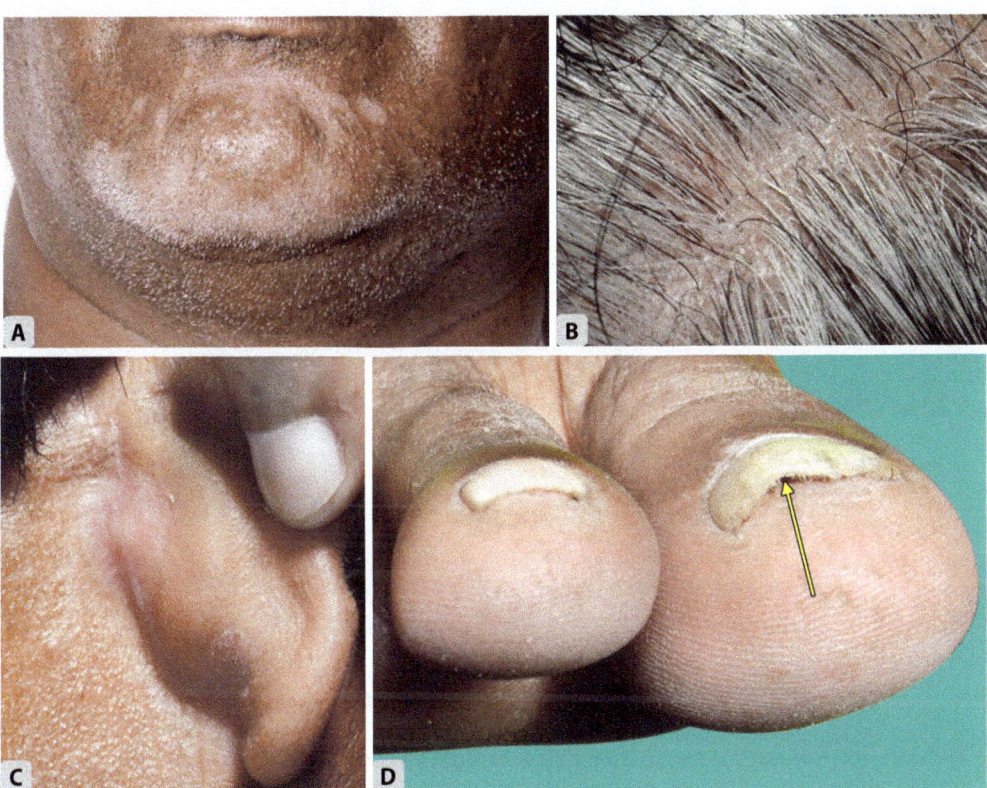

PATIENT 25: A 49-year-old male—a peasant—15 years history of scaling of scalp and 6 months history of itchy lesions in beard region. (A) Beard region—multiple thin scaly plaques with subtle erythema; (B) Vertex—silvery white scaly papules; (C) (Right) retroauricular area—erythematous scaly plaques; and (D) (Right) great toenail (GTN)—onycholysis and angulation (yellow arrow).

Patient 26

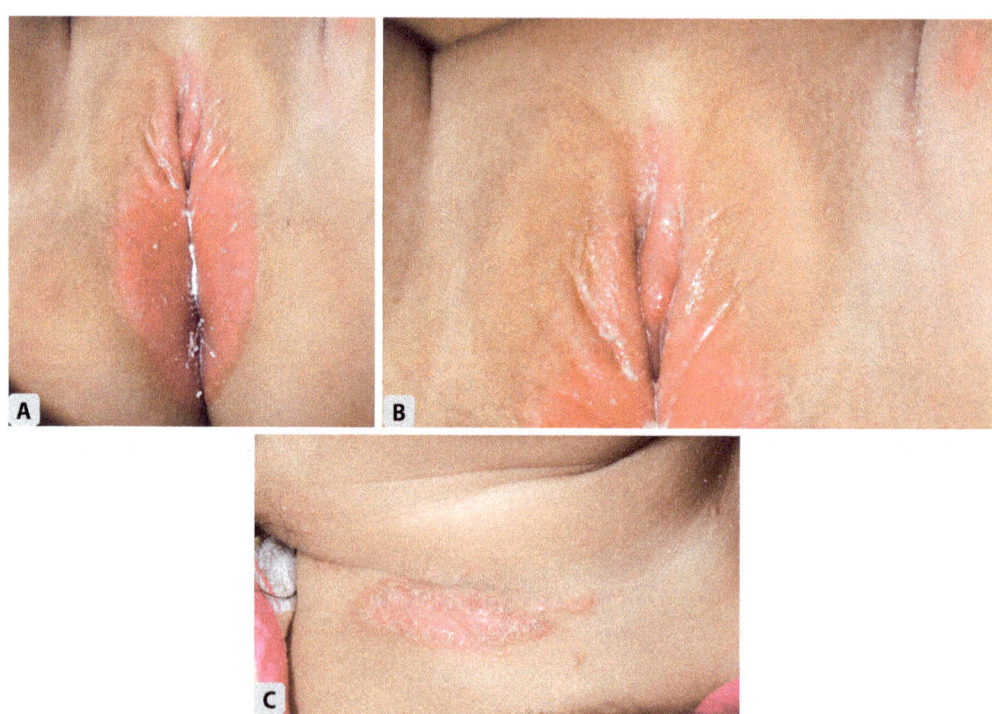

PATIENT 26: A 1-year-old female (NRI) child—brought by her grandparents—3 months history of irritable lesions. (A and B) Vulval, perianal skin, and groins folds—sharply demarcated erythematous plaques; groins—posttreatment (use of topical medicament) hypopigmentation; and (C) Anterior neck fold—elliptical erythematous psoriatic plaque with smaller lesions in the close vicinity.
A junior dermatologist may get tempted to diagnose this case as diaper dermatitis.

Patient 27

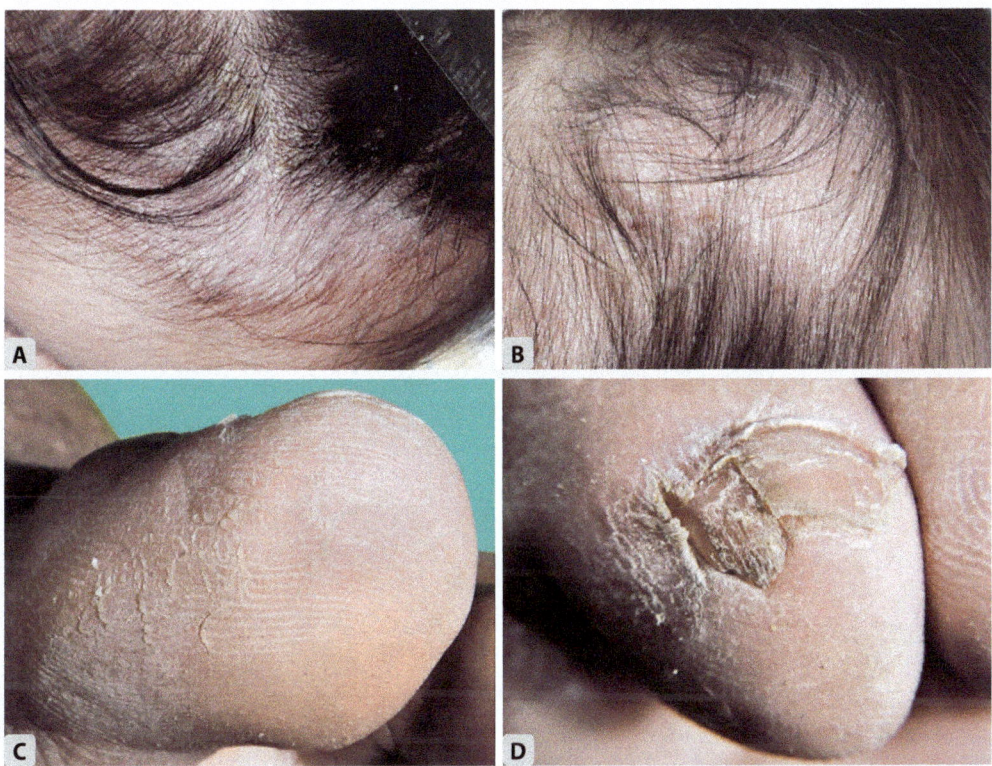

PATIENT 27: A 3-month-old male baby—brought by his maternal grandfather—with the complaint of scaly patches over scalp. (A) At a glance, the lesion over frontal scalp appeared like cradle cap; but on stroking, the lesion turned out to be a psoriatic plaque; (B) Vertex—similar lesion as in (A) maternal grandfather; (C) Outer aspect of (right) great toe (GT)—an ill-formed psoriatic plaque; and (D) (Right) little toenail (LTN)—split.

In every child with cradle cap, one has to look for clues to psoriasis either in the baby or in genetically-related accompanying subject.

Patient 28A

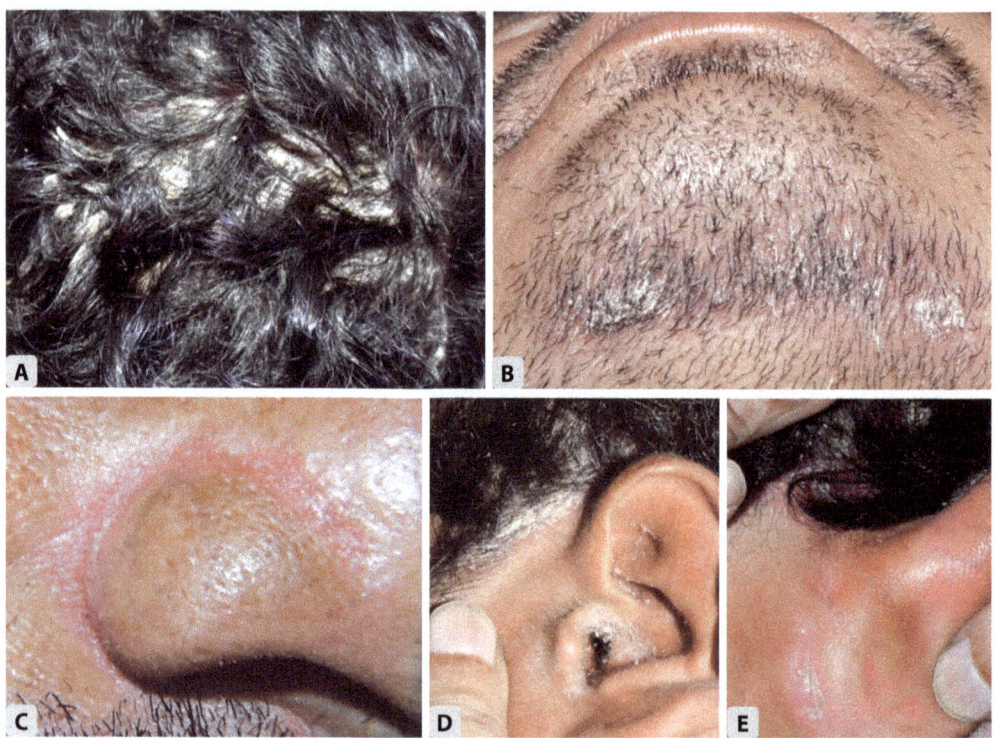

PATIENT 28A: A 36-year-old male—a cloth merchant—6 years history of dandruff. (A) Scalp—pityriasis amiantacea; (B) Submental skin—coalescent, erythematous, and scaly plaques; (C) Retro ala nasi—erythema with mild scaling; (D) Interior of (left) external earlobe—scaly, erythematous patches; and (E) (Right) retroauricular area—erythema and scaling.

Patient 28B

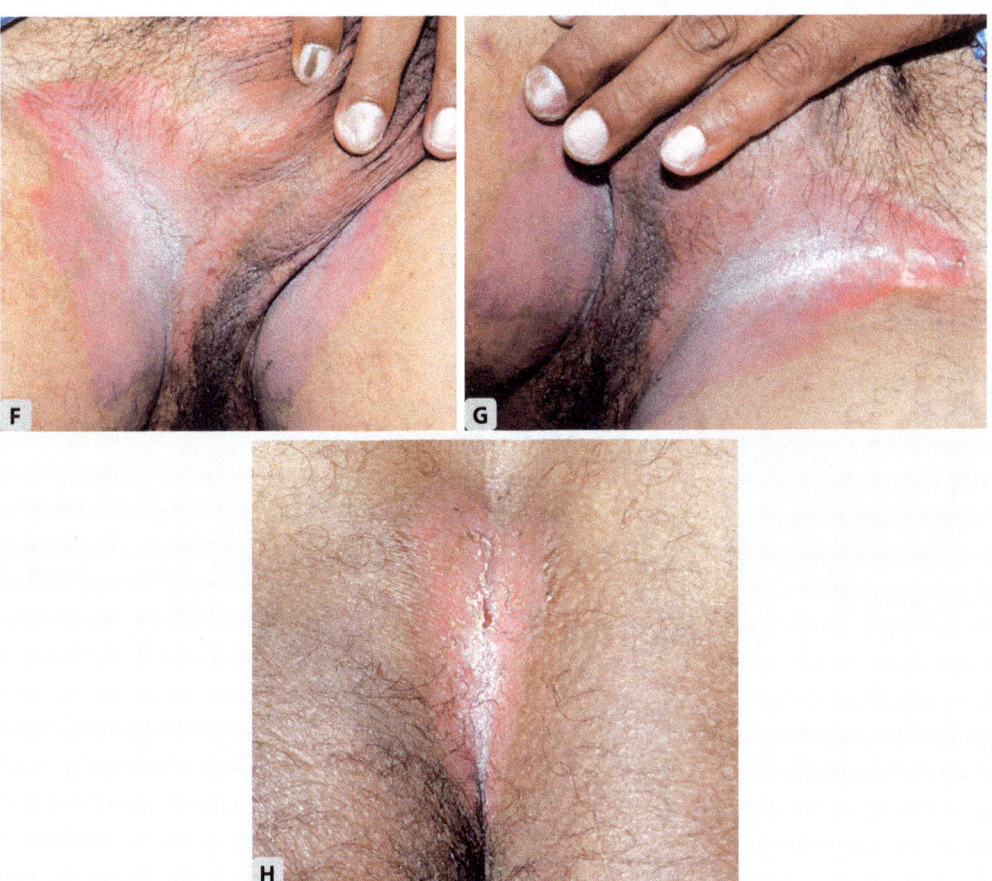

PATIENT 28B: (F and G) Both the groins—sharply demarcated nonscaly erythema with subtle maceration; involvement of scrotal sac may be noted; and (H) Upper natal cleft—similar picture as in F and G.

Photos A, B, C, D, and E may be mistaken to seborrheic dermatitis (SD) at a glance; I did search various areas of the body to pick up clues to psoriasis and I succeeded; thus, this case is a combination of sebopsoriasis and flexural psoriasis.

V. Patients Complaining of Dandruff with Scaly Plaques on Scalp

(No. of Patients Depicted—9)

Patient 1

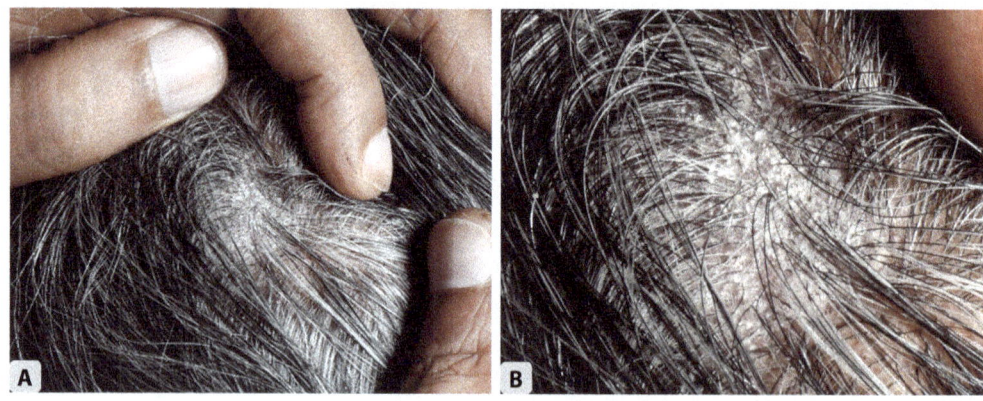

PATIENT 1: A 60-year-old female—an agricultural laborer—11 years history of itching and scaling of scalp; itching reported to be worse on occiput. (A) A well-defined plaque with silvery white scales; and (B) Close-up view of "A".

Patient 2

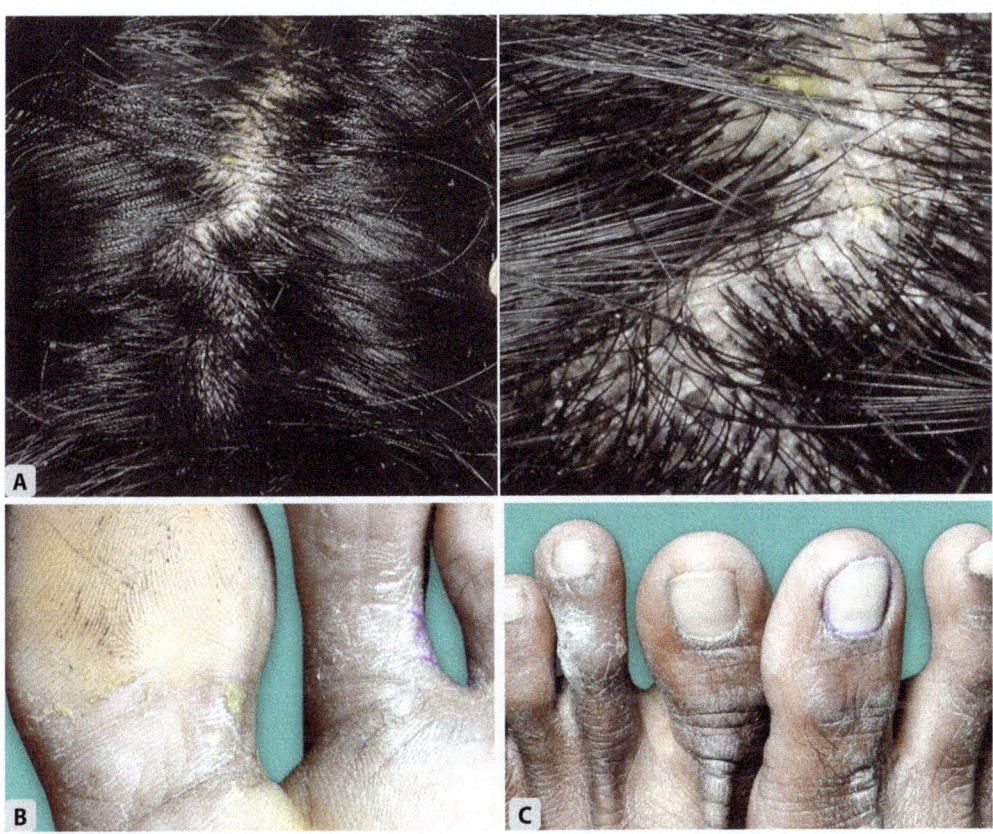

PATIENT 2: A 19-year-old male—doing his graduation—1 year history of itching and scaling of scalp. (A) Vertex—silvery white scales; (B) Under toes (left) foot—hyperkeratosis (HK) and scaling; and (C) Dorsum of second toe (left) foot—a scaly plaque; linear lichenified plaques over the tendons of both GTs.

Linear lichenified plaques over tendons of GTs are reliable diagnostic clues for psoriasis.

Patient 3

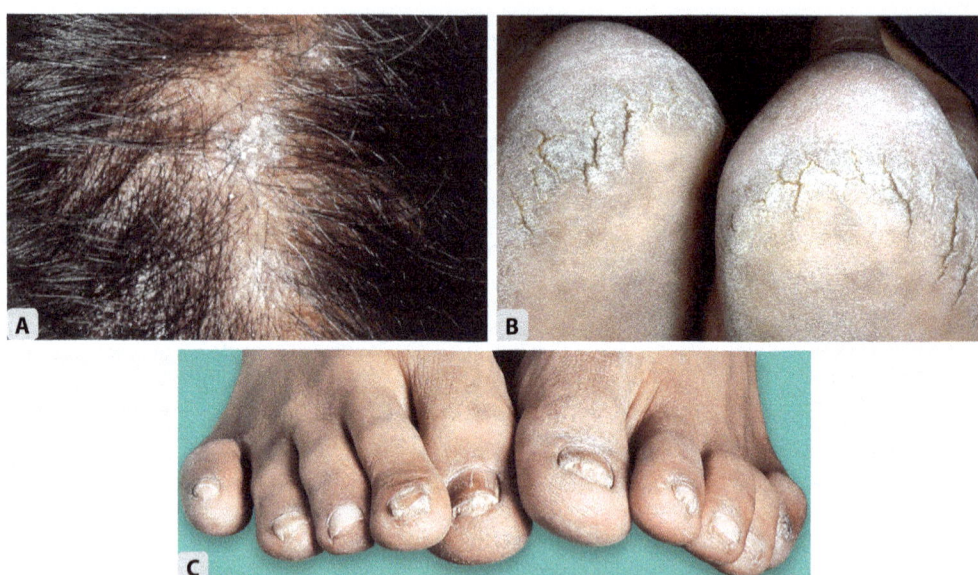

PATIENT 3: A 42-year-old male—an agriculturist—14 years history of dandruff. (A) Vertex—discrete well-defined silvery white scaly plaques; (B) Heel borders—remarkable hyperkeratosis (HK) and fissuring; and (C) All the toenails of both feet—are abnormal.

The most common cause of abnormal nails, in this region, is psoriasis (not fungus) as per my clinical experience (APMCE).

Patient 4

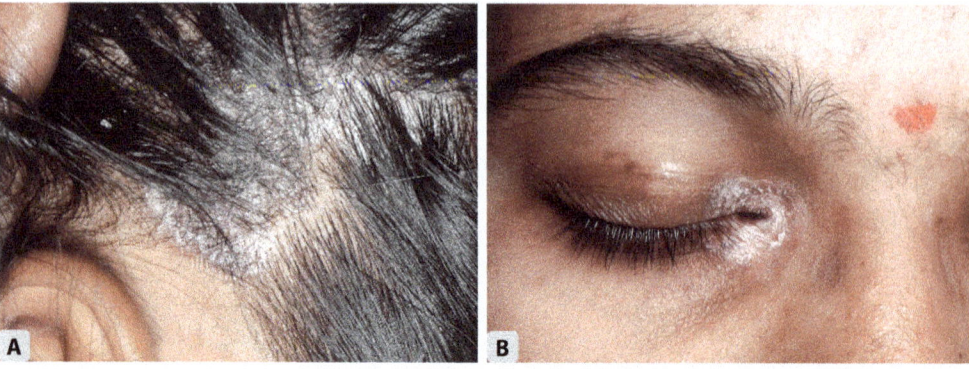

PATIENT 4: An 18-year-old female—a first year engineering student—6 months history of dandruff and 1 month history of (right) eye involvement. (A) (Left) parieto-occipital scalp—silvery white scaly plaques; and (B) (Right) inner canthus—a typical psoriatic lesion.

Patient 5

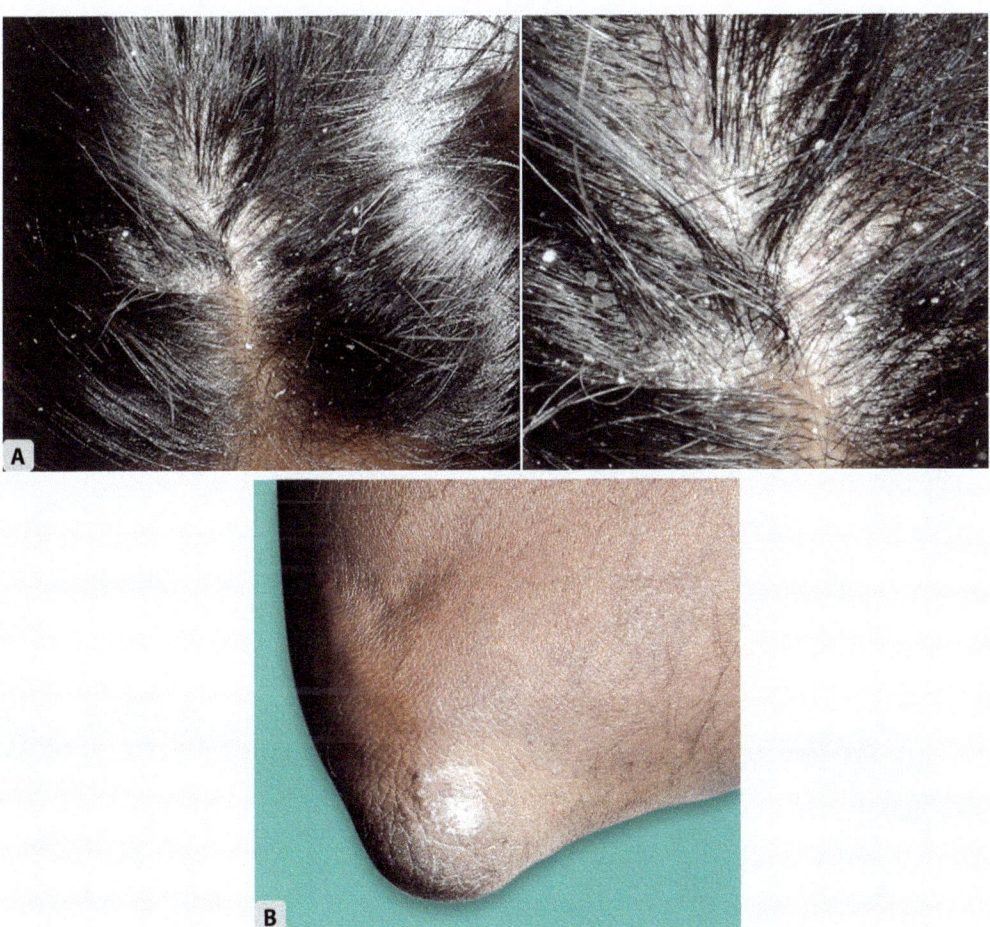

PATIENT 5: A 17-year-old female—a student—1 month history of dandruff. (A) Frontal scalp—visible desquamation and scaly plaques with silvery white scale; and (B) A 40-year-old male—father of "A"—(left) elbow—typical psoriatic lesion.

Looking beyond the patient—results in discovery of a psoriatic lesion.

Patient 6

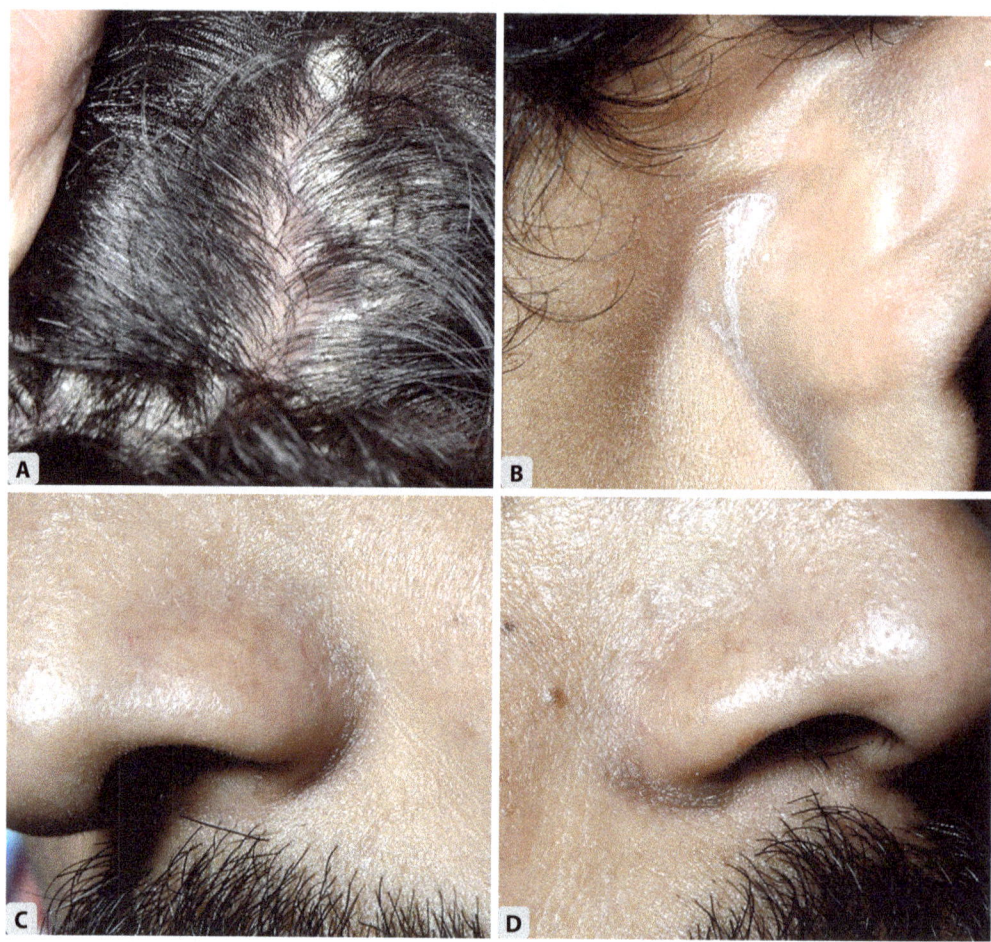

PATIENT 6: A 31-year-old male—a software engineer—6 years history of dandruff. (A) Occipital scalp—plaques with silvery white scales; (B) (Right) RAF—scaly plaque; and (C and D) Both the RAN—subtle erythema and scaling.

This case is, in fact, a case of sebopsoriasis.

Patient 7

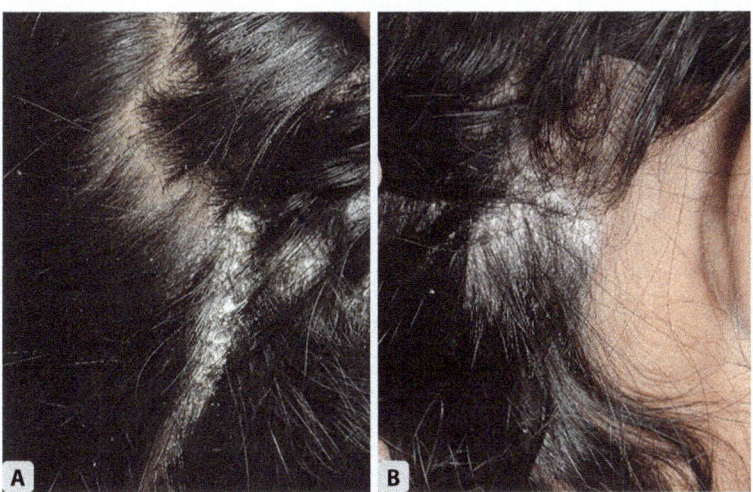

PATIENT 7: A 17-year-old female—a student/a hosteller—1 year history of dandruff. (A and B) Occipital scalp having multiple large plaques covered with silvery scales.

In this region, it is almost always on scalp that a dermatologist finds silvery white scales when compared to other regions of the body.

Patient 8

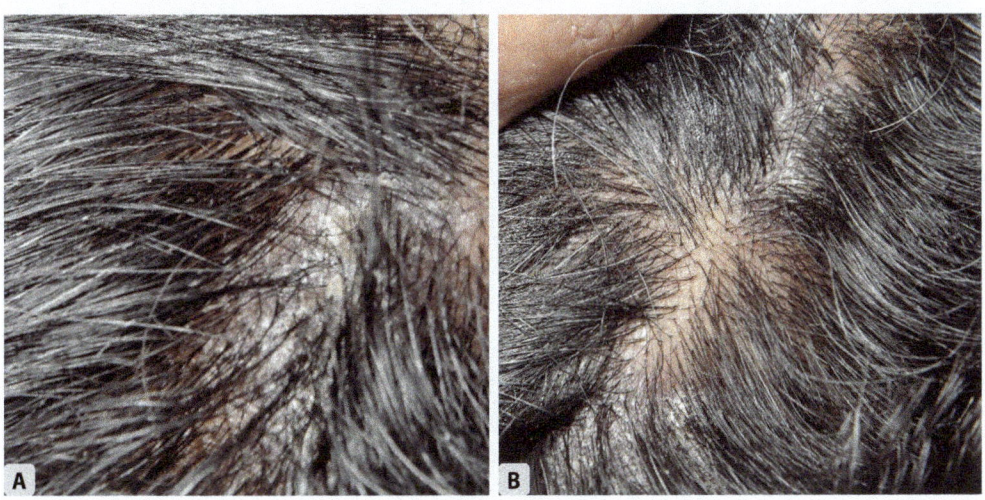

PATIENT 8: A 46-year-old male—a banker—3 months history of dandruff. (A and B) Scalp—discrete silvery white scaly plaques.

Patient 9

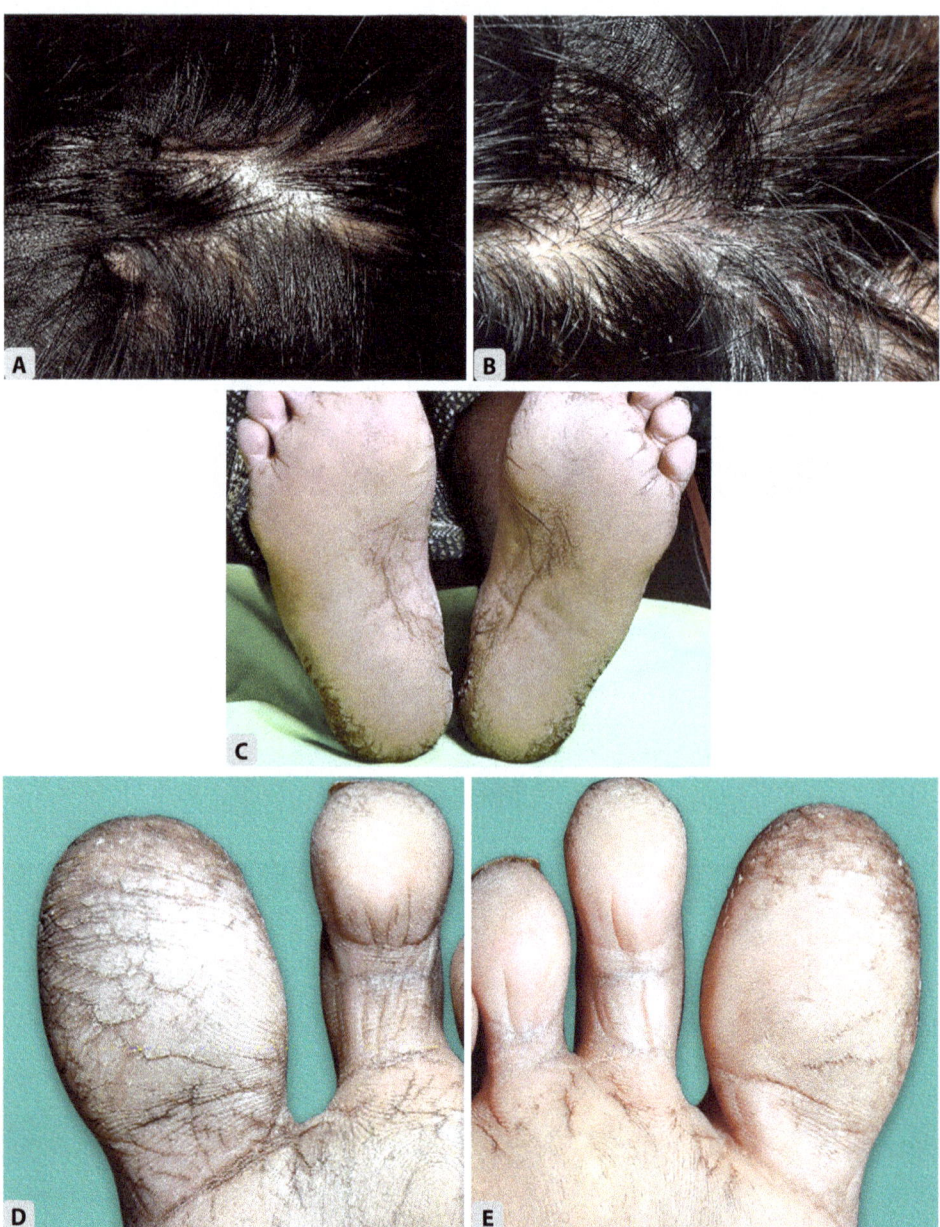

PATIENT 9: A 15-year-old female—a student—an inmate of school hostel—2 years history of dandruff. (A and B) Scalp—many silvery white scaly plaques—more in the occipital region; (C) Her 40-year-old father—an agriculturist—heavy fissuring of borders of hindfeet and insteps; and (D and E) Under toes—cracking and scaling.

This kind of extensive fissuring of borders of feet and soles cannot be considered physiological, psoriatic origin, because of impaired barrier function due to absence of granular layer.

REFERENCES

1. Wakelin S. Seborrheic dermatitis. In: Griffiths C, Barker J, Bleiker T, Chalmers R, Creamer D (Eds). Rook's Textbook of Dermatology, 9th edition. United Kingdom: Blackwell Publishing Ltd.; 2016. pp. 401-6.
2. Berth-Jones J. Eczema, lichenification, prurigo and erythroderma. In: Burns DA, Breathnach SM, Cox NH, Griffiths CE (Eds). Rook's Textbook of Dermatology, 8th edition. United Kingdom: Blackwell Publishing Ltd.; 2010. pp. 2329-34.
3. Burton JL, Holden CA. Eczema, lichenification and prurigo. In: Champion RH, Burton JL, Burns DA, Breathnach SM (Eds). Rook/Wilkinson/Ebling Textbook of Dermatology, 6th edition. United Kingdom: Blackwell Publishing Ltd.; 1998. pp. 629-80.
4. Collins CD, Hivnor C. Seborrheic dermatitis. In: Goldsmith LA, Katz SI, Gilchrest BA, Paller AS, Lefell DJ, Wolff K (Eds). Fitzpatrick's Dermatology in General Medicine, 8th edition. USA: MacGraw Hill Companies, Inc.; 2008. pp. 259-66.
5. Pinkus H, Mehregan AM. The squirting papilla. J Invest Dermatol. 1966;49:109-15.
6. Kligman AM, McGinley KJ, Leyden JJ. Dandruff: Its causes and treatment. In: Orfanos CE (Ed). Haar Und Haar Krank Heiten. Stuttgart: Springer Verlag; 1979. pp. 663-9.
7. O'Neil JL, Chan YH, Rapp SR, Povitch GY. Differences in itch characteristics between psoriasis and atopic dermatitis patients: results of a web-based questionnaire. Acta Derma Venereol. 2011;91:537-40.
8. Abramovits W, Cockerell C, Stevenson LC, Goldstein AM, Ehrig T, Menter A. PsEma—a hitherto unnamed dermatologic entity with clinical features of both psoriasis and eczema. Skinmed. 2005;4:275-81.
9. Rook A, Wilkinson DS. Eczema, lichen simplex and prurigo. In: Rook A, Wilkinson DS, Ebling FJG (Eds). Textbook of Dermatology, 3rd edition. United Kingdom: Blackwell Scientific Publication; 1986. pp. 299-348.
10. Findley K, Oh J, Yang J, Conlan S, Deming C, Meyer JA, et al. Topographic diversity of fungal and bacterial communities in human skin. Nature. 2013;498:367-70.
11. Cui I, Morris A, Ghedin E. The human mycobiome in health and disease. Genome Med. 2013;5:63.
12. Grice EA, Segre JA. The skin microbiome. Nat Rev Microbiol. 2011;9:244-53.
13. Sugita T, Suzuki M, Goto S, Nishikawa A, Hiruma M, Yamazaki T, et al. Quantitative analysis of the cutaneous Malassezia microbiota in 770 healthy Japanese by age and gender using a real-time PCR assay. Med Mycol. 2010;48:229-33.
14. Wu G, Zhao H, Li C, Rajapakse MP, Wong WC, Xu J, et al. Genus-wide comparative genomics of Malassezia delineates its phylogeny, physiology, and niche adaptation on human skin. PLoS Genet. 2015;11:e1005614.
15. Malassez L. Note sur le Champignon du pityriasis simple. Arch Physiol. 1874;1:451-9.
16. Hay R. Malassezia, dandruff and seborrheic dermatitis: an overview. Br J Dermatol. 2011;165:2-8.
17. Shuster S. The aetiology of dandruff and mode of action of therapeutic agents. Br J Dermatol. 1984;111:235-42.
18. Hay RJ, Ashbee HR. Fungal infections. In: Griffiths C, Barker J, Bleiker T, Chalmers R, Creamer D (Eds). Rook's Textbook of Dermatology, 9th edition. United Kingdom: Blackwell Publishing Ltd; 2016. pp. 321-96.
19. Parekh C, Min BH, Golberg L. Experimental studies of sodium pyridinethione. I. Percutaneous absorption in laboratory animals. Food Cosmet Toxicol. 1970;8:147-60.
20. Alexander S. Do shampoos affect dandruff? Br J Dermatol. 1967;79:92-5.
21. Aron-Brunetière R, Dompmartin-Pernot D, Drouhet E. Treatment of pityriasis capitis (dandruff) with econazole nitrate. Acta Derm Venereol. 1977;57:77-80.
22. Duffill M, Wright N, Shuster S. The cell proliferation kinetics of psoriasis examined by three in vivo techniques. Br J Dermatol. 1976;94:355-62.
23. Weinstein GD. On the cell cycle of psoriasis. Br J Dermatol. 1975;92:229-30.
24. Bhawan J, Bansal C, Whren K, et al. IL-11 Psoriasis study Group. K16 expression in uninvolved Psoriatic skin: A possible marker of pre-clinical Psoriasis. J Cutan patho. 2004;31(7):471-6.
25. Thaler M, Fukuyama K, Epstein WL, et al. Comparative studies of keratins isolated from psoriasis and atopic dermatitis. Invest Dermatol. 1980;75(2):156-8.

26. Thewes M, Stadler R, Korge B, et al. Normal Psoriatic epidermis expression of hyper proliferation-associated keratins. Arch Dermatol Res. 1991;283(7):465-71.
27. Galvin S, Loomis C, Manabate M, et al. The major pathways of keratinocyte differentiation as defined by keratin expression: an overview. Adv Dermatol. 1989;4:277-99.
28. Ljosaa TM, Mork C, Stubhaug A, Moum T, Wahl AK. Skin pain and skin discomfort is associated with quality of life in patients with psoriasis. J Eur Acad Dermatol Venereol. 2012;26:29-35.
29. Reich A, Hrehorow E, Szepietowski JC. Pruritus is an important factor negatively influencing the well-being of psoriatic patients. Acta Derm Venereol. 2010;90:257-63.
30. Tegner E. Seborrheic dermatitis of the face induced by PUVA treatment. Acta Derm Venereol. 1983;63:335-9.
31. Birnbaum RY, Zvulunov A, Havel-Halevy D, Cagnano E, Finer G, Ofir R, et al. Seborrhea-like dermatitis with psoriasiform elements caused by a mutation in ZNF750, encoding a putative C2H2 zinc finger protein. Nat Genet. 2006;38:749-51.
32. Lomholt G. Psoriasis: Prevalence, Spontaneous Course, and Genetics: A Census Study on the Prevalence of Skin Diseases on the Faroe Islands. GEC Gad. 1963;196:31-3.
33. Ackerman AB, Kligman AM. Some observations on dandruff. J Soc Cosmet Chem. 1969;20:81.
34. Plewig G, Kligman AM. The effect of selenium sulfide on epidermal turnover of normal and dandruff scalps. J Soc Cosmet Chem. 1969;20:767-75.
35. Plewig G, Kligman AM. Zelkinetische untersuch ungen bei. Kopfschyppenerk rankung (Pityriasis simplex capittilli). Arch Klim Exp Dermatol. 1970;236:406.
36. Kligman AM, Marples RR, Lantis LR, McGinley KJ. Appraisal of efficacy of antidandruff formulations. J Soc Cosmet Chem. 1974;25:73.
37. Leyden JJ, McGinley KJ, Kligman AM. Role of microorganisms in dandruff. Arch Dermatol. 1976;112:333-8.
38. Leyden JJ, Kligman AM. Dandruff cause and treatment. Cosmet Toilet. 1979;94:23.

SOUTH INDIAN'S FOOT: A STOREHOUSE OF DIAGNOSTIC CLUES FOR PSORIASIS

The "Program" Underlying Epidermis

INTRODUCTION

The epidermis is vested with a tremendous responsibility of pursuing a barrier activity against various environmental hazards and thus protects the organism. This is achieved by what is known as the terminal differentiation program (TDP) that ultimately results in the formation of the outermost layer of the epidermis called stratum corneum, which is composed of dead corneocytes. The TDP is a journey that begins from the living and proliferating cells of stratum basale with daughter cells moving outward toward the surface of the epidermis, meanwhile, punctated by halts under different strata, which form as a result of structural (morphological) changes and biochemical changes; during its transit from granular cell layer to stratum corneum, the living keratinocyte starts losing all its organelles, cytoplasm, and even nucleus; in spite of having lost all its "wealth", the dead corneocytes remain attached to the human body as stratum corneum only to safeguard its health for sometime, before getting shed into the environment.

TERMINAL DIFFERENTIATION PROGRAM (EPIDERMAL DIFFERENTIATION OR KERATINIZATION)

Terminal differentiation program is a genetically programmed and a tightly regulated process brilliantly orchestrated by a series of morphologic changes and metabolic events the endpoint of which being the transformation of a proliferating cell in the basal layer into a terminally differentiated, dead keratinocyte (corneocyte) that is composed of keratin filaments, matrix protein, and a protein-reinforced plasma membrane (cornified envelope, i.e., CE) with surface-associated lipids (i.e., cornified lipid envelope or CLE).

Thus, this tightly regulated process of TDP broadly results in the formation of a stratified cornified epidermis, the thickness of which may range from 0.4 to 1.5 mm as compared with the 1.5–4.0 mm of full-thickness skin.

This genetically programmed process, for it to be flawlessly executed, requires some key events to occur:

- The various strata that form as part of TDP can be categorized into four layers on simple morphological grounds. Each layer is specified by a few keratins. Thus, stratum basale has K14 and K5 mainly and also K15. For the keratinocytes to move suprabasally into spinous layer, the K14 and K5 have to be downregulated and induction of K1 and K10 specific for spinous layer also occurs simultaneously.[1] Thus, downregulation of the keratins specific for lower stratum in conjunction with induction of keratins specific for the overlying stratum results in fixing the order of the strata from stratum germinativum to the outer surface of the epidermis.

- *Genes*: These may be classified into two types: (1) genes that establish and maintain basal keratinocytes: Knockout mouse model discovered that p63 to be a transcription factor and its expression was shown to induce expression of K14, the first keratin unique for the epidermal lineage.[2] Further studies demonstrated that p63 not only enables basal keratinocytes stay committed to a basal proliferative state, but also prevents the onset of terminal differentiation[2] and (2) genes required for terminal differentiation: The gene/s involved in this step enable basal keratinocytes to withdraw from cellcycle irreversibly after basal keratinocytes undergo a few rounds of cell division. This is controlled in part by an isoform of ΔNp63 which mediates cellcycle exit by inducing cellcycle inhibitors and by repressing genes that promote cellcycle progression.[2,3]
- Notch signaling activity promotes terminal differentiation by inducing K1/K10 expression in spinous layer and by mediating cellcycle withdrawal as well.[2] The role of Notch activity in TDP was established by both in vitro studies and mouse model studies.[4] Ablation of Notch signaling in mouse model led to formation of a very thin spinous layer. Intact Notch signaling, on the contrary, resulted in full-thickness spinous layer. The K1/K10 is also referred to as terminal differentiation-specific complex or keratinization-specific complex.
- Ca^{2+}/protein kinase C (PKC) family: An increase in extracellular Ca^{2+} concentration acts as an important trigger for keratinocyte differentiation. There is an increasing gradient of extracellular Ca^{2+} concentration from the basal layer to the cornified layers in mature epidermis.[5] A number of calcium-responsive proteins that play key role in the formation of granular layer were identified in epidermis and a particular group of such proteins that function specifically in the transition from spinous to granular cells belongs to PKC family.[6,7]
- This family performs two functions: (1) This group of proteins downregulates K1 and K10 expression and (2) It induces markers of granular keratinocytes, which include loricrin, filaggrin and transglutaminases, and K2, a reinforcement keratin.[6] A number of epidermal keratins make it interesting to note that they have a more restricted anatomic distribution pattern. K9, for example, is specifically expressed in the suprabasal cells of palmoplantar skin. Another subset of keratins, K6, K16, and K17, are expressed in keratinocytes of the nail bed, sweat glands, hair follicles, and sebaceous glands in addition to palmoplantar epidermis.[8] Further maturation of granular cells into corneocytes is characterized by eventual loss of their cytoplasmic organelles and even nucleus and corneocytes meet their final destiny by getting shed into the environment. In addition to PKC family, there are several Ca^{2+}-binding proteins of which the calcium sensing receptor is specifically expressed in granular keratinocytes. Interestingly, either absence or overexpression of Ca^{2+}-sensing receptor determines the thickness of granular and even spinous layer.

KERATINOCYTES

All mammalian cells including epidermal keratinocytes have a cytoskeleton made of keratin filaments.

Keratins are obligate heterodimers which assemble to form polymers in the cells and thus they constitute members of intermediate filament family of proteins.[9,10] These keratins are categorized into three types based on their diameter:

1. Actin containing microfilaments (7 mm in diameter).
2. Tubulin containing microtubules (20–25 nm).
3. Filaments of intermediate size (7–10 nm).

The third category filaments are also known as keratin intermediate filaments (tonofilaments), which are of six types:

1. Keratin in epithelial cells.
2. Vimentin within mesenchymal cells.
3. Glial fibrillary acidic protein (GFAP) in glial cells.

4. Neurofilaments in neurons.
5. Desmin in muscle cells.
6. Peripherin in peripheral nerves.

The peripheral lamins A, B, and C, which represent the nuclear matrix proteins, are also intermediate filaments.

The genes encoding keratins, desmins, and lamins number about 70, which are now known to be associated with at least 72 distinct human diseases that include skin blistering diseases, premature aging syndromes, cardiomyopathy, etc.

Keratin Intermediate Filaments (Tonofilaments)

Keratin intermediate filaments provide resilience to keratinocytes, which constitute the major (95%) component of epidermis (rest of the cells include melanocytes, Langerhans cell, and Merkel cell). Some immune cells, in particular, lymphocytes, inhabitate epidermis, but only for a short while and they are extremely sparse in normal skin. Keratins are >50 individual members and represent the largest group of intermediate filament (tonofilaments) proteins. This large family of proteins shows tissue and cell type-specific expression. In the epidermis, the tonofilaments play a critical role in cell-cell adhesions (desmosomes) and cell-substratum adhesions [hemidesmosomes (HDs)].

The genes encoding individual keratins numbering about 54 are classified into three categories as per the new systemic nomenclature: (1) Epithelial keratin genes, (2) Hair keratin genes, and (3) Keratin pseudogenes. The keratin-coding genes are grouped into two families such as type I (basic) and type II (acidic). Type I and type II keratins form obligatory heteropolymers (i.e., a pair of one from each group) that represent the basic building blocks of epithelial intermediate filaments, albeit, in a cell and tissue-specific manner.

Thus, while, simple epithelia are characterized by the keratin heterodimer K8/K18, the stratified squamous epithelia are characterized by K5/K14, and K6a and K16, which offer a possible explanation for the heterogeneity seen in epidermolytic hyperkeratosis (HK), epidermolysis bullosa simplex, and pachyonychia congenita, respectively.

EPIDERMAL LAYERS

- *Stratum basale*: It is generally a mitotically active, one-cell thick continuous layer consisting of columnar-/cuboidal-shaped keratinocytes that have large dark-staining nuclei and dense cytoplasm that contains many ribosomes and dense tonofilament bundles. Keratin filaments (K5 and K14) help these basal keratinocytes attach to the basement membrane zone (BMZ) via HDs and to the surrounding cells through desmosomes.[10] In this layer, K15 is also expressed, but less abundantly. K15 can assemble with K5 in the absence of K14.

Cell kinetic studies and in vivo and in vitro studies suggest that there exist cells with different proliferative potentials in stratum basale, i.e., stem cells, transit-amplifying cells, and postmitotic cells. Though it is suggested by some studies that the basal layer is composed of a single unipotent stem cell, evidence for at least two types of progenitor cells that defer in proliferation dynamics and expression of markers is provided by other studies.[11-15]

STEM CELLS

These are the cells with extensive proliferative potential located not only at the base of epidermal proliferating units, in the interfollicular epidermis of the basal layer, and also in the hair follicle bulge. These are the cells that mediate the continuous program of self-renewal, which results in TDP that enables the epidermis to provide a barrier between the organism and the environment.

During embryogenesis itself, the barrier function is established and it is maintained in mature epidermis through continuous self-renewal program. The hair follicles bulge stem cells, though, become active following epidermal injury, they do not participate in normal tissue homeostasis, unlike the other stem cells.

Interfollicular epidermal stem cells, through asymmetric or symmetric cell division,[16] produce transit-amplifying stem cells (TASCs) and postmitotic cells. Before initiating TDP, TASCs undergo a few cell divisions. Next, for the beginning of TDP, it is mandatory that committed cells should withdraw from cellcycle. This requires inactivation of integrin extracellular matrix receptors which anchor basal cells to the basement membrane. As part of epidermal homeostasis, the production of cells in the suprabasal layers is guided by mitotic spindle orientation and asymmetric cell divisions during embryonic development.[16] Irrespective of their position, the progenitor cells in the basal layer largely produce differentiated progeny that form strata directly above them.[15,17] Consequently, the newly formed keratinocytes move suprabasally to become the first suprabasal layer of spinous keratinocytes of the epidermis. The minimum time taken for a basal cell from the point of time since it detaches from basal layer and travels across epidermis to enter stratum corneum is 14 days. Another 14 days are required for its transit through stratum corneum and to get shed into the environment. These periods vary according to the proliferative state of the epidermis.

SPINOUS LAYER

This layer is composed of cells whose cell margins offer a spine-like appearance in histologic sections. The "spines" of spinous cells are highly rich in desmosomes which promote cell-cell adhesion through a Ca^{2+}-dependent mechanism. Two conditions highlight the importance of calcium as a mediator of adhesion between epidermal cells and they include: (1) Darier disease and (2) Hailey–Hailey disease,[18] both being characterized by dyscohesion between keratinocytes. As part of TDP, these spinous cells differentiate and move upward through the epidermis. During this movement, they progressively become flatter and develop organelles known as lamellar organelles and keratin filaments get organized into large bundles around the nucleus to get inserted into desmosomes peripherally.

While the keratin pair K1/K10 characterizes the spinous layers (and these keratins are also referred to as differentiation-specific or keratinization-specific keratins), the basal layer-specific keratins K5/K14 can make their appearance in these spinous cells, when new messenger ribonucleic acid (mRNA) for these proteins is synthesized such as in hyperproliferative disorders. Similarly, synthesis and translation of messages for K6 and K16 are also favored in hyperproliferative conditions such as psoriasis, actinic keratosis, and wound healing (mRNA for K6 and K16 are normally present throughout the epidermis, but the message for mRNA for this keratin pair is translated, when required only). But, at the same time, mRNA for the synthesis of K1 and K10 is downregulated in hyperproliferative disorders.

While the progeny of progenitor cells differentiates into various strata, the composition of desmosomes also varies. In the basal cells, although rich in the desmosomal cadherin desmoglein-3 (Dsg3), the levels of this protein keep decreasing, as the strata keep moving toward the outer side of epidermis whereas Dsg1 is upregulated.[19]

Secretory granules, i.e., lamellar granules are also made in this spinous layer. In addition to upper spinous layer, the cytoplasm of the granular cell layer also contains smaller (than keratohyalin granules) lamellated granules, known as lamellar granules or bodies (also known as membrane-coating granules or Odland bodies). They are seen in abundance, particularly, in upper spinous layers and also in granular cell layer, but more peripherally located in the cytoplasm. Now, this location of these granules enables them to discharge their lipid contents into the intercellular space that play an important role in barrier function and intercellular cohesion within the stratum corneum.

GRANULAR LAYER

Spinous layer is succeeded by the granular cell layer or stratum granulosum. It acquires its name because of the presence of intracellular basophilic keratohyalin granules, which are primarily composed of profilaggrin, keratin filaments, and loricrin. Thus, cells in this layer harbor two types of granules, i.e., smaller lamellar granules and larger keratohyalin granules.

Keratinocyte TDP culminates in the conversion of plasma membrane to cornified CE, a composite of several covalently cross-linked proteins. CE assembly begins within this layer with the conversion of profilaggrin to filaggrin. The various components employed in the making of this envelope include loricrin, involucrin, filaggrin, keratins, desmosomal proteins, cystatin, envoplakin, XP-5/late envelope proteins, etc.

Filaggrin is responsible for aggregation of keratin filaments into macrofilaments. Subsequently, filaggrin is degraded into certain molecules such as urocanic acid and pyrrolidone carboxylic acid. These amino acids in addition to acting as natural moisturizing factors within corneocytes, they also provide photoprotection by filtering ultraviolet (UV) radiation. Loss-of-function mutations involving gene that codes for the protein, filaggrin, result in ichthyosis vulgaris, increased risk for atopic eczema, atopic asthma, and systemic allergies. Loricrin, a cysteine-rich protein and a major component of the CE, upon its release from keratohyalin granules, binds to desmosomal structures and is subsequently cross-linked to the plasma membrane by tissue transglutaminases to form the CE which reinforces the plasma membrane. Subsequently, the extracellular surface of the CE is covered by lipids which form the CLE. Now, the stratum corneum is better suited to perform the function of barrier activity effectively along with the intercellular lipid compartment. *The fact that granular layer is absent in psoriatic lesions speaks volumes of why psoriatics develop a dry skin, why most of the psoriatics also happen to be asthmatics, and why the lesions readily develop fissures (i.e., due to lack of cohesion between corneocytes as a result of absence of lipid coating). For the same reason, it is no surprise that the barrier function is also impaired in the skin of psoriatics.*

STRATUM CORNEUM

It is composed of stacked layers of anucleate flattened, cornified cells which are the consequence of complete differentiation of granular cells. The formation of this layer is the ultimate objective of KTD program. Apart from providing mechanical protection to the skin, the primary function of this layer is to act as a barrier to water loss and permeation of soluble substances from the environment into the skin.[20]

Functions of Stratum Corneum

While hydration, resilience, initiation of cytokine-mediated inflammation, and protection against UV damage are the various functions performed by the corneocytes, the primary functions of extracellular lipid matrix include desquamation, regulation of permeability toxin exclusion, antimicrobial, and selective chemical absorption.

STRATUM LUCIDUM

This layer is exclusive to palmoplantar skin; in addition to the other four layers, located between stratum granulosum and stratum corneum, is composed of cells that are still nucleated. These cells may be referred to as transitional cells. Keratin 9 is exclusively expressed in palmoplantar epidermis. K6, K16, and K17 are also expressed in palmoplantar epidermis in addition to skin appendages. *This is all about stratum lucidum found in major textbooks meaning that no further research whatsoever was done on this layer which is found nowhere else except palms and soles*: The skin over palms and soles is much thicker than elsewhere and this is the skin that is subjected to repeated trauma in day-to-day life.

Then, how this layer, it is very surprising and also shocking, failed to arouse interest among our esteemed Caucasian researchers!!?? Nothing that is found in this macrocosm is meaningless; everything that is created by *Bhagavan* (almighty) that is part of this universe has one or the other purpose: What has been hither to believed to be a vestigial organ, i.e., the appendix, in the recent past was found to carry out an important function, i.e., it (appendix) acts as reservoir for gut flora.[21] What was written off as a useless and a nuisance, i.e., appendicitis, creator is now found to serve an important function (kudos to those researchers who focused on it, instead of erasing its presence from their minds!). Stratum lucidum is no exception.

Against this backdrop of philosophy, they should have tried to explore the character of the cytoskeleton of the keratinocytes in this layer and the composition of CE and nature of lipids in CLE.

The progeny of proliferating cells in the basal layer cannot afford to get accumulated in the basal layer. The progeny must keep moving upward: They must get assembled into different layers.

There should be ensured proper adhesiveness between keratinocytes. As they move outward (i.e., cell polarity), the cell shape should change, i.e., from cuboidal to a flattened cell, i.e., corneocyte (i.e., morphogenetic movements). When there is injury to the skin, the basal keratinocyte should proliferate to repair the wound. When inflammation is going on, the immune and inflammatory cells should be accommodated in the epidermis. Unless there is no communication between cells as to what should be their next function, subsequent changes are bound to be chaotic. Hence, there should be a process of communication and signaling among various cells in a synchronized fashion. To enable various required changes to occur in an orderly and a flawless fashion, the epidermis is vested with various structural components which include the desmosomes, adherens junctions, gap junctions, and tight junctions.

DESMOSOMES

The desmosomes are multiprotein complexes, the ingredients of which belong to three gene superfamilies: (1) The desmosomal cadherins, (2) The armadillo family of nuclear and junctional proteins, and (3) The plakins.[22] Desmosomes (the major adhesion complex in the epidermis) are also found in meninges, myocardium, and cortex of lymph nodes. The biochemical composition of desmosomes varies from tissue to tissue, yet the core of the desmosome comprises of transmembrane glycoproteins that belong to the Dsg and desmocollin (Dsc) subfamilies of calcium-dependent cell adhesion proteins (cadherins). The critical role of calcium as a mediator of adhesion is highlighted in the case of two conditions which exhibit characteristic epidermal dyscohesion: (1) Darier disease and (2) Hailey–Hailey disease.[23]

Functions

The intracellular parts of these glycoproteins are attached to the cytoskeleton (composed of keratin filament network) via a complex of several proteins including desmoplakin, plakoglobin, one of several plakophilin (Pkp) isoforms, and not infrequently additional accessory proteins. Thus, desmosomes are the major adhesion complex in the epidermis anchoring keratin intermediate filaments to the cell membrane and bridging adjacent keratinocytes. Thus, this cell-cell coupling is believed to be facilitated by heterophilic interactions between Dsg and Dsc proteins. Adhesiveness of junctions is effected by changes in the protein composition or through protein modifications. This kind of regulation of adhesiveness between keratinocytes is a key factor in regulating cell migration, cell sorting, and the formation of proper tissue histoarchitecture during embryonic development.[24]

Plakoglobin, a protein that belongs to the armadillo protein family, is a core component of desmosomes. It relays signals to the nucleus and can also control gene expression within nucleus by forming complexes with T-cell factor/lymphoid enhancer factor (TCF/LEF)proteins. Additionally, plakoglobin can influence other biological properties of a cell such as proliferation, migration, and apoptosis. Pkp can also play a role in stimulating cytoplasmic signaling pathways and Pkp1 and Pkp2 have nuclear functions as well.[25] Desmosome proteins may also serve as antigens in many autoimmune blistering skin diseases.

ADHERENS JUNCTIONS[10]

Adherens junctions are electron-dense transmembrane structures that get linked to the actin microfilament cytoskeleton via classical cadherins, in particular, P-cadherin and E-cadherin, as well as a complex of armadillo family of proteins (cytoplasmic plaque proteins) that include α-catenin, β-catenin, and ϒ-catenin which is also known as plakoglobin.[20] It is interesting to note that plakoglobin can bind to both desmosomal cadherins and classical cadherins.

While P-cadherin is expressed mainly in the basal layer of mouse epidermis, E-cadherin is expressed throughout interfollicular epidermis. Mouse model experiments suggest that loss of E-cadherin can affect tight junctions and in turn skin barrier function.[26] It has also become evident that abnormal expression of cytoplasmic plaque proteins, i.e., the armadillo family of proteins (α-catenin, β-catenin, and plakoglobin) does affect normal epidermis function.

Apart from cadherin-catenin units, adherens junctions also comprise of nectin-afadin complexes. The nectins connect to the actin cytoskeleton via afadin.

Functions

Epithelial assembly, barrier function, adhesion, cell motility, and changes in cell shape are the various functions served by adherens junctions. The precise incorporation of nectins and cadherins seems to determine the adhesive specificity and other functions. The cadherin-catenin complex not only mediates adhesion, but also cell signaling. Several Wnt pathways are activated via β-catenin suggesting that adherens junctions coordinate morphogenetic movements with cell fate determination. Mutations occurring in genes that encode for various components of these junctions can result in autosomal recessive hypotrichosis, juvenile macular dystrophy, hypodontia, and various limb defects.

GAP JUNCTIONS

Gap junctions are formed by clusters of intercellular channels. These channels, also known as connexons, directly form connections between the cytoplasm of not only adjacent keratinocytes, but also with other cells.[27] Connexons result from the assembly of six connexin subunits in the Golgi apparatus which is finally transported to the plasma membrane. At the plasma membrane, connexons associate with other connexons to form gap junctions.

Connexins, the components of connexons, fall into three groups (α, β, and ϒ), based on their gene structure and other related factors.[28] Connexons can be homotypic (if formed from one type of connexin) and heterotypic (if formed from >1 type of connexin). Other than connexins, in vertebrates, another class of gap junction proteins, called pannexins, can be formed. Innexins, found in nonchordate animals, are related to pannexins.[29] The formation and stability of gap junctions can be regulated by various factors that include PKC, Src kinase, calcium concentration, local pH, etc.[30]

Functions

Gap junctions allow intercellular coordination and uniformity to maintain tissue/organ homeostasis in multicellular organisms by permitting sharing of low-molecular mass metabolites and ion exchange between neighboring cells.[29] Other essential functions include cell synchronization, cell growth, cell differentiation, and metabolic coordination of avascular organs such as epidermis.

TIGHT JUNCTIONS

Claudins constitute the main structural proteins of tight junctions. There are about 24 subtypes of claudins of which seven are expressed in human epidermis. Of these seven, the principal claudins include one and four. Apart from claudins, the other component, transmembranous proteins include immunoglobulin G (IgG)-like family of junctional adhesion molecules (JAMs) and the occludin group of proteins. Though these transmembranous proteins do not bind to one another, they can bind to the intracellular zonula occludens proteins (Z0-1, Z0-2, and Z0-3). These proteins provide a direct link with cytoskeleton by interacting with actin.[24,31]

Functions

These tight junctions play a key role in skin barrier integrity, as they are thought to "seal" the intercellular space. They form a seal in the granular layer of epidermis also which is very much crucial for maintaining the water barrier function of the epidermis. These junctions also help to maintain cell polarity.[24] Tight junctions regulate the paracellular flux of water-soluble molecules between adjacent cells.[32] When mutations occur in the components of tight junctions, in particular the claudin proteins, resulting in various diseases, all of which are autosomal recessive in nature, the key role played by tight junctions play in the skin, liver, eye, ear, and kidney becomes very clear.

Now, let us have a look at how the epidermis is anchored to dermis (how dermis gets bound to the underlying subcutis is beyond the scope of this book).

DERMAL-EPIDERMAL BASEMENT MEMBRANE

The space between the overlying epidermis and underlying dermis is referred to as BMZ or dermoepidermal junction (DEJ) and is filled with a number of extracellular matrix molecules, many of them being glycoproteins, secreted by epidermal keratinocytes, in particular, basal keratinocytes and dermal fibroblasts.[33] Transmission electron microscopy differentiates this zone into two layers, i.e., the upper layer, lamina lucida, is a less electron-dense region and directly abuts the overlying plasma membranes of basal keratinocytes and the lower layer, lamina densa, an electron-dense region, is anchored to the underlying dermis.

The basement membrane is an agglomeration of various agents produced by keratinocytes and fibroblasts. These agents include proteins in HDs [i.e., plectin 500 kDa, bullous pemphigoid antigen 1 (BPAG1) 230 kDa, BPAG2 180 kDa, integrin subunit α6 120 kDa, and integrin subunit β4 180 kDa], tetraspan, types IV and VIII collagen, laminins 5 and 6, and heparan sulfate proteoglycans whereas fibroblasts produce nidogen (entactin) and other proteins. Subsequently, these dermal fibroblast-derived proteins are translocated to the plasma membranes of basal keratinocytes where they condense and thereupon get incorporated into the epidermal basement membrane. This is largely facilitated by organizational cues, which are provided by integrins in basal keratinocyte plasma membranes.

The chain of components that secures adherence of keratinocytes to dermis and thus shoulder the crucial and critical responsibility of maintaining structural and functional integrity of skin and also protecting the skin against sharing forces is as follows.

Broadly speaking, these ultrastructurally recognizable components include HDs, anchoring filaments, and anchoring fibrils.

Hemidesmosomes are, ultrastructurally, electron-dense attachment complexes that extend from the intracellular compartment of the basal keratinocytes to the lamina lucida. Thus, each HD has an inner intracytoplasmic plaque and an outer plaque which extends to the lamina lucida. Originally, HDs were designated as HD1 to HD5 with their respective molecular masses (see above). Further studies have identified the proteins represented by the five components of HDs (i.e., HD1 to HD5).

Thus, while the intracellular domains of the HDs within the basal keratinocytes attach to the keratin intermediate filament network (i.e., K5 and K14 keratins, sometimes keratin 15 in the absence of K14), in the extracellular space within the lamina lucida, the HDs are contiguous with the laminin 332 in the anchoring filaments: This unit is referred to as HD-anchoring filament complex.

Anchoring filaments are thread-like structures that coalesce below the extracellular part of the HD plaque. While the presence of other molecules cannot be ruled out, the major component of anchoring filaments may be 332 (i.e., α3, β3, and ϒ2), earlier known as laminin 5: The laminin 332 in the anchoring filaments gets complexed with α6β4 integrin in the HD above and with type VII collagen in the anchoring fibrils below.

Almost all the components of this biological chain that anchors keratinocytes, in particular, the basal keratinocytes, to the underlying dermis, have their respective gene or genes that code for them including intracellular cytoskeleton. Therefore, any loss-of-function mutation hitting any of these genes reflects the importance of this chain in the maintenance of structural and functional integrity of the skin, especially in the epidermolysis bullosa group of diseases.[34]

I wonder rather get shocked by looking at these changes along heel borders and soles. Why should epidermis give in this way to trauma/external threats? After all, millions of years ago, the human body was built. Since then, skin must have faced many epidermal disruptive problems/fatal hazards from environment. Long ago, it must have mastered the art of maintaining its structural integrity and thus it's most important function of skin barrier activity. After all, the formation of epidermal barrier is one of the most crucial functions of keratinocyte that it owes to the human organism.

Absent granular layer in psoriatic lesions means absence of keratohyalin granules, tight junctions, and lamellar granules (Odland bodies). The later extrude their lipid contents into the intercorneocyte space. These lipids help not only cohesion between corneocytes, but also play an important role in barrier activity.

Thus, not only stratum corneum, tight, gap, adherens junctions, desmosomes but also cytoskeletal elements too enable nucleated epidermis to contribute to barrier activity of the epidermis. Lipids are actively synthesized, by keratinocytes, during epidermal differentiation and get extruded into the extracellular domains where they lay extracellular lipid-enriched layers formation and maintenance of barrier function is also influenced by cytokines, cyclic adenosine monophosphate (cAMP), or calcium.[21] Therefore, changes in epidermal differentiation and lipid composition lead to disturbed skin barrier which may be involved in the pathogenesis of different skin diseases such as psoriasis, atopic eczema, contact dermatitis, ichthyosis, etc., by paving way for the entry of environmental allergens, microbes, etc.

Therefore, it is no surprise at all that in psoriasis, the increased epidermal cell turnover which comes in the way of normal keratinocyte differentiation program and the rapid proliferative state cannot spare time for formation of a very important epidermal layer, i.e., granular layer. Therefore, this results in poor cohesion between corneocytes and also impaired barrier activity. This is the reason why, perhaps, the psoriatic plaques initially begin as dry scaly patches which finally evolve into thickened inflammatory plaques which exhibit marked tendency for cracking, i.e., fissuring as a result of poor cohesion between corneocytes. The xerotic beginning of a psoriatic plaque is because of absent tight junctions due to absent granular layer and also due to lack of lipid mantle which contribute to ready loss of water from the epidermis.

Feet are the most trauma-prone parts of human body, more so in India as 70% of its population lives in villages, most of which are still in need of good roads; villagers still make use of nonmotorized bicycles for transport and almost all of them indulge in field (farming) activities, thus making their soles susceptible to trauma.

In genetically predisposed individuals, the areas regularly subjected to physical trauma coupled with mental trauma and intercurrent (throat and cutaneous) infections readily develop HK in feet. This jeopardizes the structural integrity and due to lack of intercorneocyte lipids (secondary to absent granular layer) which help cohesion, stratum corneum gives in resulting in cracks which become deeper due to continued trauma.

Trauma to feet is not exclusive to ruralites, urbanites too are susceptible to trauma. These days, health consciousness is on rise in India. Urbanites, including men and women, in addition to their routine activities in their day-to-day life, they also go for either morning or evening walk wearing shoes or sandals. Footwear is, I opine, bound to inflict trauma to dorsae and soles of the feet. The severity of trauma inflicted, may vary from site to site in feet and also from individual to individual, based on their pedal biomechanics. Therefore, entire skin covering over feet may not become hyperkeratotic, except few areas. Hence, the areas that become hyperkeratotic with or without fissures (fissuring, i.e., superficial or deep associated with HK is fairly common) constitute diagnostic signs for psoriasis. These are as follows:

- Hyperkeratosis with superficial fissures involving the toe pulps or toe pads of either great toe or toe pulps of rest of the toes or any one toe of either foot or both feet.
- Hyperkeratosis and superficial fissuring of lateral aspects of great toes.
- Hyperkeratosis with or without fissuring of undertoes.
- Hyperkeratosis of one or few or rarely all intertriginous areas of either foot.
- Hyperkeratosis, maceration with or without candidiasis of fourth webspace of either foot.
- Well-circumscribed, dark HK, and scaly plaques on dorsae of the toes or dorsum of one of the toes.
- Multiple cracks all over the soles or any part of the sole.
- Marked HK and a typical pattern of fissuring of heel borders.
- Hyperkeratosis and scaling of borders of feet.
- Eroded skin of borders of feet or web spaces or balls of feet.

I assume that psoriasis is the predisposing factor for candidiasis of any part of hand or foot, i.e., paronychia or intertrigo of the web spaces. I may put the events leading to candidiasis this way. *HK is the prerequisite for maceration which occurs due to free entry of water molecules in to the epidermis due to impaired barrier function secondary to absent granular layer; macerated skin enables Candida species to become pathogenic.* Macerated skin enables the resident *Candida albicans* (*C. albicans*) to become pathogenic. So, I may say that candidiasis should always arouse suspicion as to psoriasis in a given patient. Nonpsoriasis-prone skin does not develop HK because granular layer is intact as there is no increased cellturnover. So, also barrier function which is a two-way activity. The tight junctions in granular layer do not let the intraepidermal water molecules out. Similarly, the lipid mantle in between corneocytes does not let water molecules, allergens, irritants, and microbial pathogens to gain entry into epidermis. In psoriasis affected skin, thus, the barrier activity is impaired. As a result, water molecules from within and outside cause maceration. As a result, *C. albicans*, an opportunistic pathogen, fishes in troubled waters.

- A linear, lichenified plaque on the dorsum of either great toe, extending onto the dorsum of the foot over the tendon.
- Dark, warty HK of one or more of the four malleoli.
- Subtle changes of lichenification involving ankle flexures (may be mistaken to chronic atopic eczema); looks, as if, it is being treated with a topical agent.
- Candidal paronychia or candidal intertrigo.

REFERENCES

1. Ishida-Yamamoto A, Tanaka H, Nakane H, Takahashi H, Iizuka H. Inherited disorders of epidermal keratinization. J Dermatol Sci. 1998;18:139-54.
2. Koster MI, Kim S, Mills AA, DeMayo FJ, Roop DR. p63 is the molecular switch for initiation of an epithelial stratification program. Genes Dev. 2004;18:126-31.
3. Westfall MD, Mays DJ, Sniezek JC, Pietenpol JA. The Delta Np63 alpha phosphoprotein binds the p21 and 14-3-3 sigma promoters in vivo and has transcriptional repressor activity that is reduced by Hay-Wells syndrome-derived mutations. Mol Cell Biol. 2003;23:2264-76.
4. Blanpain C, Lowry WE, Pasolli HA, Fuchs E. Canonical notch signaling functions as a commitment switch in the epidermal lineage. Genes Dev. 2006;20:3022-35.
5. Dlugosz AA, Yuspa SH. Coordinate changes in gene expression which mark the spinous to granular cell transition in epidermis are regulated by protein kinase C. J Cell Biol. 1993;120:217-25.
6. Dlugosz AA, Yuspa SH. Protein kinase C regulates keratinocyte transglutaminase (*TGK*) gene expression in cultured primary mouse epidermal ketatinocytes induced to terminally differentiate by calcium. J Invest Dermatol. 1994;102:409-14.
7. Kirfel J, Magin TM, Reichelt J. Keratins: a structural scaffold with emerging functions. Cell Mol Life Sci. 2003;60:56-71.
8. Langbein L, Schweizer J. Keratins of the human hair follicle. Int Rev Cytol. 2005;243:1-78.
9. Pan X, Hobbs RP, Coulombe PA. The expanding significance of keratin intermediate filaments in normal and diseased epithelia. Curr Opin Cell Biol. 2013;25:47-56.
10. Niessen CM. Tight/adherens junctions: basic structure and function. J invest dermatol. 2007; 127:2525-32.
11. Clayton E, Doupé DP, Klein AM, Winton DJ, Simons BD, Jones PH. A single type of progenitor cell maintains normal epidermis. Nature. 2007;446:185-9.
12. Gomez C, Chua W, Miremadi A, Quist S, Headon DJ, Watt FM. The interfollicular epidermis of adult mouse tail comprises two distinct cell lineages that are differentially regulated by Wnt, Edaradd, and Lrig1. Stem Cell Reports. 2013;1:19-27.
13. Rampolas P, Mesa KR, Kawaguchi K, Park S, Gonzalez D, Brown S, et al. Spatiotemporal coordination of stem cell commitment during epidermal homeostasis. Science. 2016;352:1471-4.
14. Sada A, Jacob F, Leung E, Wang S, White BS, Shalloway D, et al. Defining the cellular lineage hierarchy in the interfollicular epidermis of adult skin. Nat Cell Biol. 2016;18:619-31.
15. Sánchez-Danés A, Hannezo E, Larsimont JC, Liagre M, Youssef KK, Simons BD, et al. Defining the clonal dynamics leading to mouse skin tumor initiation. Nature. 2016;536:298-303.
16. Lechler T, Fuchs E. Asymmetric cell divisions promote stratification and differentiation of mammalian skin. Nature. 2005;437:275-80.
17. Williams SE, Beronja S, Pasolli HA, Fuchs E. Asymmetric cell divisions promote Notch-dependent epidermal differentiation. Nature. 2011;470:353-8.
18. Fuchs E. Scratching the surface of skin development. Nature. 2007;445:834-42.
19. Carofoli E, Brini M. Calcium pumps: structural basis for and mechanism of calcium transmembrane transport. Curr Opin Chem Biol. 2000;4:152-61.
20. Steinert PM. The complexity and redundancy of epithelial barrier function. J Cell Biol. 2000;151:F5-8.
21. Simpson CL, Patel DM, Green KJ. Deconstructing the skin: cytoarchitectural determinants of epidermal morphogenesis. Nat Rev Mol Cell Biol. 2011;12:565-80.
22. Girard-Madoux MJH, de Agüero MG, Ganal-Vonarburg SC, Mooser C, Belz GT, Macpherson AJ, et al. The immunological functions of the Appendix: An example of redundancy? Semin Immunol. 2018;36:31-44.
23. Al-Jascar C, Bikker H, Overduin M, Chidget M. Mechanistic basis of desmosomes-targeted diseases. J Mol Biol. 2013;425:4006-22.
24. Runswick SK, O'Hare MJ, Jones L, Streuli CH, Garrod DR. Desmosomal adhesion regulates epithelial morphogenesis and cell positioning. Nat Cell Biol. 2001;3:823-30.
25. Schmidt A, Jäger S. Plakophilins—hard work in the desmosome, recreation in the nucleus? Eur J Cell Biol. 2005;84:189-204.
26. Tunggal JA, Helfrich I, Schmitz A, Schwarz H, Günzel D, Fromm M, et al. E-cadherin is essential for in vivo epidermal barrier function by regulating tight junctions. EMBO J. 2005;24:1146-56.
27. Mese G, Richard G, White TW. Gap junctions: basic structure and function. J Invest Dermatol. 2007;127:2516-24.
28. Richard G. Connexin disorders of the skin. Clin Dermatol. 2005;23:23-32.
29. Velasquez S, Eugenin. EA. Role of pannexin-1 hemi-channels and purinergic receptors in the pathogenesis of human diseases. Front Physiol. 2014;5:96.

30. Scott CA, Kelsell DP. Key functions for gap junctions in skin and hearing. Biochem J. 2011;438:245-54.
31. Gupta IR, Ryan AK. Claudins: unlocking the code to tight junction formation during embryogenesis and in disease. Clin Genet. 2010;77:314-25.
32. Morita K, Miyachi Y. Tight junctions in the skin. J. Dermatol Sci. 2003;31:81-9.
33. El Ghalbzouri A, Jonkman MF, Dijkman R, Ponec M. Basement membrane reconstruction in human skin equivalence is regulated by fibroblasts and/or exogenously activated keratinocytes. J Invest Dermatol. 2005;124:79-86.
34. Salam A, Proudfoot LE, McGrath JA. Inherited blistering skin diseases: underlying molecular mechanisms and emerging therapies. Ann Med. 2014;46:49-61.

2

Anatomy of Normal Nail and Toenail in Psoriasis

NAIL UNIT

An analogy may be drawn between a female's mammary gland development and nail matrix formation: While the former is a modified apocrine gland, the latter is the result of modified proximal nail fold (PNF).

The nail apparatus begins to form during the 9th embryonic week, i.e., first trimester, from the epidermis of the dorsal tip of the digit and nail matrix development becomes complete by the 15th week and from then onward nail plate production begins which continues till the death in the absence of disease.

The proximal border of the nail fold extends downward and proximally into the dermis to form the nail matrix primordium. In the process of further development, it offers a wedge shape in longitudinal sections, consisting of a proximal (dorsal), an intermediate matrix or germinative matrix or matrix, and a distal (ventral) section. Ultimately, except the dorsal section, the other two sections of the nail matrix remain as if inserted between nail plate above and periosteum of the distal phalanx bone below.

Components of Nail Unit

By extending downward and proximally, the objective of PNF is to enable its ventral portion evolve into nail matrix, the sole function of which is to keep producing a horny "dead" product, i.e., the nail plate. Thus, while the nail plate is the main component of nail unit, others include four specialized epithelia, i.e., (1) The PNF, (2) The nail matrix, (3) The nail bed, and (4) The hyponychium.

Proximal Nail Fold

A dorsal and a ventral portion together form a skin fold in the nail apparatus, referred to as PNF. Except for being thinner and devoid of pilosebaceous units, the dorsal portion of PNF is anatomically similar to the skin of the dorsum of the digits. The ventral portion, which cannot be seen from the exterior, extends downward and proximally and takes a bend to progress distally to complete nail matrix and nail bed formation.

From the junction of the two portions of the PNF projects a horny layer that gets firmly attached to the superficial nail plate, called cuticle. The main function of the cuticle is to prevent separation of the nail plate from the PNF. A noteworthy feature is that the granular layer formation stops at the junction of the dorsal matrix (ventral portion of the PNF) and intermediate matrix, i.e., germinative matrix or matrix. Thus, the limit between the PNF and the nail matrix can be histologically established at the site of disappearance of the granular layer.

The horizontal orientation of the numerous capillaries in the form of fine regular loops with arterial and the venous limbs, with a small space in between, provides a wonderful clinical opportunity to the dermatologist to discern systemic lupus erythematosus (SLE), scleroderma, and dermatomyositis (the diseases in which the morphology of these loops are typically altered) with the help of capillary microscopy.

Nail Wall

The lateral nail folds (LNFs) and tissue adjacent to them are referred to as nail wall by some authorities. The LNFs are in continuity with the skin on the sides of the digit laterally whereas, medially they are joined by the nail bed.

Nail Matrix

While the definition of nail matrix appears to be controversial,[1] the description of the nail matrix is confusing. Nevertheless, the author makes an attempt to enable the reader gain a clear idea as to nail matrix through the following lines: The matrix can be subdivided into dorsal (the ventral aspect of the PNF), intermediate (germinal matrix or matrix), and ventral (nail bed) sections.

The most major contribution for nail plate formation comes from intermediate matrix/germinal matrix/matrix followed by dorsal section of matrix. The contribution made by ventral matrix (nail bed), according to some authorities, is nil or unclear. Hence, the nail bed (ventral section of matrix) is referred to as sterile matrix meaning that the major contributor to nail plate ends where the intermediate matrix, i.e., between the dorsal and ventral sections of matrix, joins the ventral section of matrix, i.e., nail bed (sterile matrix). Therefore, the most nail forming section of matrix is given the following names, i.e., (1) Germinative matrix, (2) Intermediate matrix, and (3) Matrix (matrix is further divided into proximal and distal regions).

The matrix is not completely covered by PNF in all the digits: A white half-moon-shaped area, the lunula, is visible through the proximal part of the nail plate and it represents the most distal region of the matrix and is most conspicuous on the thumb and great toe.[2]

Does matrix epithelium differ from epidermis elsewhere?

Matrix is devoid of granular layer and pilosebaceous units. Apart from this, in addition to normal epithelial keratins,[3-5] matrix cells differentiate with the expression of trichocyte hard keratins (K31–40 and K81–86) which get incorporated into the nail plate, concomitantly with normal epithelial keratins.[6-8] Thus, the nail matrix cells are capable of synthesizing both "soft" or skin type and "hard" or hair type keratins. Of the various components of nail apparatus, it is only the nail matrix that is capable of synthesizing hard keratins, in particular Ha1 keratin. Other than these, there is no difference between intracellular activities of matrix epithelium and epidermis elsewhere from the "viewpoint" of electron microscopy.

Other Cells in Nail Matrix

Melanocytes: Though nail matrix cells possess the key enzymes necessary for melanin production, they usually remain inactive and this is the reason why they are not detectable in pathologic sections, but a large number of physiologic and pathologic conditions can activate them. If these melanocytes are activated, it may result in either diffuse or banded nail plate pigmentation. Such changes most commonly occur in Blacks and Japanese than in Caucasians. DOPA-negative melanocytes are sparsely present in matrix and nail bed. The DOPA-positive melanocytes occur in clusters in suprabasal location of the matrix epithelium, unlike in epidermis.

Langerhans cells: These cells occur more abundantly in the proximal region than in the distal matrix and are detected by CD1a staining. Their location is the same as in normal epidermis, i.e., in the suprabasal layers, but occasionally within the basal layer of the distal matrix epithelium.

Merkel cells: These cells are demonstrable in nail matrix and they are numerous in fetus than in adult nails possibly as a result of influence of the age.

Nail Plate

A fully keratinized structure that it is, the nail plate is produced throughout life without any break, provided the nail matrix remains intact and the nail plate progressively thickens from its origin to its distal margin.

Nail plate is made of three different layers. While the PNF gives origin to superficial nail plate, the matrix gives origin to the middle layer and the nail bed gives origin to deep ventral layer of the nail plate.[9] Till now, the view held was that matrix alone is responsible for nail plate production. In support of this, the studies done by Zais and Alvarez[10] in squirrel monkeys, and similar studies by others[11] conducted on human volunteers, and studies by Berker and Angus[12] led to the proposal that nail matrix alone is responsible for nail plate formation, but other studies,[13,14] though, proposed that bulk of the nail plate was produced by matrix cells, the nail bed also contributes to the nail plate based on nail thickness and mass; nevertheless, there appears to be a general consensus that it is, in conclusion, matrix cells that produce nail plate.

The nail plate, though smooth, often displays longitudinal ridges which increase with aging and the pattern of these ridges can be used for forensic identification. The bottom of the nail plate is longitudinally ridged corresponding to the rete ridges of underlying nail bed.

When the intact nail plate is viewed from above, two distinct areas may be noticed: The proximal part of the fingernails, especially of the thumb and great toe, display a whitish, translucent, and half-moon-shaped area, called the lunula, while the distal zone appears pink because of nail bed epithelium being thinner and hence nail bed blood vessels are rather the blood flow in these vessels is readily visible as pink color. A keen observation of the nail plate discloses the distal white/yellowish white margin and immediately proximal to this is the isthmus which signifies the most distal and strongest attachment of nail bed to the undersurface of the nail plate. If this attachment is breached in diseases such as psoriasis, it results in onycholysis, i.e., separation of the distal nail plate from nail bed that progresses proximally.

Nail thickness depends on the length of the nail matrix and nail bed and it increases with age in the first two decades. While thinning of the nails is usually a sign of nail matrix disorders, nail thickening is most commonly a consequence of nail bed disorders. Using either ultrasound or optical coherence tomography, nail plate thickness can be measured in health and disease.[4]

How the nails are able to keep themselves continuously growing?

This question pertains to all the bodily tissues and the answer is stem cells which display a unique ability of differentiating into various cell types. Because stem cells are required for tissue homeostasis and tissue regeneration in the event of injury,[15] throughout life, they obviously possess the ability of long-term cell-renewal capacity. According to recent discoveries, stem cells in nail organs exist in two different activation modes—slow cycling and actively proliferating once—to fulfill the demands of continuously growing nails.[16,17] Thus, it has been demonstrated that nail organ contains a gradient of slow-to-fast cycling stem cells. In the nail proximal folds are found slow-cycling stem cells [nail proximal fold stem cells (NPFSCs)], more active cells in the intermediate zone (IZ or matrix), and finally rapidly proliferative nail stem cells (NSCs) in the nail proximal matrix regions.

Why stem cells with different proliferative potentials need to be present in nails?

In the absence of one group of stem cells, the other group takes up the role of absent group of stem cells,[3] according to the studies on normal turnover in small intestines. Perhaps, such backup is needed in every tissue of different organs including nail unit.

Nail Bed

The nail bed is that part of the nail unit which extends from the distal margin of the lunula (lunula represents the distal region of germinative matrix/matrix) to the isthmus and is completely visible through the nail plate. The nail bed epithelium is thinner than that of nail matrix and is usually two to five layers thick. The underlying connective tissue, i.e., the dermis is closely opposed to the periosteum of the distal phalanx. Thus, the nail is intimately connected to the bone and this appears to be responsible for the common occurrence of bone alterations in nail disorders and vice versa.

Nail bed keratinization, like nail matrix, is not characterized by formation of granular layer. Nevertheless, it may form when nail bed is exposed as in avulsion.

Hyponychium

At the tip of the digit, the nail plate separates from the underlying tissues and it marks the anatomic area between the nail bed and the distal groove. While its anatomic structure is similar to that of plantar and volar skin, granular layer is a normal component.

The horny layer of hyponychium partially occurs under the nail plate. Though hyponychium is normally covered by the nail plate, it may become visible in nail biters.

In contrast to the horizontal arrangement of the capillaries in PNF, the capillaries are arranged in a perpendicular fashion in the hyponychium; hence, they are visible as red dots with dermoscopy.

BASEMENT MEMBRANE ZONE

Neither there are differences in the antigenic composition of the basement membrane zone (BMZ) in different portions of the nail apparatus, nor does it differ with that of epidermis elsewhere.

Clinical significance: This may explain the involvement of nails in diseases caused by mutations of BMZ-associated genes as well as in autoimmune skin diseases involving the BMZ antigens.

DERMIS

Whereas, dermis in nail apparatus is devoid of pilosebaceous units, no subcutaneous tissue is found in nail unit. The proximal nail matrix is anchored to the periosteum of the proximal phalangeal bone through posterior ligament which forms as a result of condensation of dermal connective tissue beneath proximal nail matrix. Underneath the nail matrix, the rete ridges of the dermis are characteristically long and root-like in shape whereas the dermis under the nail bed consists of a loose network of connective tissue containing of numerous blood vessels and glomus bodies.

Longitudinal grooves and ridges characterize the nail bed dermis and they run from the lunula to the hyponychium. The longitudinal orientation of the capillaries within the nail bed grooves explains the linear pattern of nail bed hemorrhages (splinter hemorrhages). Connective tissue bundles form abundant connective tissue networks in the nail bed dermis that radiate to the phalangeal periosteum. The nail bed dermis contains numerous glomus bodies.

BLOOD AND NERVE SUPPLY

Both the nail matrix and nail bed derive rich arterial blood supply from paired digital arteries, which are supplied from the large superficial and deep palmar arcades[18] and a small dorsal digital artery on either side: While on their way, they produce branches that supply the matrix and PNF and also produce arches that supply the matrix and the nail bed. Thus, the nail matrix has two different sources of blood supply, i.e., (1) branches from paired arteries on either side and (2) from the arches.

The nail bed is richly supplied by encapsulated neurovascular structures containing one to four arteriovenous anastomoses and nerve endings. These are also known as glomus bodies and are involved in the regulation of blood supply to the digits during adverse thermoregulatory conditions. Thus, the glomus bodies are important in maintaining microcirculation. Under cold conditions, arterioles constrict, but glomus bodies dilate.[19]

Nerve Supply

The cutaneous sensory nerves, which originate from the dorsal branches of the paired digital nerves, run parallel to the digital vessels.

HOMEOSTASIS OF THE NAIL APPARATUS

The nail apparatus is protected by two structures which are, perhaps, solely responsible for homeostasis of the nail apparatus: Proximally, it is cuticle, a horny layer that projects onto the surface of the nail plate, from the junction of the two epithelial surfaces of PNF and is firmly attached to the nail plate and prevents the separation of the nail plate from the nail fold and thus protects the structures at the base of the nail, particularly the germinal matrix (matrix) from environmental hazards such as irritants, allergens, and bacterial and fungal pathogens. Distally, the guard for nail unit is isthmus (onychocorneal band); if it is breached, the onycholysis progresses proximally, separating the distal nail plate from the nail bed. Such a development in the nail unit endangers the homeostasis of the nail apparatus the same way when the cuticle is disrupted.

CHEMICAL AND PHYSICAL PROPERTIES

The nail plate, like hair, is made of mainly low-sulfur filamentous proteins (keratins) that get embedded in an amorphous matrix composed of high-sulfur proteins rich in cysteine. Nail keratins consist of 80–90% hard hair type keratins and 10–20% soft skin type keratins. The hardness and strength of the nail plate are due to its high content of hard keratins and cysteine-rich high-sulfur proteins.

Other nail plate constituents include water, lipids, and traces of several inorganic elements, in particular, iron, zinc, and calcium. The noteworthy feature is, contrary to the popular belief, they do not contribute to nail hardness. The nail plate's flexibility depends on its water content and increases with nail plate hydration. In addition to water, significant amounts of phospholipid, present mainly in the dorsal and intermediate layers, also contribute to nail plate's flexibility.[20]

The high porosity of the nail plate allows it to be rapidly hydrated and dehydrated—hence, the average water content of the nail plate is significantly lower in winter compared to summer. Under normal conditions, the water content of the nail plate is almost 18% and it is the intermediate nail plate that harbors most of the water. Long nails are more prone to dehydration. Nail becomes brittle when its water content falls below 18%; when the water content rises above 30%, the nail becomes opaque and soft.

NAIL GROWTH

The production of nail plate begins as early as 15th week of fetal life and it continues till death in the absence of disease. The growth progresses in a proximal to distal manner throughout life. Nail growth in psoriasis-related studies found an inhibitory effect of cytostatic drugs[5,21] which suggest that cell kinetics and linear growth have a direct correlation. Nail growth varies from age to age; it is slow at birth, increases a little during childhood to reach its peak between second and third decades of life and decreases significantly after the age of 50 years. While conditions that have been associated with a slow growth rate include systemic illness, malnutrition, peripheral vascular and neurologic diseases, antimitotic drugs, onychomycosis, and yellow nail syndrome (arrest of nail growth), conditions that have been associated with accelerated nail growth include pregnancy, finger trauma, psoriasis, and treatment with oral retinoids or itraconazole. Longitudinal ridging of the nail plate (nail beading) is a feature of accelerated nail growth.

The slow growth rate of nail is advantageous, from the viewpoint of a forensic expert, as the nails may furnish information as to the pathologic condition that had occurred many months before the time of observation. Drugs, chemicals, and biologic substances which exhibit their affinity to get deposited in nail plates can be detected and measured. Noninvasive way of collection of the nail sample is the major advantage. The big toe is the most promising one for investigators because of its bigger size and slow growth.

NAIL APPARATUS IN PSORIASIS

When nail unit is affected by psoriasis, various changes occur, which may be categorized as specific and nonspecific nail signs. As per the literature, contained in the major textbooks authored and edited by Caucasians, there are only three cardinal signs of nail psoriasis that are supposed to occur only in fingernails and these include large, deep, irregular pits, the presence of an erythematous border along the onycholytic area, and Salmon patches, i.e., oil drop sign (a focal area of onycholysis with a small exudate appearing as yellow-red areas of discoloration occurring in the center of the nail or bordering an onycholytic area).

While any component of the nail unit may be affected, it is nail matrix and nail bed that are most commonly affected in psoriasis.

The rest of the nail changes described such as subungual hyperkeratosis (SUHK), nail plate discoloration, uneven nail surface, splinter hemorrhages, acute and chronic paronychia, and transverse midline depression in the thumbnails may be considered nonspecific and occur in descending order of frequency.

TEXTBOOK FACTS ABOUT NAIL PSORIASIS

Nail psoriasis occurs only in 50% of patients with skin psoriasis—in 83% of those with psoriatic arthritis. The three cardinal signs described and supposed to occur only in fingernails are meant for diagnosing nail psoriasis only, i.e., in rest of the 50% of psoriatics who do not display fingernail signs, it must be understood that laboratory (histopathology) alone can come to the rescue of the consultant dermatologist when he/she confronts a puzzling dermatitis, practicing overseas, i.e., in America and Europe. As per overseas literature, psoriasis always presents as well-defined erythematous plaques covered with silvery white scales, excepting some bodily locations such as flexures. Is it so in India, my dear learned colleagues practicing in India? Well, coming back to the overseas theory on this subject.

What happens in nail unit affected by psoriasis?

The nail bed is closely attached to the undersurface of the nail plate leaving no gap whatsoever. When psoriasis-affected nail bed produces scales, they cannot be shed in a normal way; hence, they accumulate between nail plate and nail bed resulting in SUHK and onycholysis; as a consequence, invasion by microbes, allergens, and irritants which may cause nail plate discoloration and other changes.

In recent times, high-resolution MRI has enabled the researchers to unfold the clinical significance of close proximity of the nail unit to the distal phalanx. In other words, what does the close relationship between the soft-tissue attachments of the distal interphalangeal joint and the matrix signify?

The fibers of the extensor tendon of the distal interphalangeal joint insert to the periosteum and then are directed to the proximal nail matrix, which they envelope and link to the bone. The collateral ligaments of the digit anchor the lateral sides of the nail to the interphalangeal joint. Consequently, any acute inflammation of the interphalangeal joint necessarily affects the nail and vice versa.

PITS

These are due to proximal nail matrix disease. The abnormal keratinization that occurs, consequently, in the proximal region of nail matrix produces foci of parakeratotic cells that fall off the upper surface of the superficial nail plate to produce a pit. Though nail pitting is a feature of some other diseases such as alopecia areata, lichen planus, atopic dermatitis, and inflammation of PNF due to any etiology, psoriasis is characterized by large, deep, and irregularly distributed pits and such pitting is diagnostic for nail psoriasis.

ONYCHOLYSIS

Onycholysis, like pits, is caused by a number of conditions and may occur even in the absence of any known etiology (idiopathic onycholysis). In general, the two most common causes of this nail change include psoriasis and onychomycosis.

An "oil spot" or "Salmon patch" that forms as a result of focal nail bed parakeratosis, when extends to the free edge, results in onycholysis—typically a reddish-brown proximal margin runs along the onycholytic area, making a definite diagnosis of nail psoriasis easier.

Alternatively, onycholysis may begin at the distal edge, disrupting the line of strongest attachment of nail bed to nail plate, represented by the isthmus or onychocorneal band, in which case, the separation of distal nail plate from nail bed progresses proximally.

NONSPECIFIC NAIL CHANGES

- *Discoloration*: Nail thickening and SUHK are the major factors that contribute to a yellow appearance, commonly observed in toenails, nondermatophytes such as *Candida* species and bacteria such as *Pseudomonas* may be responsible for greenish discoloration of the nail plate more frequently than dermatophyte infection.
- *Subungual hyperkeratosis*: It is due to nail-bed disease which contributes to remarkable nail plate thickening that is most marked distally and progresses proximally. Onychomycosis also causes SUHK which may get superimposed on one-fifth of psoriatic nails.
- *Nail plate abnormalities*: These include superficial longitudinal splits, thin atrophic nails, and fragility. Rarely, trachyonychia or crumbling, which is rated as severe nail plate abnormalities, may be produced by nail psoriasis.
- *Splinter hemorrhages*: It is seen more commonly in the nail bed of fingernails and much less commonly in toenails. They appear as red to black, small, and thin longitudinal lines under the nail plate, i.e., in the nail bed. They are more commonly observed in the distal nail plate and occur due to rupture of the longitudinally oriented nail bed capillaries.
- *Acute and chronic paronychia*: Nail bed inflammation may be dramatic and inflammation leading to gross disruption of the nail matrix which may result in nail loss, nail bed becoming scaly, or a deep transverse furrow (Beau's lines) may form. Loss of cuticle is a usual feature of chronic psoriatic paronychia. As a consequence, nail plate can become thin and this may be countered by nail bed disease which gives rise to a thickened nail. The nail fold may turn scaly, as in psoriasis elsewhere.

AUTHOR'S VIEWPOINT/EXPERIENCE

Thus, I am given to understand that our Caucasian colleagues seem to have preferred fingernails to toenails for their research (for reasons known to them only) and paper publications in various renowned international journals and paper presentations in various national and international conferences in order to sustain their career.

While that is all about them, my story goes like this—though I started my private clinical practice a little more than three decades ago, I have no hesitation to admit that at the end of one decade's practice, I was still going wrong in my diagnosis in at least 30% of cases and I used to correct myself in their second or third visit, by which time they might have spent 100s of rupees toward their travel charges, consultation fees, and medicines prescribed and many hours spent toward travelling from far-off places to reach me and a few hours of waiting at my clinic to enter my chamber in an exhausted state and also in a furious state. Some used to control their anger, but some could not help bursting out at me, thus hurting my ego with resultant shootup of my blood pressure. I used to get drenched in their emotions driven by their frustration and dissatisfaction at my prescription. For example, i.e., a male patient in his 60s gets seated on the stool closed to my executive table and shows his legs, while complaining of severe itching, which display a picture of widespread acute eczema encircling the entire length of lower legs; he gets up from stool and turns around to show his popliteal fossae which are heavily crusted. I used to diagnose it as acute eczema with secondary impetiginization (such presentation used to be fairly common during peak harvest seasons). Accordingly, I used to pen my prescription, keeping in view his urgent need to recover from the ailment so that he could go to his fields at the earliest and thus participate in harvest activities. He was instructed to come for review after 2 weeks. But, he lands in my office in just a week's time complaining that not only his itching became worse, but the eruptions have progressed to involve even his external genitalia and other bodily regions including his web spaces of the hands. After looking at the web spaces and external genitalia, I get shocked; how could I miss his scabies in the first visit!? Then, I used to enquire by fielding certain questions to the patient only to find out how I missed his scabies in his first visit.

Doctor: Please let me know how you presented to me earlier?

Patient: Sir, I showed to you my oozing legs.

Doctor: Ok! Did I not examine your hands and external genitalia at that time!?

Patient: No sir! That time my hands were not involved, but my external genitalia were having some elevated lesions which were causing severe itching during evenings and nights.

Doctor: You fool, why you did not reveal that in your first visit; I shout at him.

Patient: Sorry sir! I felt very shy to show my private parts.

Doctor: Now you are facing the music!

My prescription to this patient consisted of a short course of systemic steroids in a tapering fashion and other supportive drugs. The systemic steroids rather my ignorance and taking things for granted played havoc with the patient. I did see infants and young children developing a widespread eczematous eruption, who were afflicted by scabies. It was for the first time that I came across an elderly patient presenting with such an extensive eczematous eruption. Unable to accept this clinical defeat after having put in 10 years of experience, I started indulging in retrospective analysis as to what went wrong with this case and whether I was at fault or the patient.

Patients' feeling shy to show their private parts is fairly common and understandable. So, I cannot throw blame on him. Therefore, it was me who was at fault for the simple reason that I failed to look beyond his lower legs. Had I done so, perhaps, I would have not missed his scabies? Then what prevented me to examine his other bodily regions? Such massive eczematous eruption in an adult did not let me think in terms of scabies. I was all the while obsessed with atopic eczema: I remember to have tried to elicit history of atopy in his family including patient himself, but in vain. Therefore, it was my obsession with another possibility and though there was no history of atopy (a history of atopy is generally available in only 70% of the cases), I took it for granted (in fact, I took mileage out of the fact that 30% of patients do not give history of atopy) that it was atopic eczema. But, I had to answer another question. Does atopic eczema present in acute form involving lower legs? It is generally the flexures that are typically affected in an adult in atopic eczema and the flexures display a picture of chronic eczema, i.e., lichenification. But, in our country, it is fairly common on the part of our patients to apply some indigenous preparation, which is highly irritant in nature and some soaps, which are too irritant in nature, have the potential to elicit an acute eczematous response from the skin. Perhaps, this logical argument too was there in the back of my mind. Thus, my failure to look beyond the lesions shown to me by the patient and taking things for granted and my obsession with atopic eczema has led to the disastrous therapeutic outcome.

Meanwhile, a middle-aged lady entered my chamber; the patient introduced her to me as his wife and he brought her as she also started complaining of severe itching in nights.

I could not forgive myself and instantly returned fees to the couple in order to buy a bit of peace of mind.

Thus, I learnt an invaluable lesson from this debacle: For a dermatologist to emerge as an astute clinician, there should be no place for obsessions and should not take things for granted and more importantly, the dermatologist should look beyond lesions in every case and must undertake a thorough examination of the entire skin, if necessary, hidden parts too.

What made Ramamurthy focus on toenails rather than fingernails?

In the first 15 years of my clinical practice, I used to be scared of a patient presenting with a fingernail abnormality. My clinical acumen was not sharp enough to interpret fingernail changes. Luckily, women with chronic paronychia of the first few fingers of their right hands were the subjects that used to seek my help. I used to advise them to avoid wet work, if possible or dry their hands as soon as the contact with water came to an end. Any amount of pure topical antifungal coupled with systemic antifungal was of no use in controlling the nail fold inflammation. I used to get their blood sugars done only to know that they were not diabetic patient. After all, candidal paronychia is caused by *Candida albicans* which is a well-known opportunistic pathogen. None of them were either diabetics or immunocompromised hosts. Then what was the predisposing factor? Wet work alone!? I used to get puzzled: If wet work and detergent agents alone were to be the predisposing factors, then crores of women in India, both ruralites and urbanites, should develop this condition. But, in my clinical practice, I used to see infrequently a woman or a hotel worker with candidal paronychia and some of them with candidal intertrigo of the web spaces of hands not uncommonly. Pure antifungal treatment used to be of no use. This was further puzzling me.

Then, came a day which brought an elderly villager to my clinic who sought my intervention for one of his great toenail abnormality. That was a clear-cut case of onychogryphosis. He was in panic as fellow villagers advised him to consult a dermatologist urgently to rule out leprosy. I tried to elicit personal and family history of Hansen's but in vain. I examined his skin thoroughly and all the major peripheral nerves and cutaneous nerves which yielded no clue to Hansen's. Sensations were intact and no motor deficits noted. Then, I assured him confidently that he had no leprosy at all. "Then why this nail is like this?" was his question; "Sir, please look at the other toenails which also appear abnormal to me." Then, I lifted his (right) leg and took his (right) foot into my hands. My keen observation of toenails revealed some unexpected rather amusing nailplate abnormalities. Some of his intertriginous areas were hyperkeratotic. Some of his toe pulps were also hyperkeratotic and some were scaly, displaying superficial cracks. His undertoes were also hyperkeratotic and fissured. Heel borders displayed fissured hyperkeratotic plaques. Insteps displayed typical psoriatic plaques.

"Sir, do not bother about all those changes. They are very common among us who regularly go to fields sometimes barefooted."

From that day onward, I started examining the toenails of all the patients, whatever may be their cutaneous disease. Interestingly, some changes were being observed frequently among psoriatics and also their genetically-related accompanying persons such as parents, uncles, aunts, first cousins, or patient's siblings. If no one was accompanying, I used to contact the patient's parents or siblings or other genetically-related subjects to elicit a history of psoriasis, through cell phone and almost all the times I used to succeed in obtaining a history of psoriasis.

Thus, over the last 12 years, my confidence levels kept escalating to the extent that I cannot, but share my observations with my learned colleagues at this juncture, i.e., at the age of 62 years having put in a little more than three decades of clinical learning/experience.

Thus, the various toenail changes that I observed, in particular, among psoriatics include onycholysis, most commonly of great toenail (though any toenail, except little toenail, may develop this change), arch-shaped curvature of the toenails with or without SUHK, pincer nail, dystrophic nail, koilonychia, thinning of the nail plate, dry nails with superficial longitudinal cracks, Beau's lines, angulation of nail plate free margin, asbestos sheet-shaped toenails, onychauxis, i.e., nail plate appears thickened because of SUHK, band-shaped melanosis more often involving lateral or outer parts of the nail plates, not uncommonly entire nail plate, full-thickness longitudinal and central fissuring of the great toenail plates (very rarely other nail plates), onychogryphosis, bilateral and linear and yellowish to whitish streaks on the nail plate running along the LNFs associated with chronic psoriatic paronychia of LNFs—this change almost always affecting the great toenails, chronic paronychia of PNF, candidal intertrigo, and last but not the least, the typical splitting of little toenail of either foot or occasionally both feet; the split occurs in such a way that medial piece is always larger and smaller piece is on lateral side which is not infrequently melanotic.

If any toenail of either foot displays any one of the changes described above, it warrants a thorough search for psoriasis in the patient or a history of psoriasis in his or her pedigree, as per my experience.

While some of the above mentioned changes are not only diagnostic of nail psoriasis, they are also diagnostic of psoriasiform dermatitis or atypical dermatitis or unclassified eczema in question, being psoriasis vulgaris.

The three cardinal signs which include pitting, onycholysis with a red line, and Salmon patch are diagnostic of nail psoriasis only and they cannot be relied upon as diagnostic clues for diagnosing an unclassified dermatitis/eczema as psoriasis and these three cardinal signs are described to occur only in fingernails in literature, but I must say, they are extremely rare in this region, except pitting.

Other nail abnormalities, displayed by psoriatics, include splinter hemorrhages, SUHK, onychauxis, trachyonychia, and paronychia, which cannot be considered as of diagnostic importance for psoriasis, as they are commonly seen in other conditions also.

The prevalence of foot psoriasis appears to be very high among patient population. Patients with lichen planus frequently exhibit foot psoriasis. Similarly, patients with vitiligo also not uncommonly display psoriasis involving their feet. Patients with alopecia areata have psoriatic feet, albeit, rarely; these observations may prove the point (psoriasis being associated with these diseases mentioned above) that psoriasis too is autoimmune in origin. Remaining patients with other diseases also exhibit feet psoriasis not uncommonly. Such patients may not display psoriatic lesions elsewhere on the body.

Then, I indulge in thorough family history. Generally, I succeed in obtaining a positive family history of psoriasis; thus, it is noteworthy that psoriasis is fairly commonly confined to feet only. As it is usually asymptomatic (except in cases of presence of painful deep fissures), it is neglected by the patient and does not seek a dermatologist's intervention. *For the same reason and also because of ignorance on the part of the consulting dermatologist, asymptomatic foot psoriasis, thus, remains an undiagnosed condition.*

Of the various nail changes that I noted, though warrant a thorough search for presence of psoriasis elsewhere on the body or in the patient's pedigree, the following toenail abnormalities are not only highly diagnostic for nail psoriasis, they also come to the rescue of the consultant dermatologist to confirm the dermatitis in question as psoriasis, and these are as follows as per my experience:

- Angulation of nail plate's free margin in one or more than one toenail of either foot.
- Arch-like curvature of the free nail margin in one or more than one toenail of either foot.
- Onycholysis of either great toe or both great toes; onycholysis may involve any toenail, but not little toenail.
- Median split, i.e., superficial or full depth involving not uncommonly great toe; this kind of split may occur in any toenail, perhaps, extremely rarely little toenail.
- Pincer nail (the most common cause of pincer nail in this region is psoriasis).
- Asbestos sheet's shape of free margin of one or more than one toenail of either foot.
- Bilateral, linear whitish to yellowish streaks running along and close to LNFs of one or both great toenails.
- Lateral nail plate dystrophy associated with paronychia of LNFs (this is more commonly noted among fingernails than toenails).
- Koilonychia of three or more than three nail plates of either one foot or both feet put together. Phospholipids confer softness on the nail plate. KLN is due to increased softness. The center of the nail plate gets depressed due to trauma reflecting increased softness. The amount of phospholipids present in psoriatic nail needs to be investigated. Perhaps, the increased softness of psoriatic nail may also be responsible for asbestos sheet abnormality and this softness could also be held responsible for nail plate getting molded into different shapes.
- Vertical splitting of any toenail plate, but most often the little toenail plate of one foot or both feet; the nail plate splits into two parts: (1) The medial larger one, and (2) The lateral small piece which is usually melanotic.
- If two or more nail plates of one foot or both feet put together display diffuse melanonychia or band-like melanonychia of lateral half of nail plate or only little toenail of either foot.
- A given toenail plate may display more than one abnormality; e.g., angulation and melanonychia.
- Complete melanonychia or partial melanonychia involving lateral half of either little toenail alone is itself diagnostic of psoriasis vulgaris or dermatitis of either one or two major flexures or any other puzzling dermatitis, i.e., acute or chronic, anywhere on the body. The nail folds, i.e., PNF and LNFs are normally soft; but in foot psoriasis, either LNF or PNF or all the three nail folds become hyperkeratotic and hard in consistency. Because of increased transepidermal water loss due to contact with bathing soaps or detergents or washing powders or frequent use of hand cleansers, they shrink, become hard, and thus get separated from the nail plate. This is also a diagnostic clue not only for psoriasis vulgaris, but also for any puzzling dermatitis anywhere on the body that is to be interpreted as psoriasis.

I could obtain a history of clear-cut trauma from almost all the patients who displayed the above mentioned nail changes.

REFERENCES

1. de Berker D, Angus B. Markers of epidermal proliferation are limited to nail matrix in normal nail. Br J Dermatol. 1996;135:555-9.
2. Cohen PR. The lunula. J Am Acad Dermatol. 1996;34:943-53.3.
3. Tian H, Biehs B, Warming S, Leong KG, Rangell L, Klein OD, et al. A reserve stem cell population in small intestine renders Lgr5-positive cells dispensable. Nature. 2011;478:255-9.
4. Mogensen M, Thomsen JB, Skovgaard LT, Jemec GB. Nail thickness measurements using optical coherence tomography and 20-MHz ultrasonography. Br J Dermatol. 2007;157:894-900.

5. Achten G. L'ongle normal. J Med Esth Chir Dermatol. 1988;15:193-200.
6. de Berker D, Wojnarowska F, Sviland L, Westgate GE, Dawber RP, Leigh IM. Keratin expression in the normal nail unit: markers of regional differentiation. Br J Dermatol.2000;142:89-96.
7. Perrin C, Langbein L, Schweitzer J. Expression of hair keratins in the adult nail unit: an immuno-histochemical analysis of the onychogenesis in the proximal nail fold, matrix, and nail bed. Br J Dermatol. 2004;15:362-71.
8. Hashimoto K. Ultrastructure of the human toenail. 1. Proximal nail matrix. J Invest Dermatol. 1971;56:235-46.
9. Lewin K. The normal fingernail. Br J Dermatol.1965;77: 421-4.
10. Zaias N, Alvarez J. The formation of the primate nail plate. An autoradiographic study in squirrel monkey. J Invest Dermatol. 1968;51:120-36.
11. Norton LA. Incorporation of thymidine-methyl-H3 and glycine-2-H3 in the nail matrix and bed of humans. J Invest Dermatol. 1971;56:61-8.
12. de Berker D, Angus B. Proliferative compartments in the normal nail unit. Br J Dermatol. 1996;135:555-9.
13. Johnson M, Comaish JS, Shuster S. Nail is produced by the normal nail bed: a controversy resolved. Br J Dermatol. 1991;125:27-9.
14. Johnson M, Shuster S. Continuous formation of nail along the bed. Br J Dermatol.1993;128:277-80.
15. Fuchs E, Tumbar T, Guasch G. Socializing with the neighbors: stem cells and their niche. Cell. 2004;116:769-78.
16. Leung Y, Kandyba E, Chen YB, Ruffins S, Chuong CM, Kobielak K. Bifunctional ectodermal stem cells around the nail display dual fate homeostasis and adoptive wounding response toward nail regeneration. Proc Natl Acad Sci USA. 2014;111:15114-9.
17. Takeo M, Chou WC, Sun Q, Lee W, Rabbani P, Loomis C, et al. Wnt activation in nail epithelium couples nail growth to digit regeneration. Nature. 2013;499: 228-32.
18. Smith DO, Oura C, Kimura C, Toshimuri K. Arterial anatomy and tortuosity in the distal finger. J Hand Surg.1991;16A:297-302.
19. Ryan TJ. The arteriovenous anastamoses. In: Jarrett A (Ed). The Physiology and Pathophysiology of the Skin. London: Academic Press; 1973. pp. 612-14.
20. Dawber RPR, de Berker D, Baran R. Science of the nail apparatus. In: Baran R, Dawber RPR (Eds). Diseases of the Nails and Their Management, 4th edition.Oxford. Blackwell Science; 2010. pp. 1-34.
21. Zaias N. The movement of the nail bed. J Invest Dermatol. 1967;48:402-3.

3(I)

Color Atlas: Abnormalities Involving the Epidermis

EPIDERMAL ABNORMALITIES OF FEET

The crucial changes involving dorsum of the skin (that are of diagnostic importance to psoriasis) may be categorized into three groups based on a rough estimate of their frequency of occurrence. These changes in the skin over dorsae and soles of feet are characterized by hyperkeratosis (HK) and fissures of variable depths that include palmar creases like cracks and variable deeper versions.

- *Most common*:
  - Heel border fissures
  - Feet border fissures
  - Fissures of soles
  - Hyperkeratosis and cracks of toe pulps/toe pad fissures
- *Not uncommon*:
  - Web spaces
  - Under toes
  - Lateral aspects of great toes (GTs)
  - Dorsum of GT
  - Malleoli
- *Rare*:
  - Skin over Achilles tendon

HEEL FISSURES

I wonder rather get shocked by looking at these changes along heel borders and soles. Why should epidermis give in this way to trauma/external threats? After all, millions of years ago, the human body was built. Since then, skin must have faced many epidermal disruptive problems/fatal hazards from environment. Long ago, it must have mastered the art of maintaining its structural integrity and thus, it's most important function of skin barrier activity. After all, the formation of epidermal barrier is one of the most crucial functions of keratinocyte that it owes to the human organism. Nevertheless, four patterns of heel border fissuring have been noted: (1) Linear fissuring, (2) Plaque with fissures pattern, (3) Tortoise-shell pattern fissuring, (4) Crisscross pattern of fissuring, and (5) Blaschko'slines pattern.

150 South Indian's Foot: A Storehouse of Diagnostic Clues for Psoriasis

A to D: These photographs depict linear fissuring.
C: A psoriatic plaque denoted by yellowish circle over (right) Achilles tendon.
E and F: Depict linear subtle fissuring.

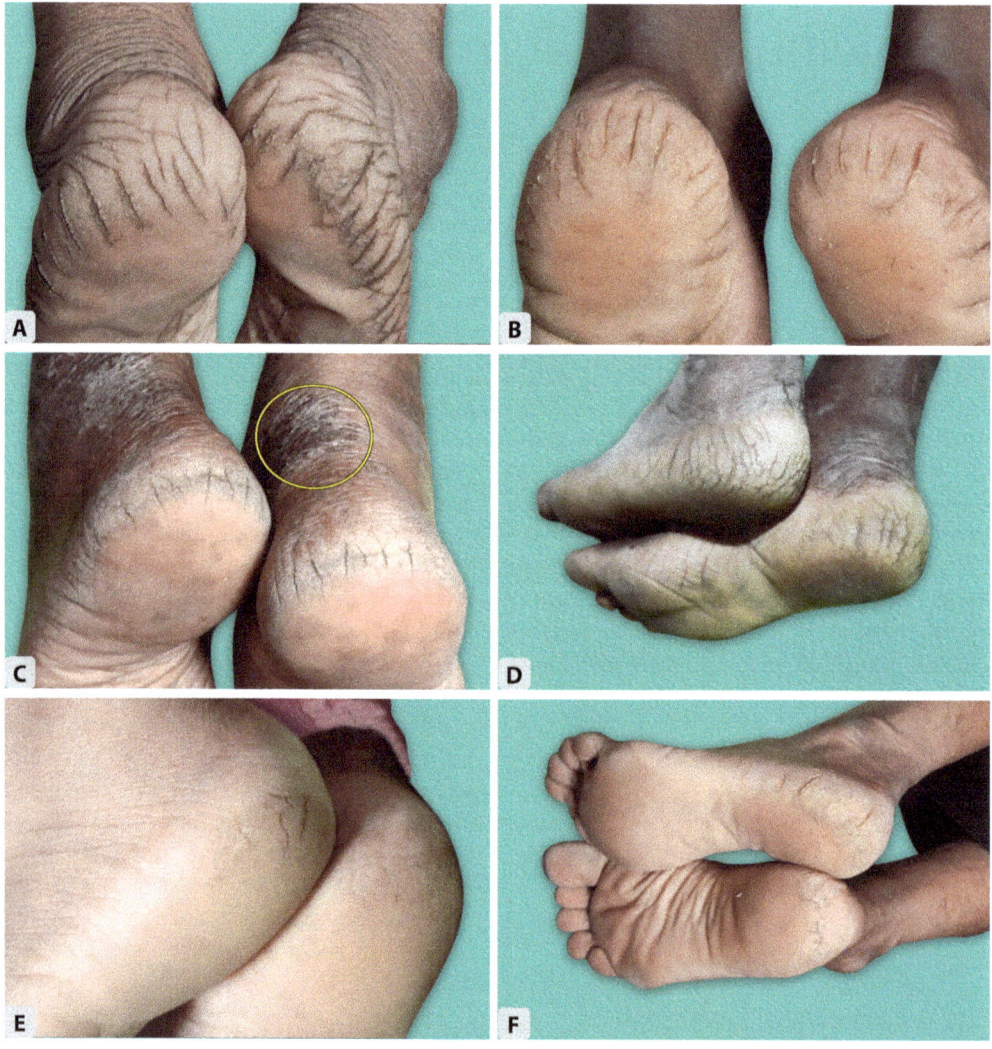

Tortoise-shell Pattern

A to F: Depict tortoise-shell pattern fissuring. "D" and "E" display hypertrophic psoriasis with deep tortoise-shell pattern fissuring.

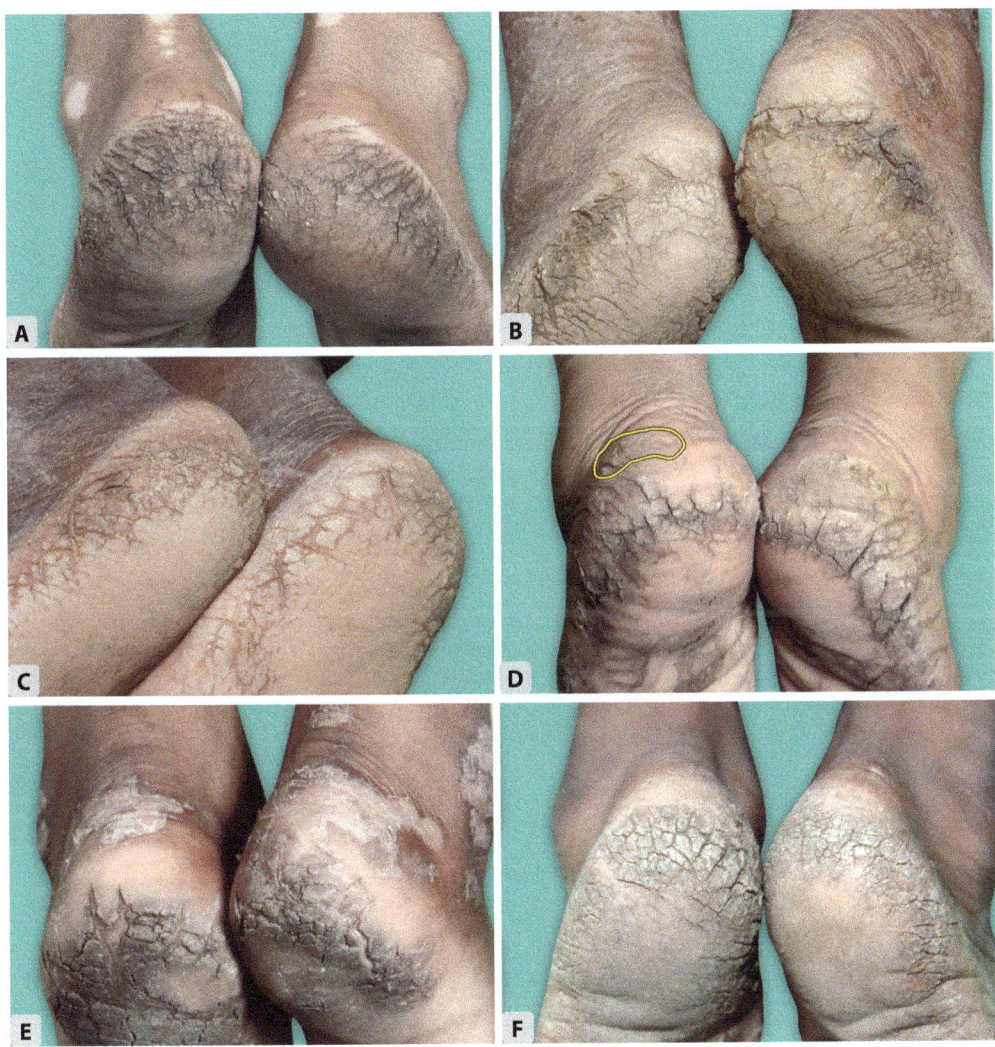

G: Also depicts tortoise-shell pattern.
H: Also depicts tortoise-shell pattern in a very subtle fashion.

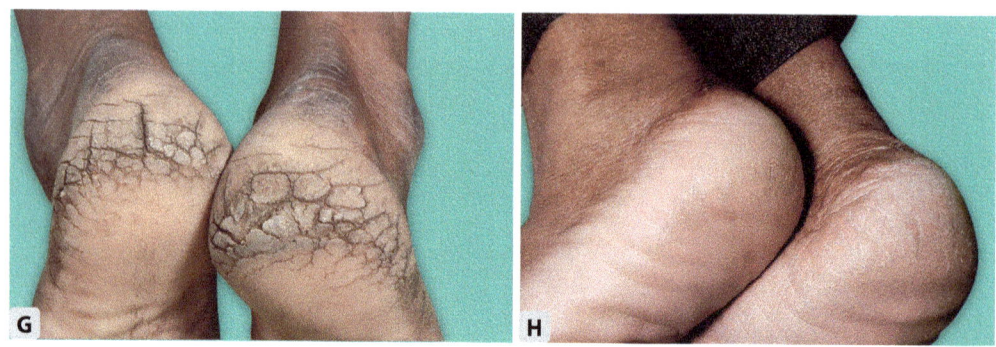

Plaque with Fissures Pattern
A to C: Depict typical psoriatic plaque formation along the heel borders with fissures.

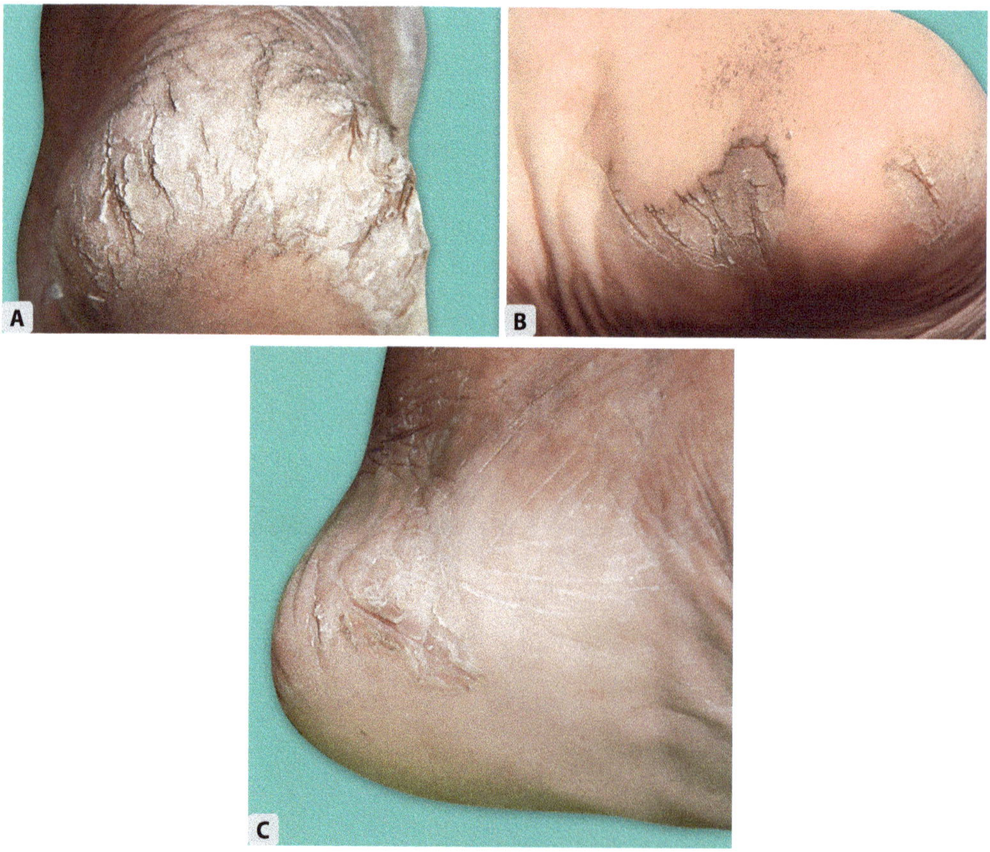

FOOT BORDERS

A and B: Depict linear fissures.

C: Heel borders display distorted psoriatic plaques. Rest of the borders display a little bizarre fissuring.

D: Inflammatory plaques extending along the borders of feet.

E: Creases mimicking palmar creases may be noted.

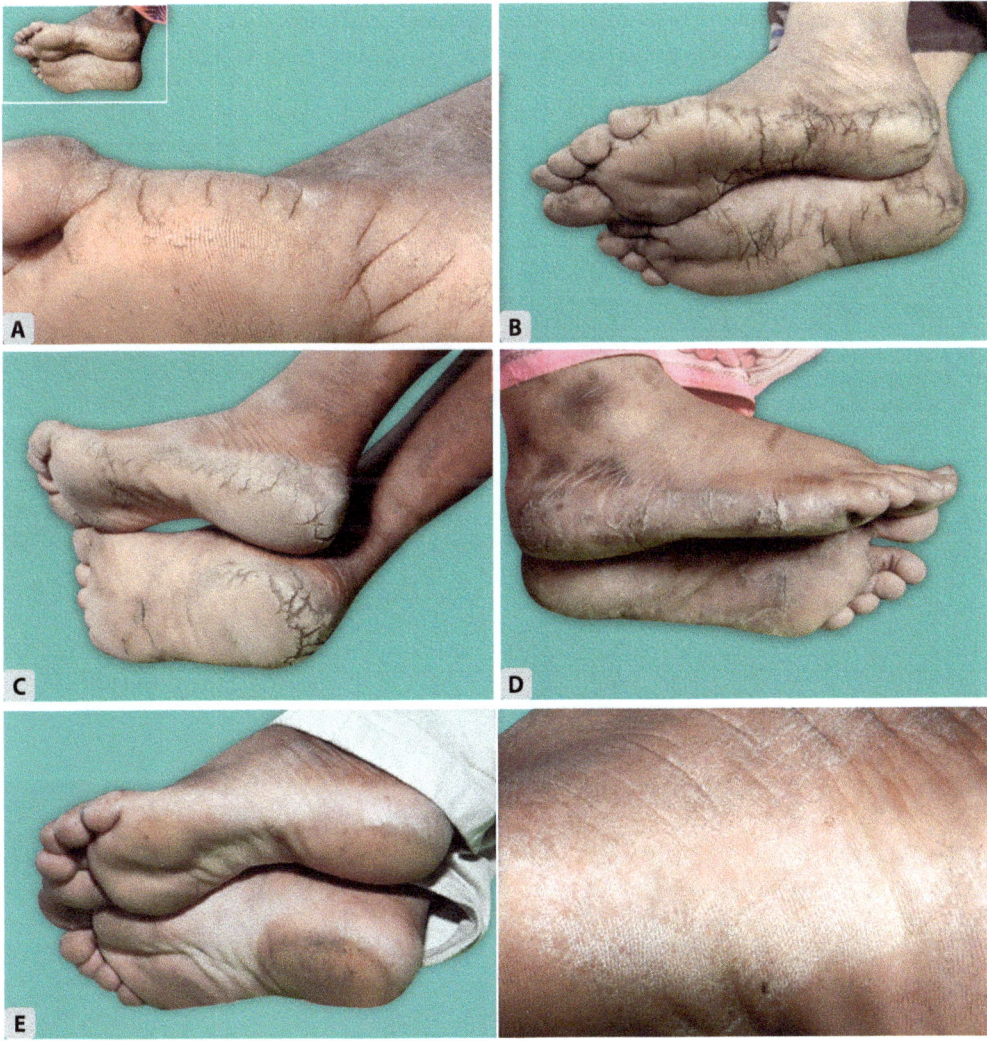

ONLY SOLES

Psoriatic fissures, along borders of feet or on soles, on toe pulps, toe pads, and under toes, may form with or without plaque formation. My assumption for formation of fissures without plaques is that there exists subclinical psoriasis in predisposed individuals; consequently, trauma to feet precipitates fissures without plaque formation.

A: Depicts ill-formed plaques with fissuring.

B: Depicts superficial fissures in a crisscross pattern.

C and D: Depict similar pattern of fissuring as in B, but fissures are a bit deeper.

E: Depicts crisscross pattern of fissuring involving insteps and under toes.

F: Depicts subtle fissuring in instep which displays psoriatic plaque in evolution; blebs may be noted indicated by arrows.

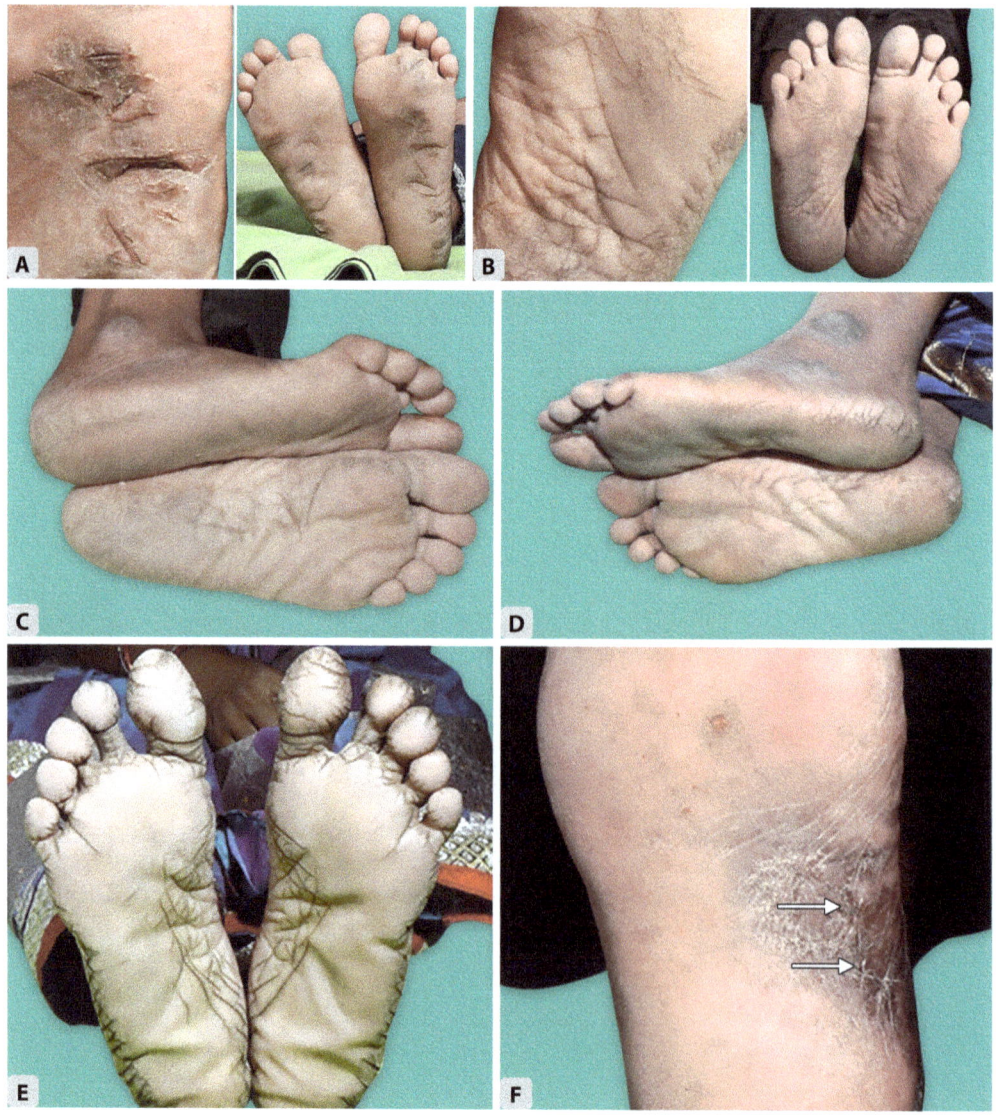

G: Depicts crisscross pattern of superficial fissuring in the insteps.
H: Depicts hypertrophic plaques with fissures.
I: Balls of both feet display linear fissures.
J: Crisscross pattern of fissuring predominantly involving insteps. Plaque formation on heel border may be noted.
K: Linear fissuring involving predominantly insteps and to some extent balls of feet.
L: Crisscross pattern of fissuring; ill-formed plaques may be noted along borders (yellow circle).

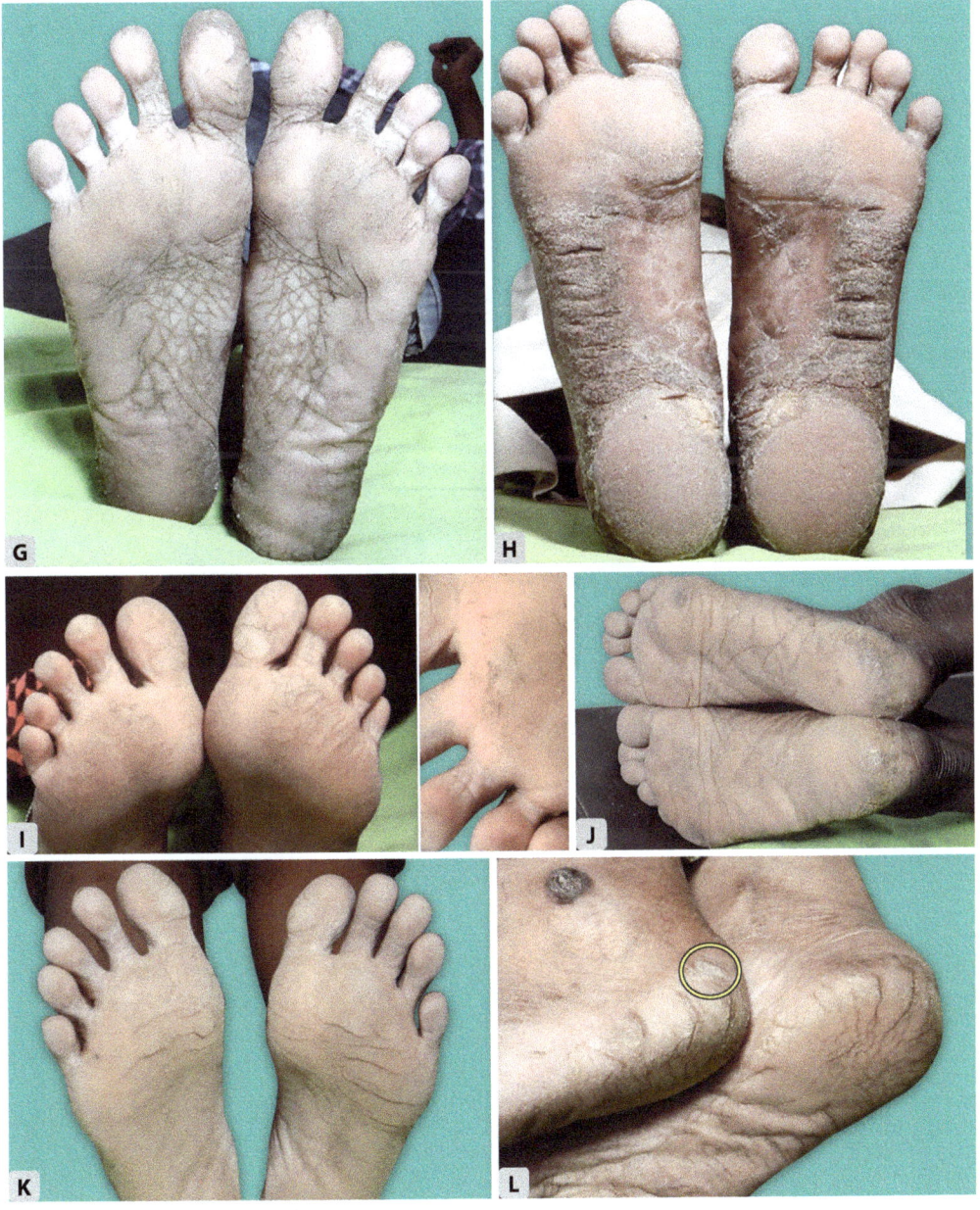

M: Crisscross pattern of fissuring.
N: Similar pattern of fissuring as in M. Lesions in yellow circles represent psoriatic plaques.
O: Blaschko's lines pattern of fissuring.

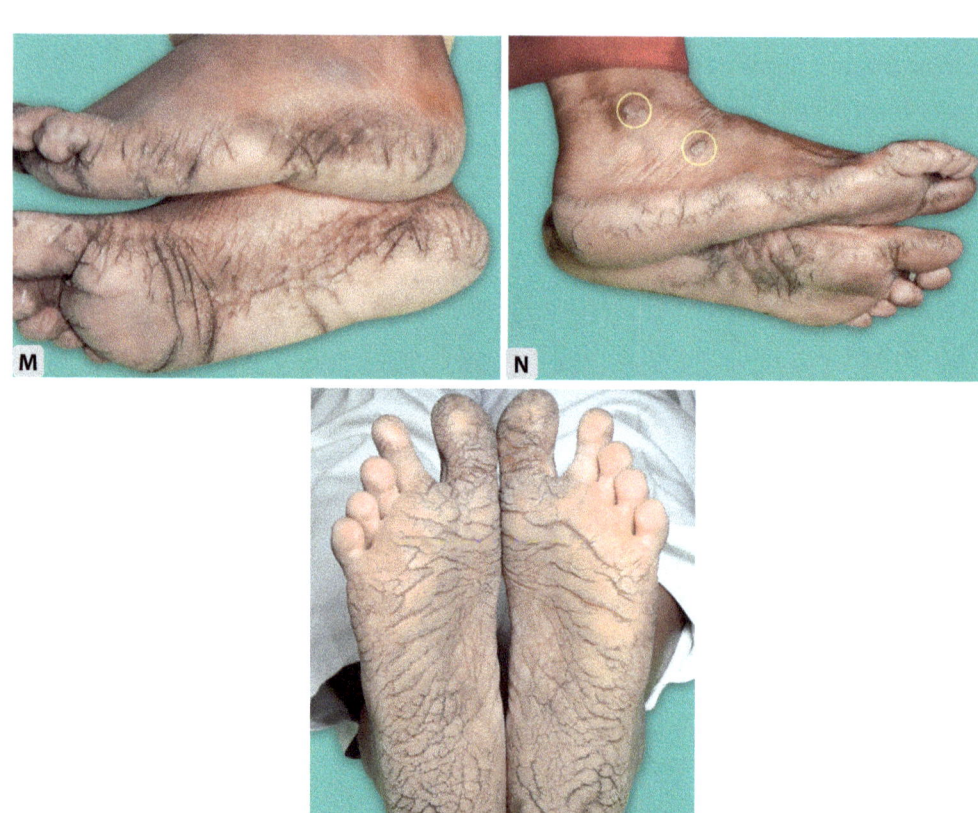

Color Atlas: Abnormalities Involving the Epidermis 157

TOE PULPS/PADS

A and B: Mild HK and scaling may be noted on toe pulps and toe pads.
C and D: Tortoiseshell pattern; fissuring and HK may be noted.
E: Remarkable HK and deep fissures may be noted.
F: Hypertrophic version of psoriatic expression involving both GT pads.

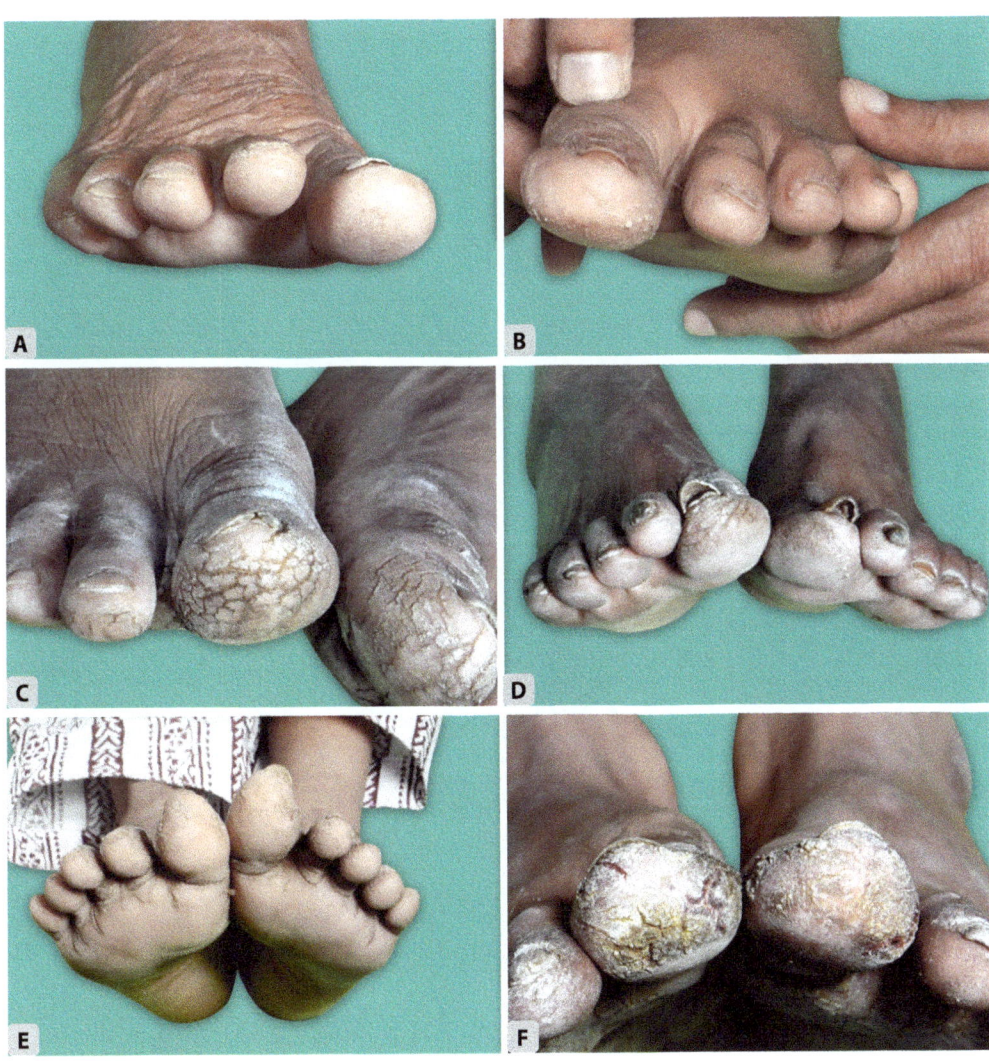

G and H: Display plaque formation over toe pulps and toe pads.

I: Plaque formation on all the toe pads of (right) foot and involvement of ball of the foot may also be noted.

J: Toe pads of both feet display HK and scaling.

K: (Right) GT displays an exfoliating scaly pad.

L: Toe pads display tortoiseshell pattern of cracking.

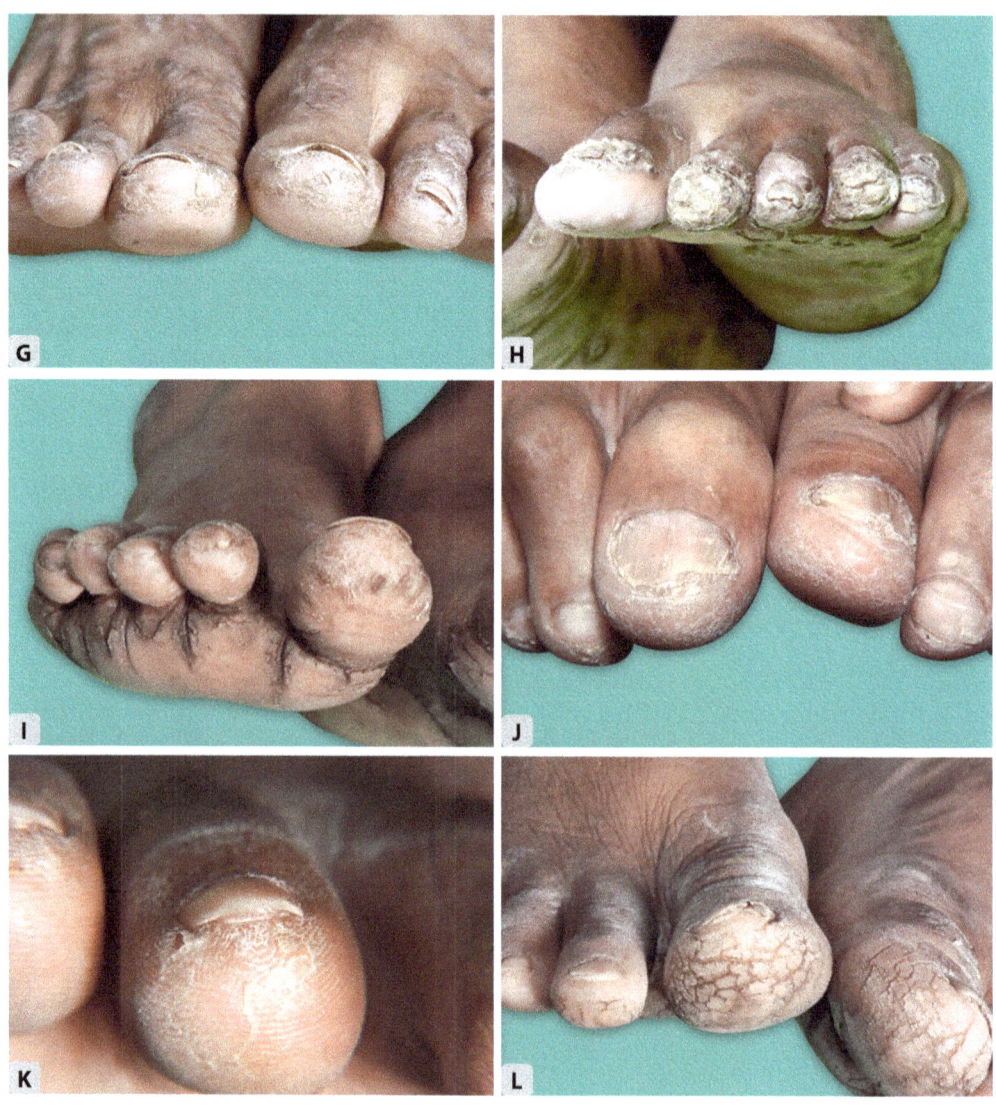

WEB SPACES

A: Hyperkeratosis and typical silvery white surface (after stroking).
B: Similar changes may be noted as in "A".
C: Marked HK; base of the adjacent toe displays typical psoriatic plaque.
D: On stroking, profuse silvery white scale demonstrated.
E: Remarkable HK with multiple superficial cracks; involvement of under toes may also be noted.
F: This web space displays a classic well-circumscribed plaque against the backdrop of diffuse HK.

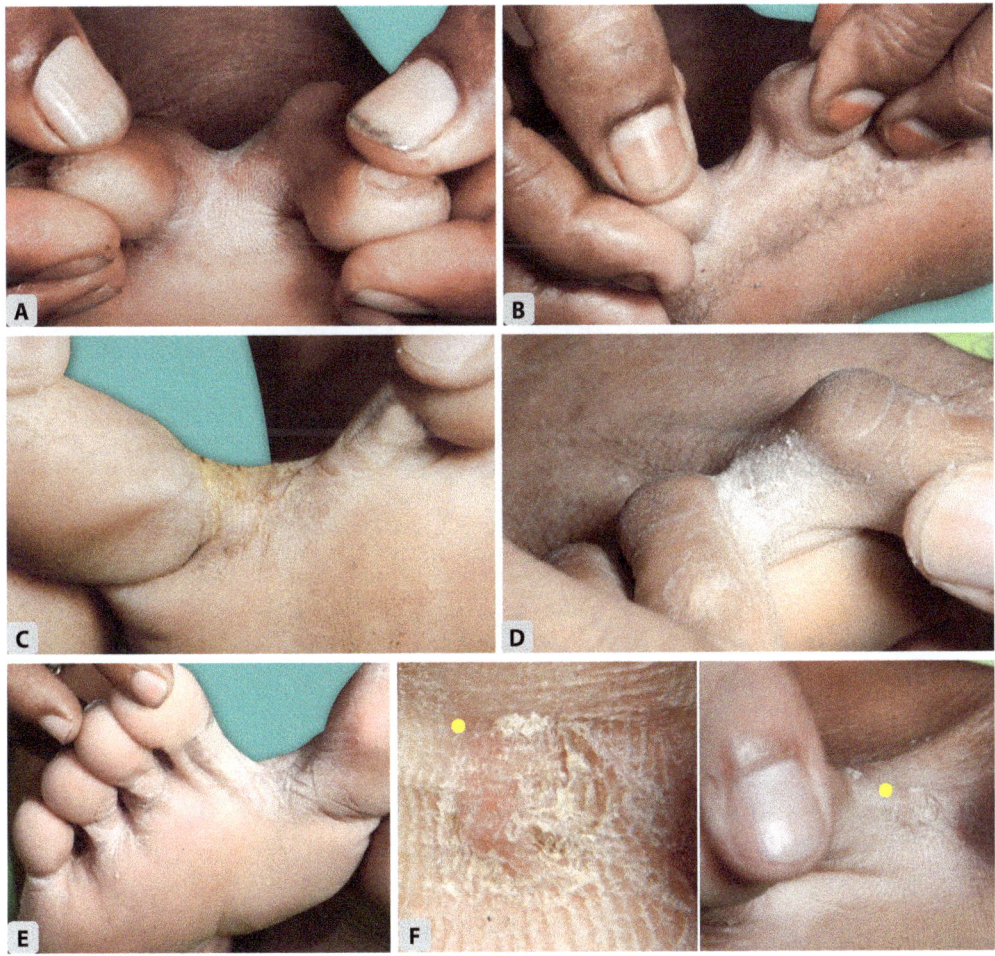

G: Maceration setting in.
H: Macerated HK lesion.
I: Maceration appears to be complete.
J: Candidiasis is setting in; suggested by the fringed out edge.

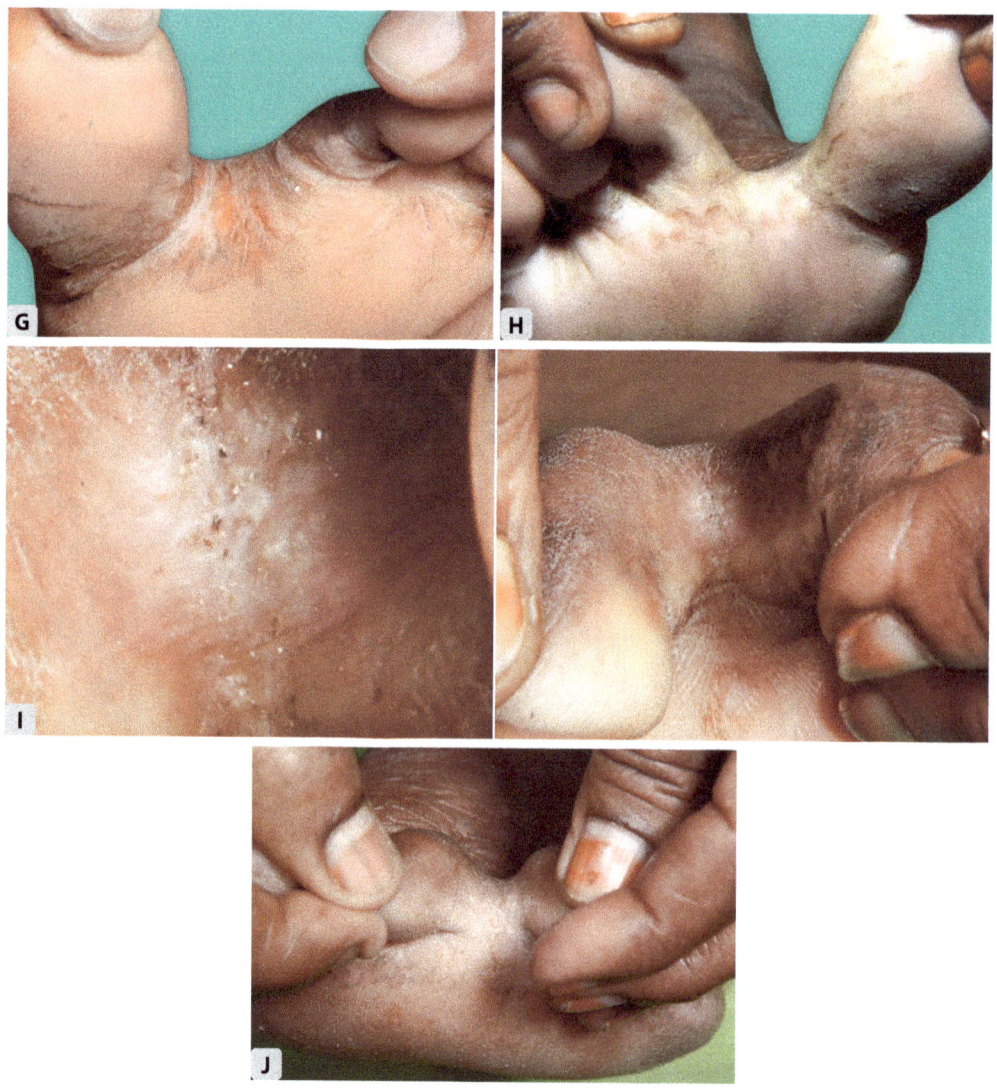

Color Atlas: Abnormalities Involving the Epidermis   161

K: Candidiasis is established against the back drop of moist, shiny, and macerated skin: Suggested by the fringed out edge lining the periphery.

L: Extensive candidal intertrigo.

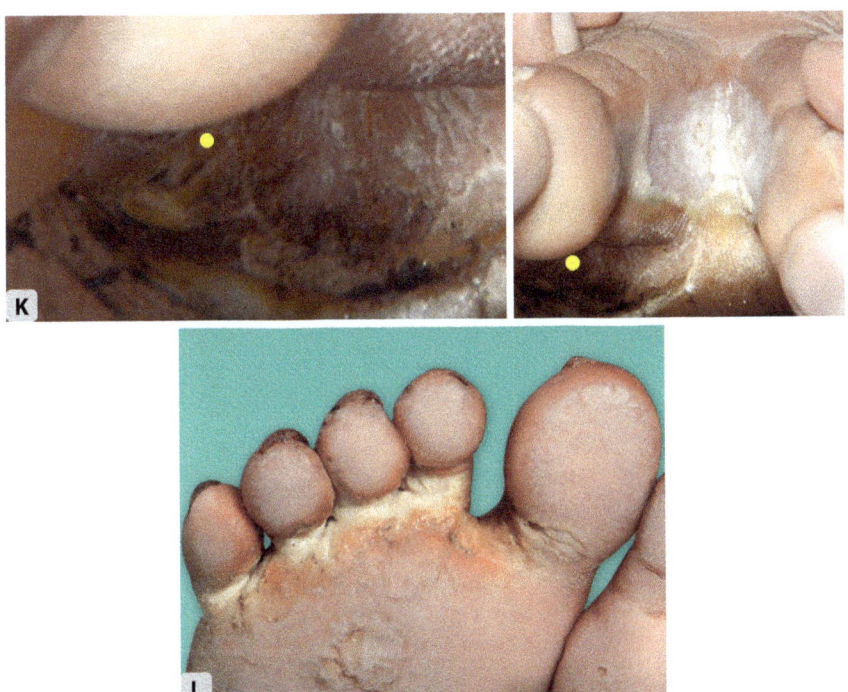

DORSUM OF GREAT TOE

A: Dorsae of GTs and other toes displaying mild/early changes of lichenification.

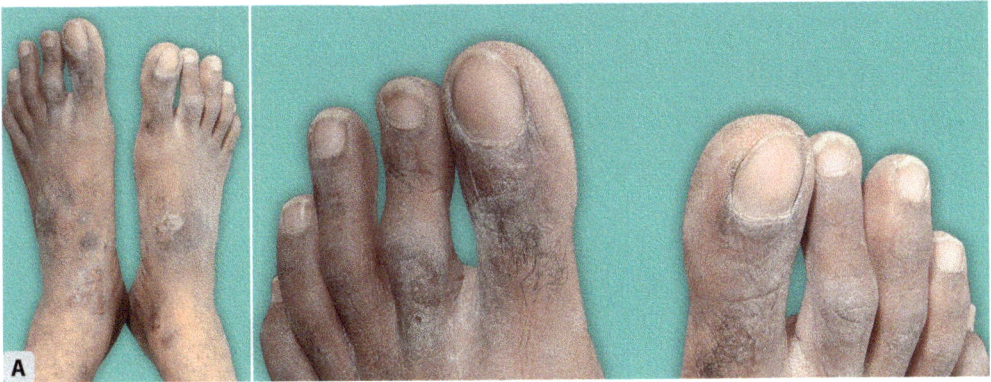

South Indian's Foot: A Storehouse of Diagnostic Clues for Psoriasis

B: Dark plaques on dorsae of GTs; a typical psoriatic plaque may be noted just above the outer border of left foot (yellow arrow).

C: Typical lichenified plaques on dorsae of GTs and some other toes.

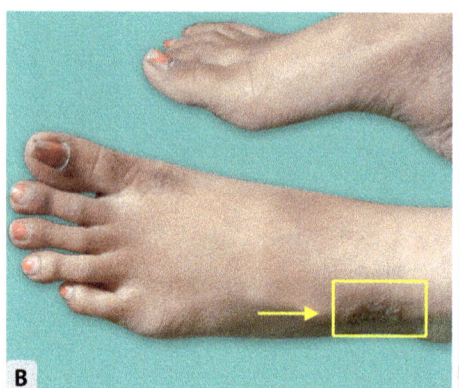
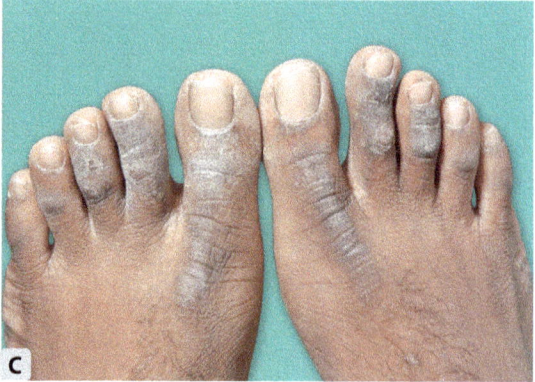

MALLEOLI

A: Dark HK fissured plaque on the dorsum of (left) lateral malleolus and a typical psoriatic plaque may be noted below the malleolus.

B: Dark HK, scaly plaque.

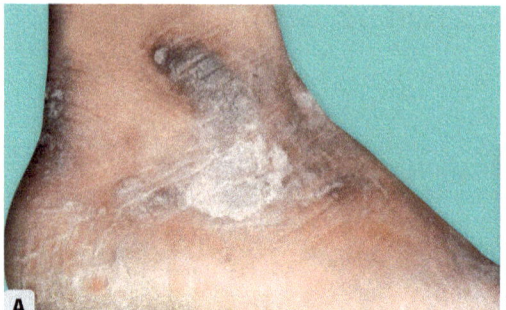
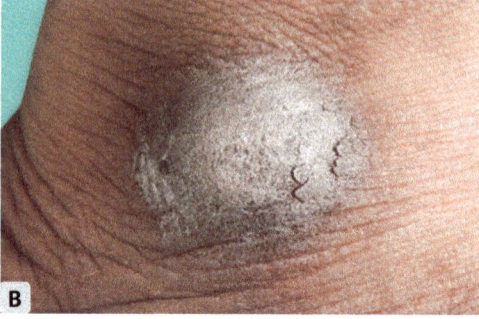

C: (Left) lateral malleolus displays a clinically noninflammatory (nonscaly) acanthotic (psoriatic) plaque.
D: Psoriatic changes may be noted on (left) lateral malleolus. A typical psoriatic plaque just above the outer border of left foot may be noted.
E: (Left) lateral malleolus displays a dark nonscaly HK plaque.
F: Psoriatic changes are evident.
G: Typical psoriatic plaque; in the ankle flexure of (L) foot.
H: (Left) lateral malleolus displays similar changes as in "G". Heel border HK with fissures may be noted.

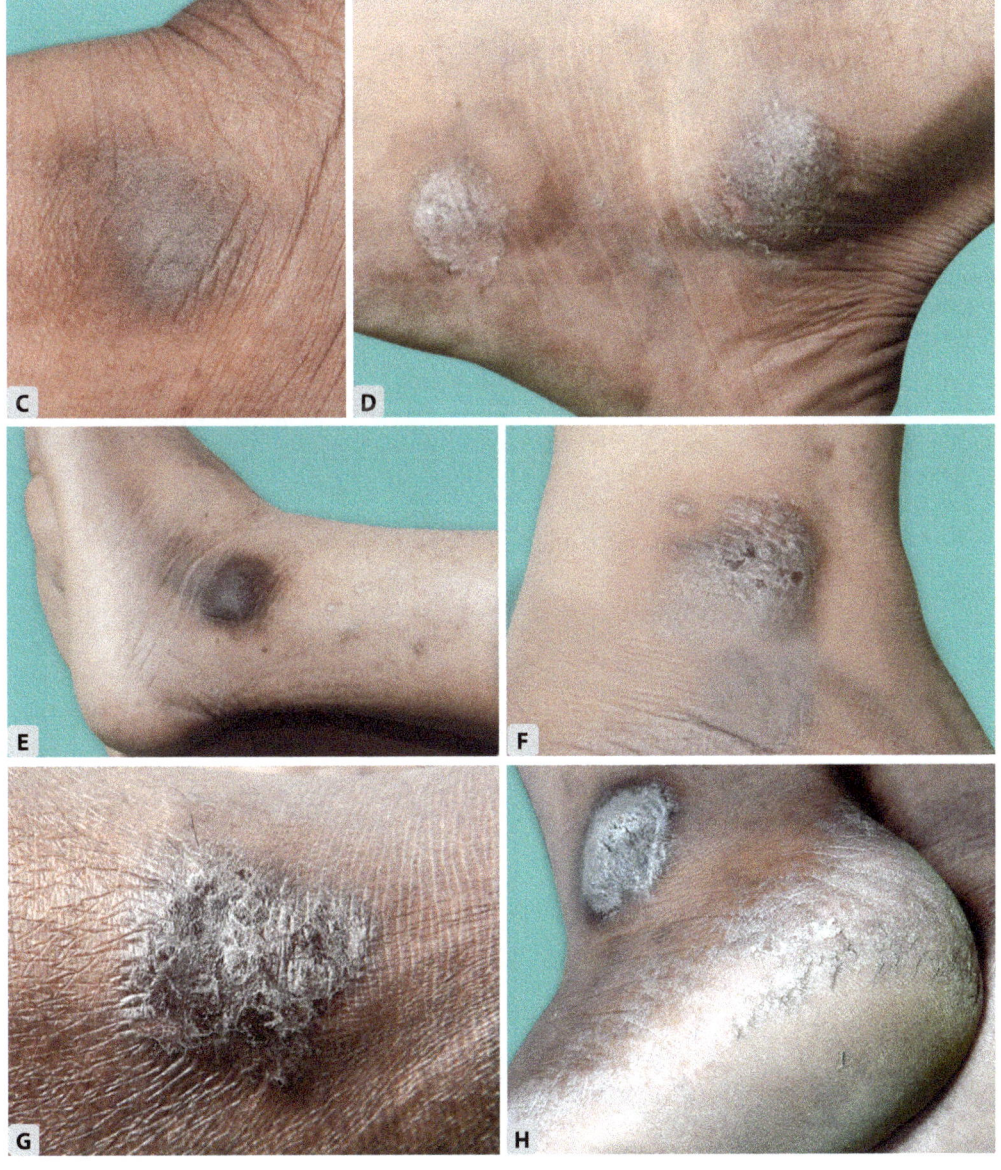

3(II)

Color Atlas: Nail Abnormalities

INTRODUCTION

The toenail abnormalities that I have noticed over the last 15 years may be categorized into the following groups based on a rough estimate of their frequency of occurrence:
- Most common
- Fairly common
- Common
- Not uncommon
- Rare
- Fairly rare
- *Most common*:
  - Angulation
  - Overcurvature
- *Fairly common*:
  - Koilonychia (KLN)
  - Melanonychia (MLN)
- *Common*:
  - Onycholysis (ONL)
  - Asbestos sheet-shaped nail
  - Dome-shaped elevation (DSE)
  - Pincer nail
- *Not uncommon*:
  - Median split of nail plate
  - More than one abnormality
  - Lateral nail dystrophy (LND)
  - Yellowish to whitish streaks
  - Tent-like elevation (TLE)
  - Psoriatic paronychia
- *Rare*:
  - Cave-like curvature (CLC)
  - Nail plate—pulp kiss sign
  - Little toenail split (LTN split)
- *Fairly rare*:
  - Unfolding carpet roll-like curvature
  - Short little toenail (SLTN)

Color Atlas: Nail Abnormalities 165

ANGULATION

A: Second and third toenails (TNs) of left foot display angulation, i.e., yellow dots.
B: Left great toenail (GTN)—typical angulation may be noted.
C: Left middle TN—angulation.
D: Left GTN displays angulation.

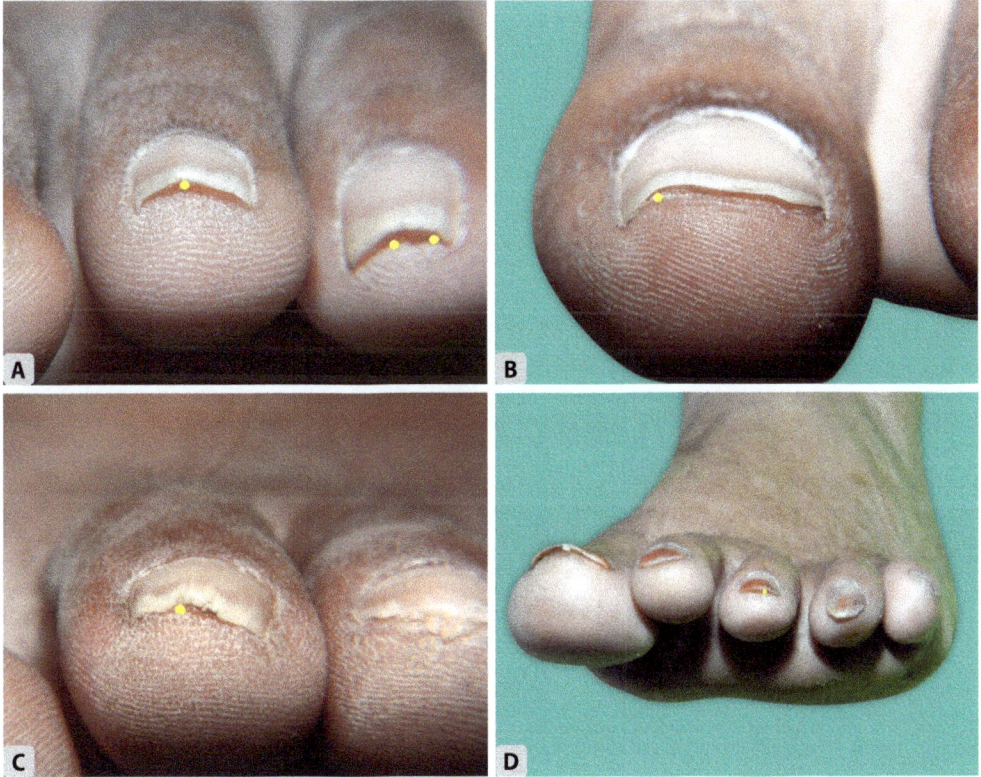

ARCH-LIKE CURVATURE

A: Left GTN displays typical arch-like curvature.
B: (R) GTN arch-like curvature.
C: (R) third and fourth TNs display two-in-one abnormality (i.e., both angulation and increased curvature).
D: (Right) second TN displays fractured arch-like curvature.

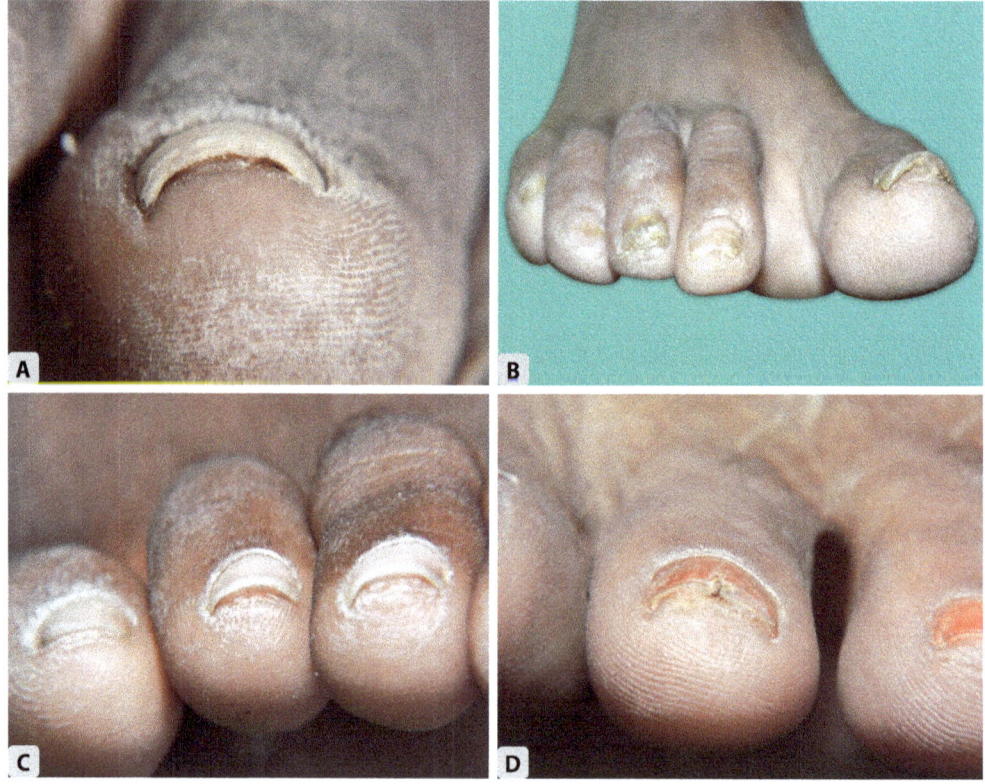

Color Atlas: Nail Abnormalities   167

KOILONYCHIA

A: (Right) third TN—typical KLN: The pulp of this TN displays a scaly, hyperkeratotic plaque; (right) fourth TN displays a distorted asbestos sheet nail due to superimposed KLN.

B: (Left) GTN and (left) second TN display KLN. So, also (right) second TN.

C: Both GTNs display KLN; toe pulps and lateral aspects of both GTNs display hyperkeratosis (HK) and scaling.

D: Almost all the TNs of (right) foot display varied degrees of KLN.

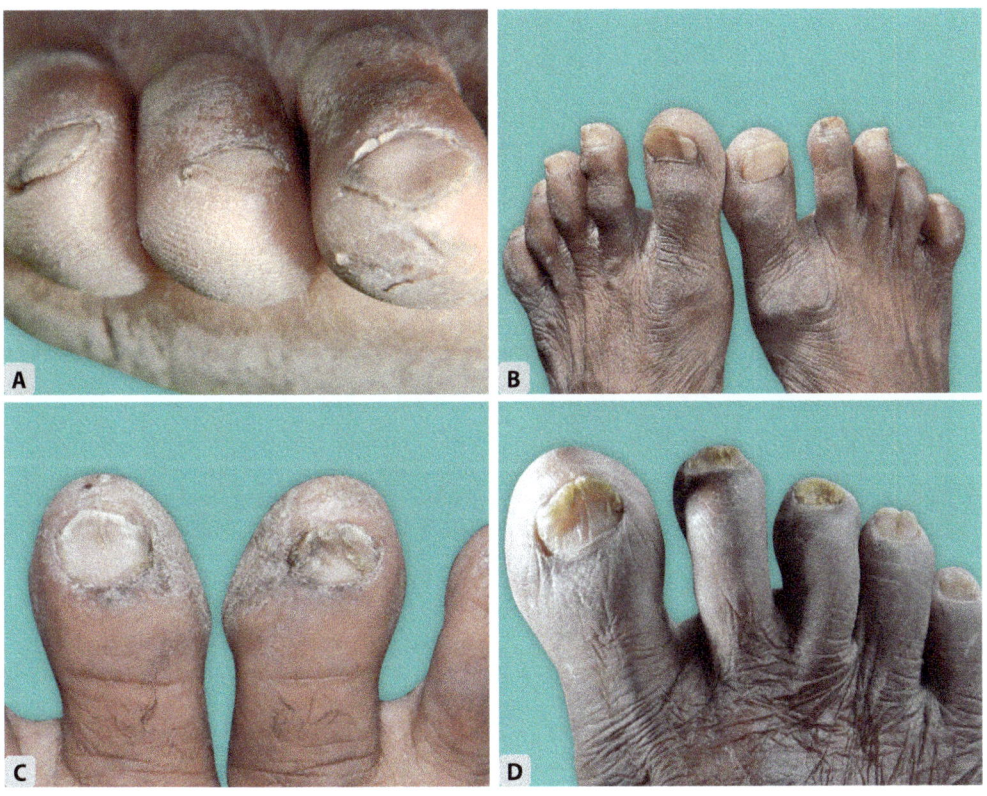

MELANONYCHIA

A: (Left) LTN displays band-like MLN involving the outer aspect of nail plate.

B: Diffuse MLN of left LTN; outer periphery of nail unit displays psoriatic scaling.

C: (Left) LTN displays diffuse MLN. Outer lateral nail fold (LNF) is scaly and hyperkeratotic and moves away from the nail plate (i.e., chronic psoriatic paronychia).

D: Except (right) GT, all the other TNs display diffuse MLN. Lichenified plaque may be noted on the dorsum of (right) GTN.

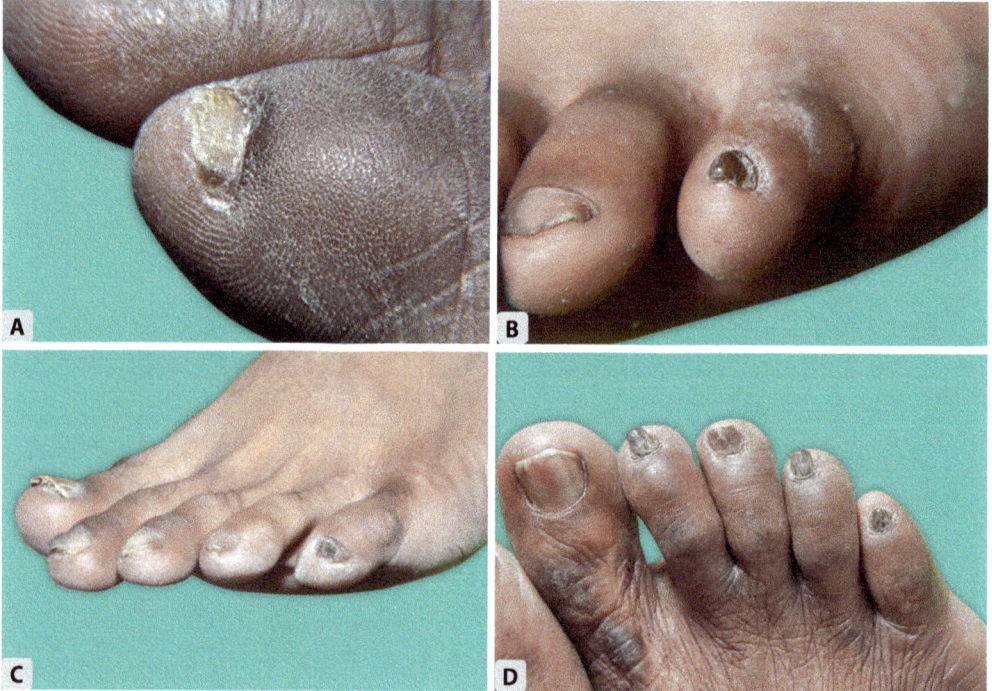

E: (Right) second TN displaying band-like MLN involving the medial nail plate: Psoriatic lesions may be noted on the toepulps, toepads, and elsewhere.
F: Second, third, fourth, and fifth TNs of left foot display band-like MLN. ONL of left GTN may be noted.
G: Band-like MLN of (R) LTN: A scaly patch close to proximal nail fold (PNF) may be noted.
H: Diffuse MLN of (left) LTN. The nail plate splitting into two unequal halves may also be noted.

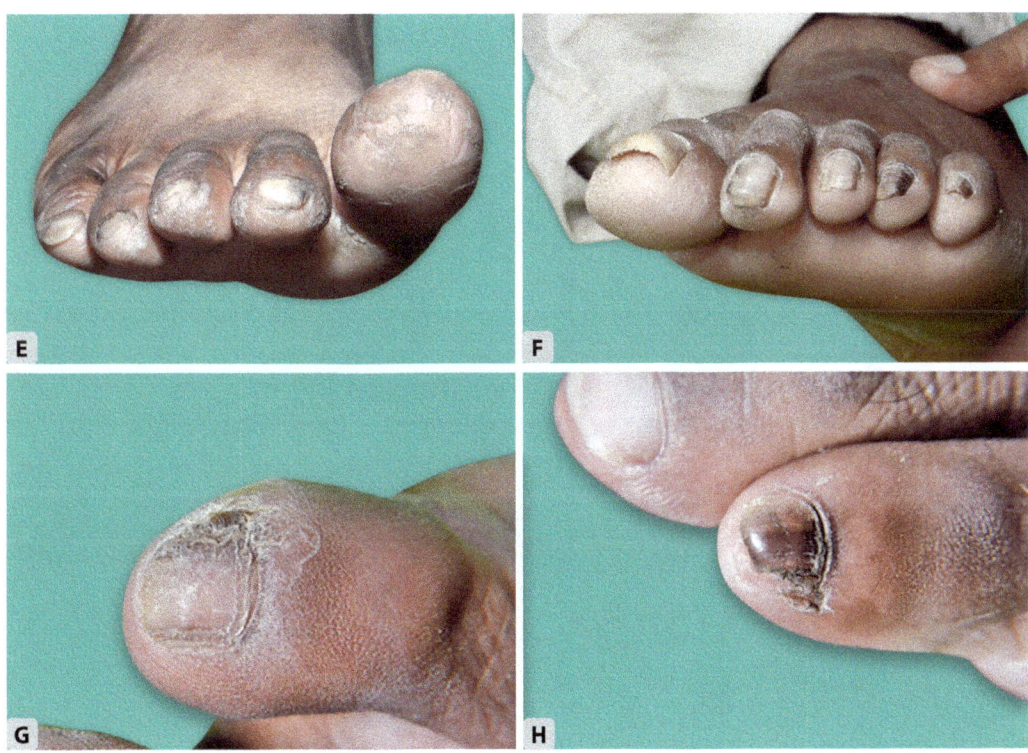

South Indian's Foot: A Storehouse of Diagnostic Clues for Psoriasis

ONYCHOLYSIS

A: (Right) GTN displays ONL; a well-defined scaly plaque may be noted on the dorsum of adjacent TN (yellow box).
B: (Left) GTN and (left) second TN display streaky ONL.
C: First three TNs of left foot display ONL of varied sizes.
D and E: Display ONL.

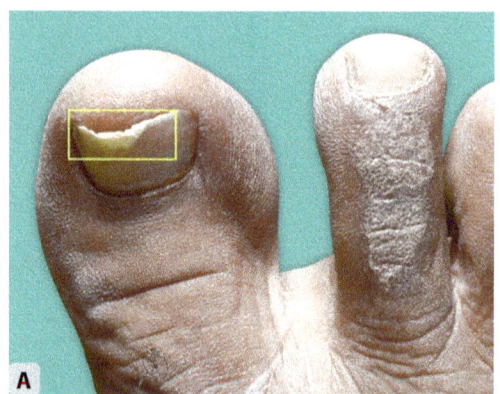
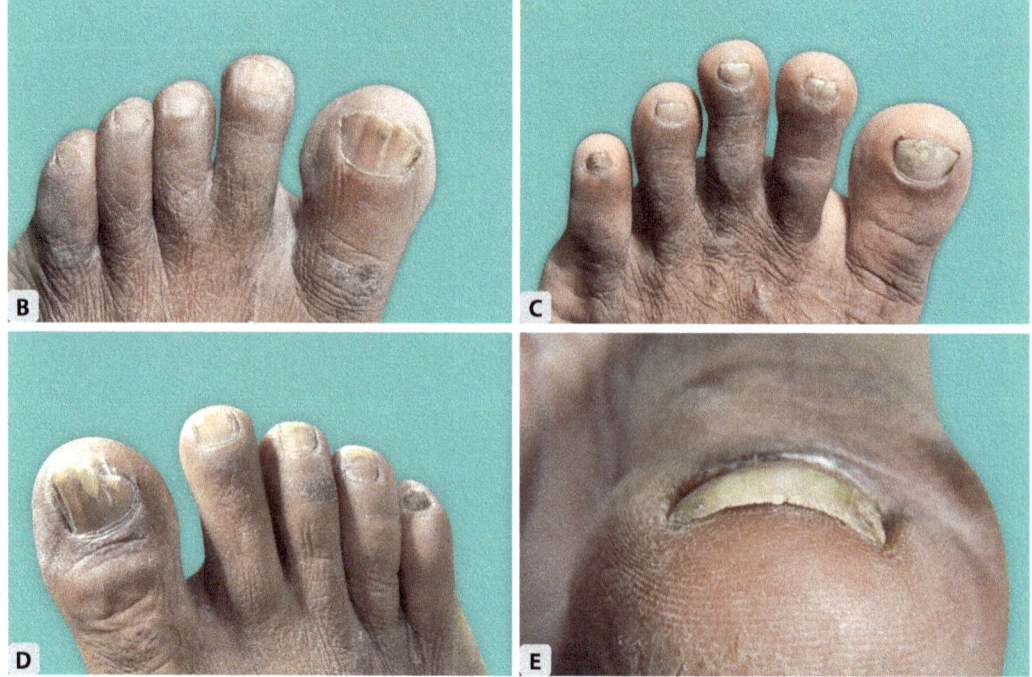

Color Atlas: Nail Abnormalities 171

F: Displays chipped off ONL portions of the both GTNs.
G: (Right) GTN displays similar feature. LNFs display psoriatic scaling.

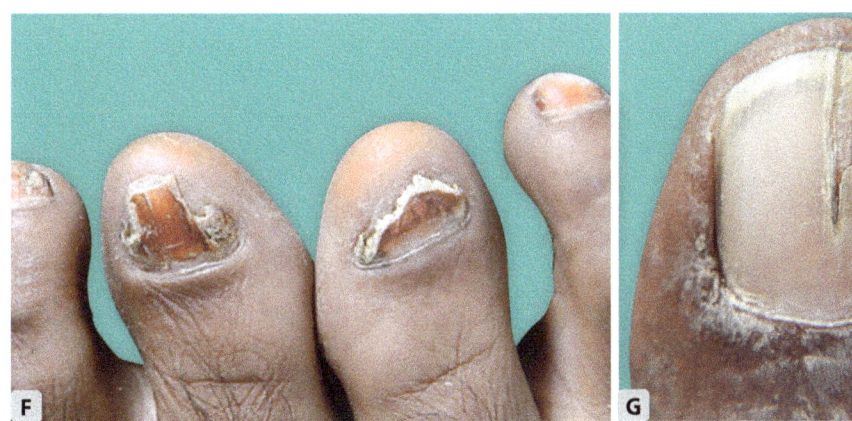

ASBESTOS-SHAPED NAIL

A: Displays a typical asbestos-shaped nail margin; (L) second TN.
B: (L) Second TN—similar feature.
C: Similar feature but very subtle.
D: Distorted asbestos sheet nail margin may be noted; second 4th TN.

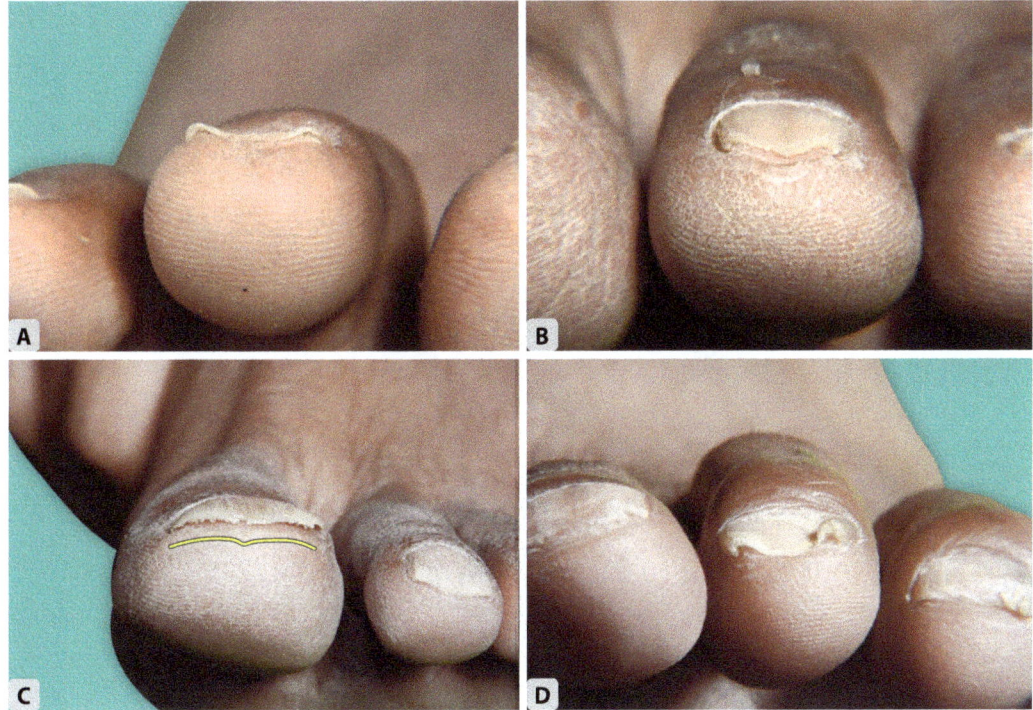

E: Right second TN displays distorted asbestos sheet margin. Toe pulps display HK and cracks.
F: Left second TN displays similar feature as in "E".
G: (Right) second, third, and fourth TNs display a bit distorted asbestos sheet abnormality, perhaps, due to superimposed KLN.

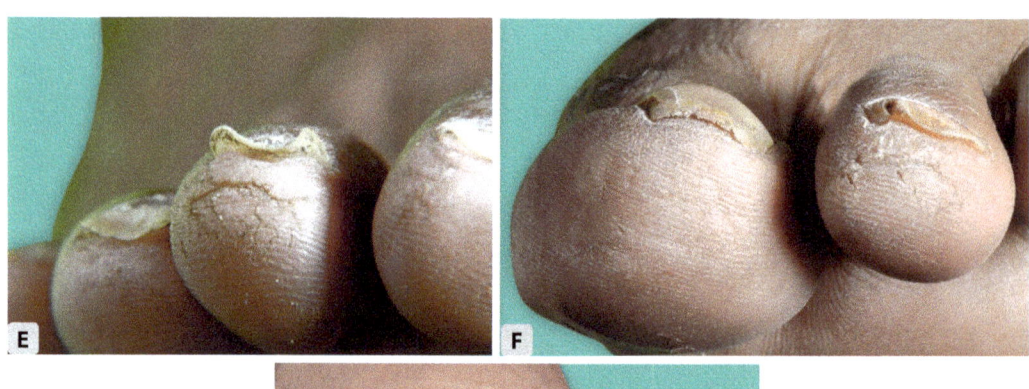

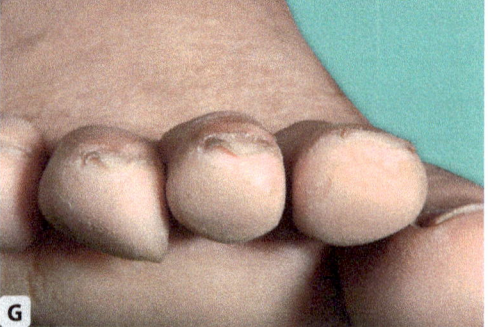

DOME-SHAPED ELEVATION WITH SUBUNGUAL HYPERKERATOSIS

A: (Right) GTN displays a typical dome-shaped elevation (DSE) with subungual hyperkeratosis (SUHK); pulp and pad are HK and scaly.

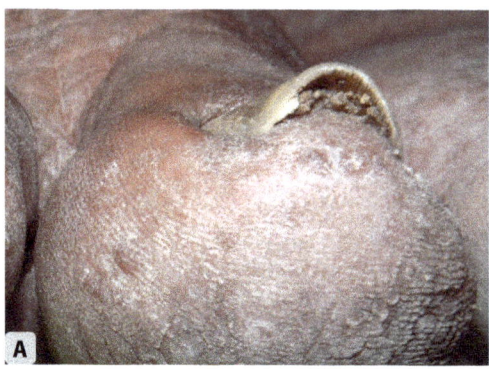

Color Atlas: Nail Abnormalities 173

B: (Right) GTN displays a slightly deformed DSE.
C: Slightly deformed DSE with onychauxis and SUHK [(right) GTN].

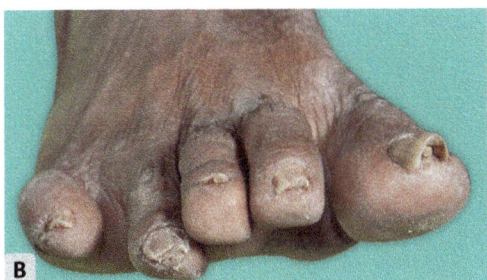
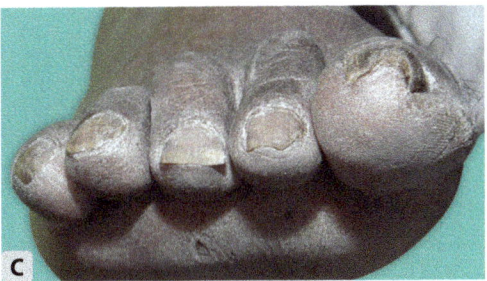

PINCER NAIL

A: Great toenail, third TN, and fourth TN of (left) foot display typical pincer nails; the remaining toes display dome-like elevation.
B: (Left) GTN—apincer nail with SUHK. Adjacent toe is diffusely melanotic and deformed. Pulp of (left) GT displays HK with superficial cracks.

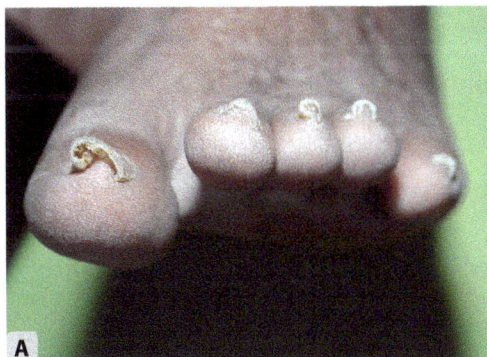
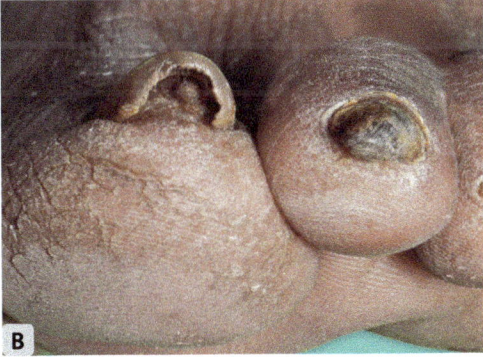

C: (Left) GTN—a typical pincer nail; toe pulps and sides of toe pads are HK and cracked.

D: Fourth and fifth TNs of (left) foot display pincer nails; ball of the (left) foot close to the base of (left) LTN displays a scaly lesion.

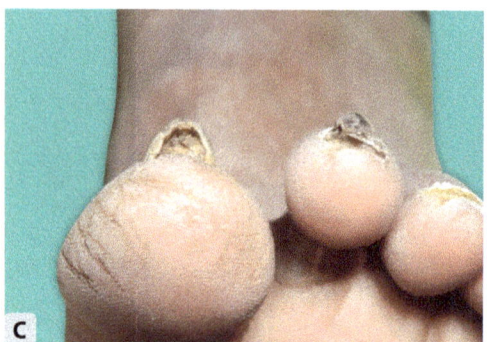
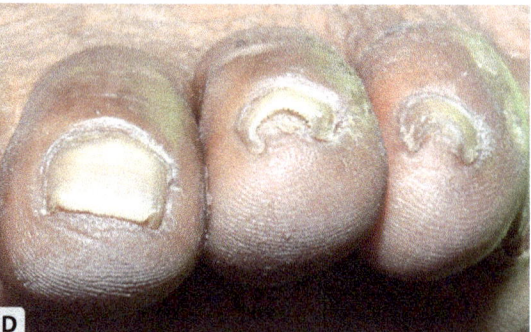

MEDIAN NAIL SPLIT

A: Partial thickness split of (left) GTN.

B: Full-thickness split of (right) GTN.

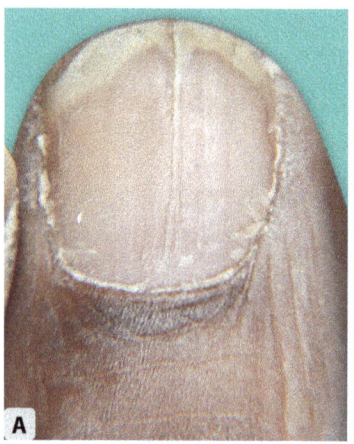
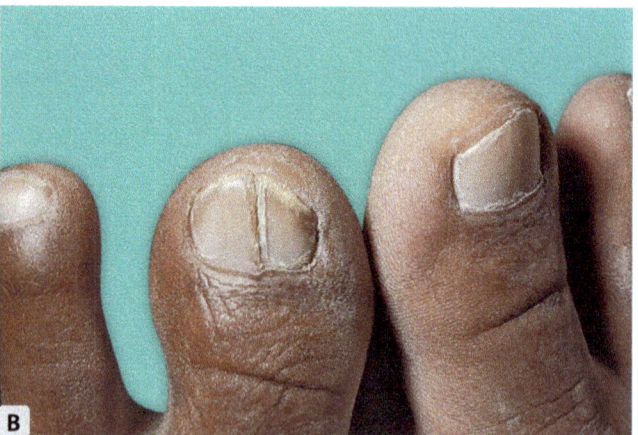

C: Similar split—(right) GTN.
D: Median split in the onycholytic area of (left) second TN.

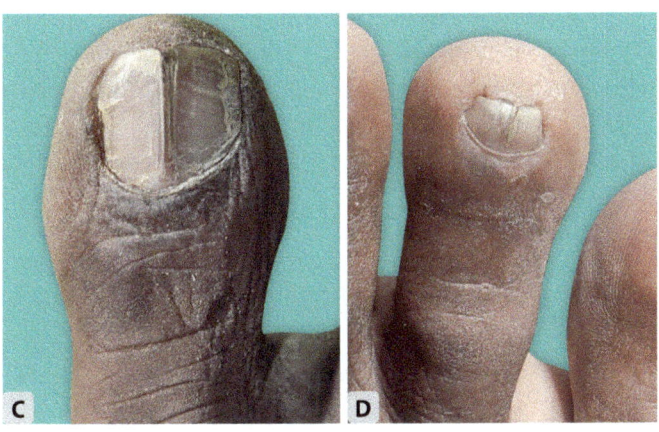

LATERAL NAIL FOLD HYPERKERATOSIS AND LATERAL NAIL DYSTROPHY

A: Chronic paronychia of both LNFs and PNFs of both GT with LND.

B: Lateral nail fold of both GTs is chronically inflamed. LNF becomes hyperkeratotic and gets everted, thus moves away from the lateral margin of nail plate. Eventually, LN dystrophy sets in.

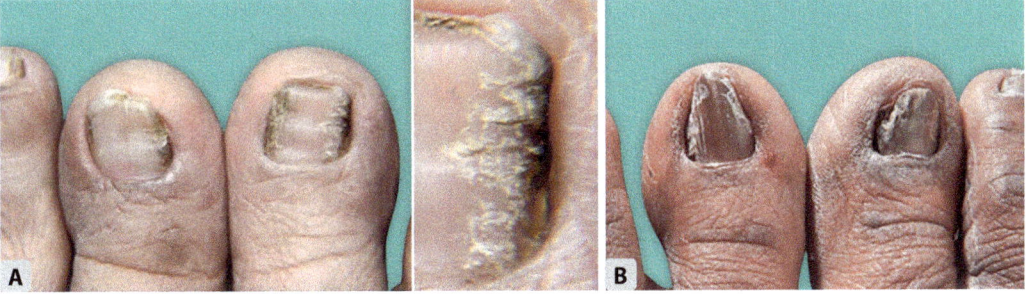

C: (Left) GTN—both LNFs chronically inflamed (a pathognomonic feature of psoriatic paronychia). (Right) LNF HK and moves away from nail margin. LND setting on both sides; normal PNF may be noted. *LNFs are medially connected to nail bed. Chronic inflammation of LNF and resultant eversion of LNFs might trigger lateral nail dystrophy (LND).*

D: Both GTNs displaying similar picture as in "C".

E: (Left) LNF of (right) thumb HK—gets everted and LND setting in. *Pseudomonas* invasion may be noted.

F: Similar picture as in "C". Yellowish streak may be noted on left side; periungual HK and scaling may also be noted.

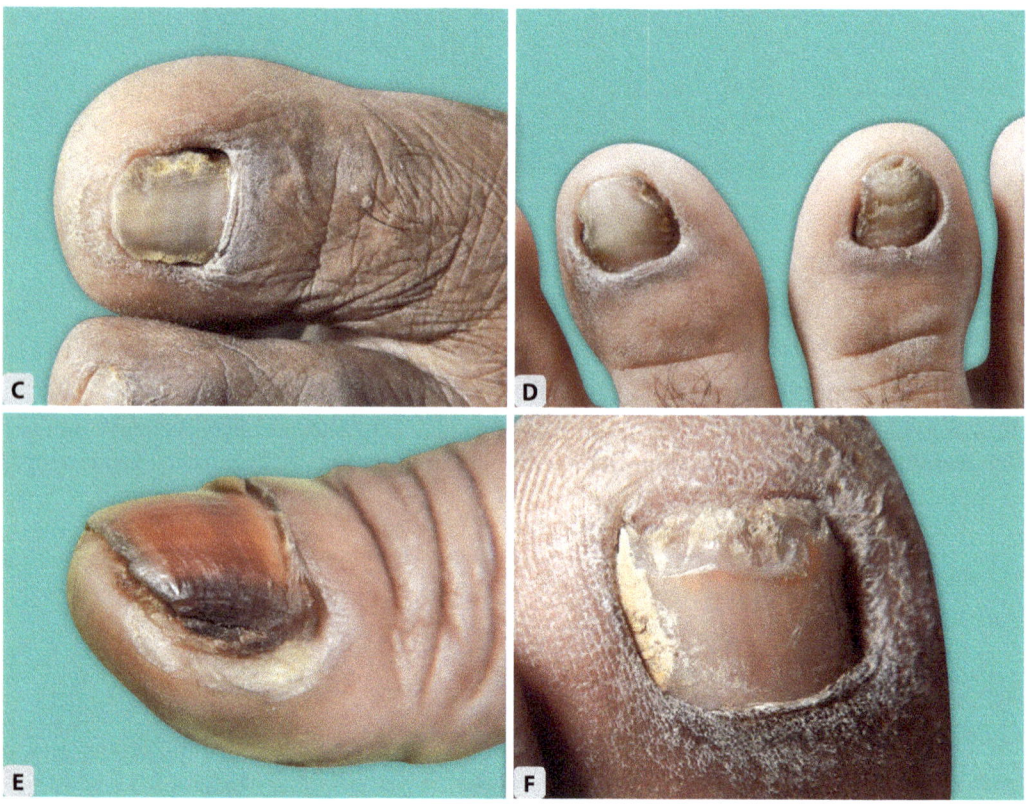

Color Atlas: Nail Abnormalities 177

YELLOWISH TO WHITISH STREAKS

A: (Right) GTN displays yellowish streaks along the lateral margins of the nail plate close to the LNFs.

B: Similar findings as in A; Beau's lines may also be noted. So, also periungual psoriatic scaling.

C: Whitish streaks along the LNFs in the nail plate of (left) GTN.

D: (Right) GTN displays similar streaks. In the inset, it may be noted a small scaly lesion on the medial LNF on (right) GT (yellow box).

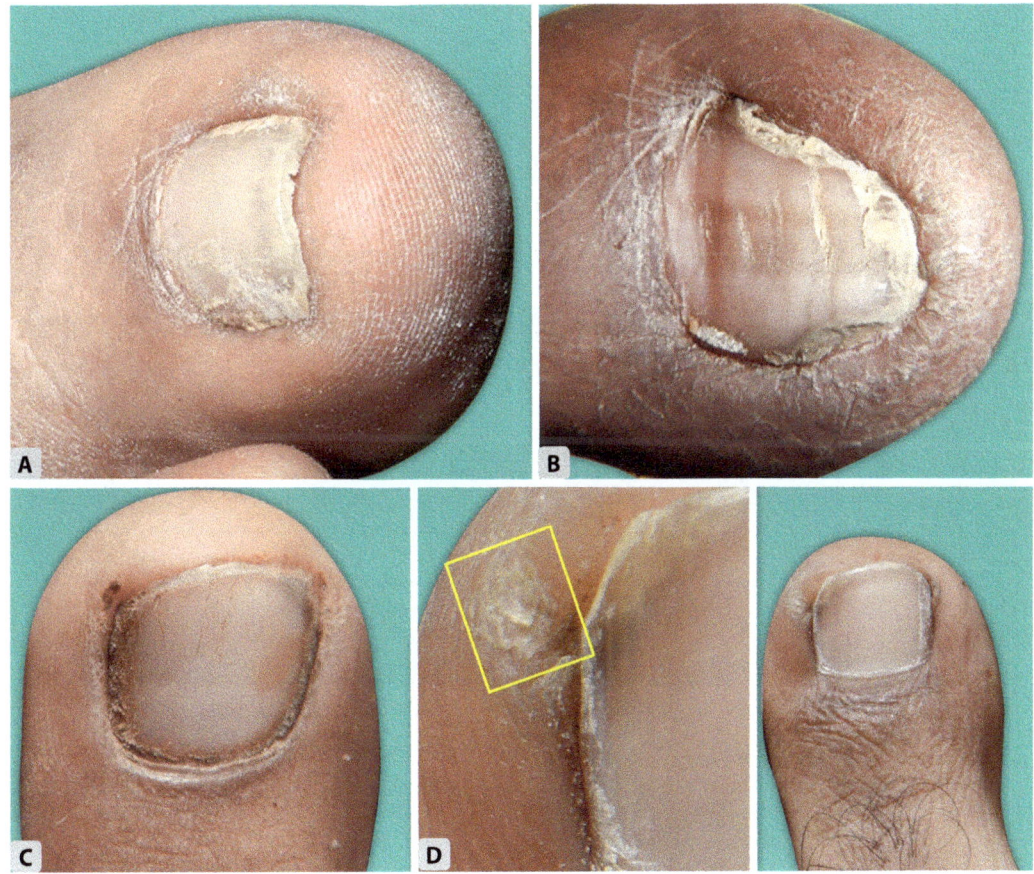

ONYCHAUXIS

A: Left LTN displaying onychauxis. The periphery of the nail unit displays psoriatic scaling.
B: (Right) GTN displays typical onychauxis.
C: (Left) LTN displaying similar change.
D: (Right) GTN displays similar change.

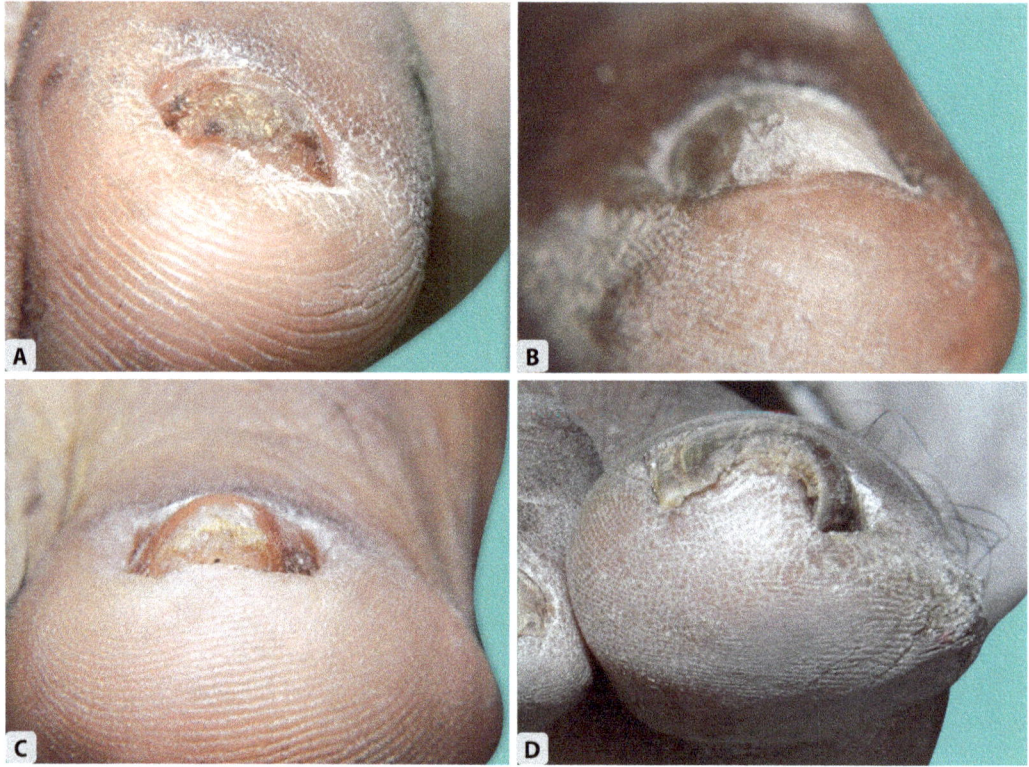

TENT-LIKE ELEVATION

A: (Right) GTN—typical TLE with SUHK.
B: (Left) second TN with typical TLE.
C: (Left) LTN with a typical similar change; (left) fourth TN displaying angulation may also be noted.
D: (Left) second TN with TLE.

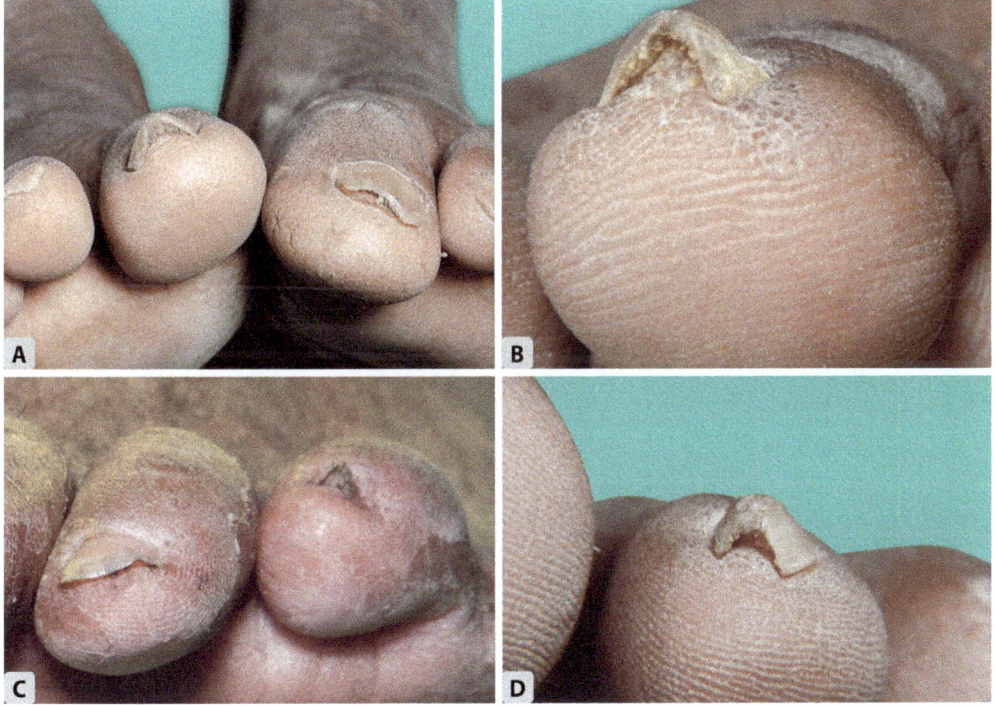

PSORIATIC PARONYCHIA

A: All the five fingers of (right) hand display chronicparonychia affecting all the three nail folds of all the fingers. The LNFs are characteristically HK and offer an everted edge-like appearance. This hand may be mistaken to a case of candidal paronychia.

B: The entire length of the nail folds is chronically inflamed with resultant HK nail folds with predominant dystrophy of lateral thirds of the nail plate.

C: (Left) index finger—both the LNFs and PNFs are inflamed: Dystrophic changes along the lateral nail margins may be noted. At a glance, it may be mistaken to candidal paronychia, but the involvement of (L) LNF clinches the diagnosis in favor of psoriasis.

D: Looks like a case of typical candidal paronychia affecting PNF; therefore, one must have a look at the LNFs; the lower portion of the (R) LNF hyperkeratotic and gets everted. Dystrophic changes involving the (R) lateral nail margin may be noted.

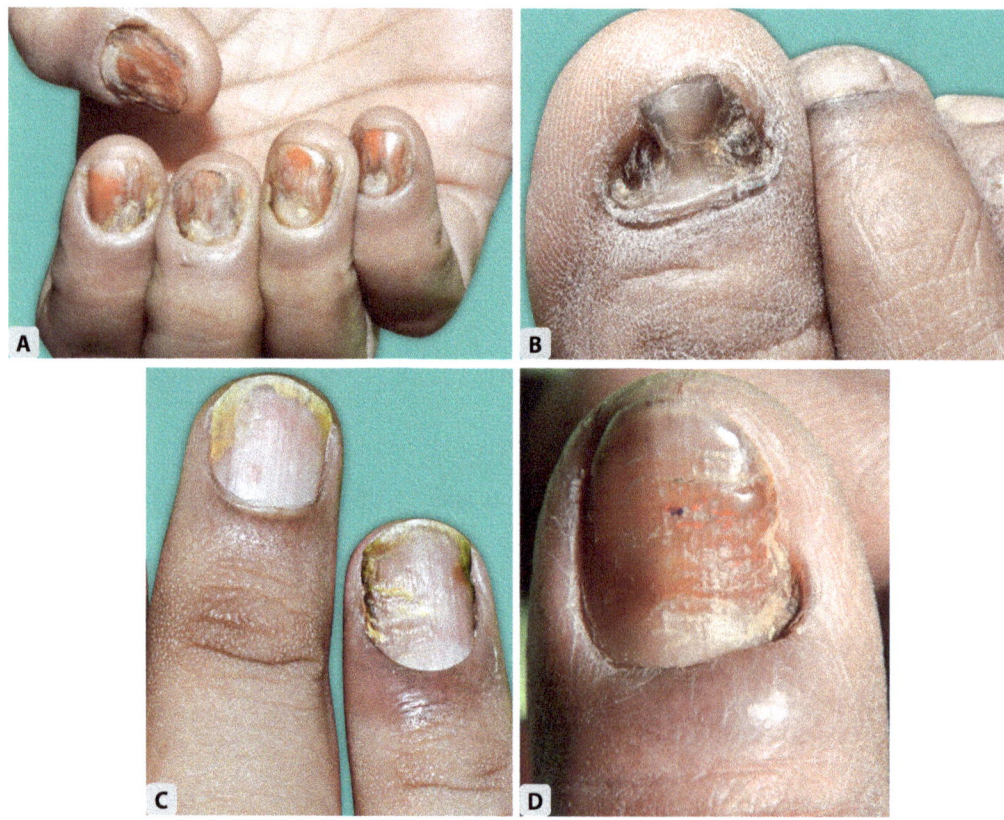

E: Like the finger nail folds, all the three nail folds of both GTs are inflamed.
F: Both the GTs LNFs are inflamed, sparing the PNFs. Both the GTNs also display streaky ONL. Yellowish to whitish streaks may also be noted. LNFs are seen moving away from the nail plates.

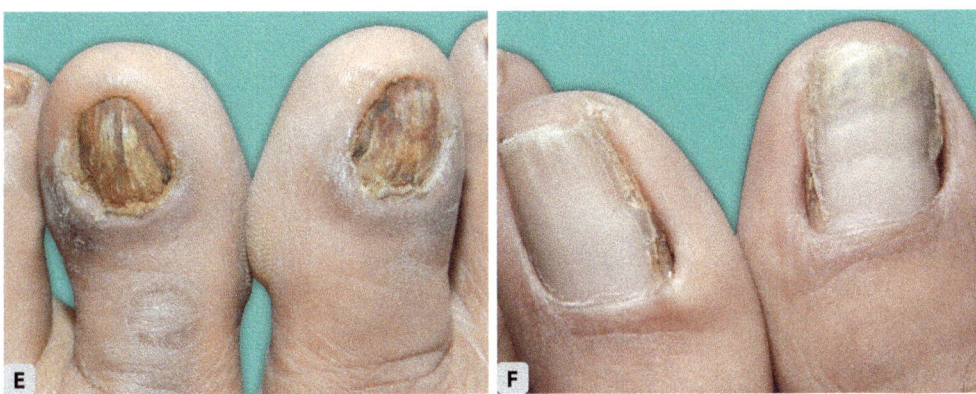

CAVE-LIKE CURVATURE

A: Cave-like curvature of (R) LTN with psoriatic scaling in the periphery of the nail apparatus.
B: Another patient with similar nail abnormality.

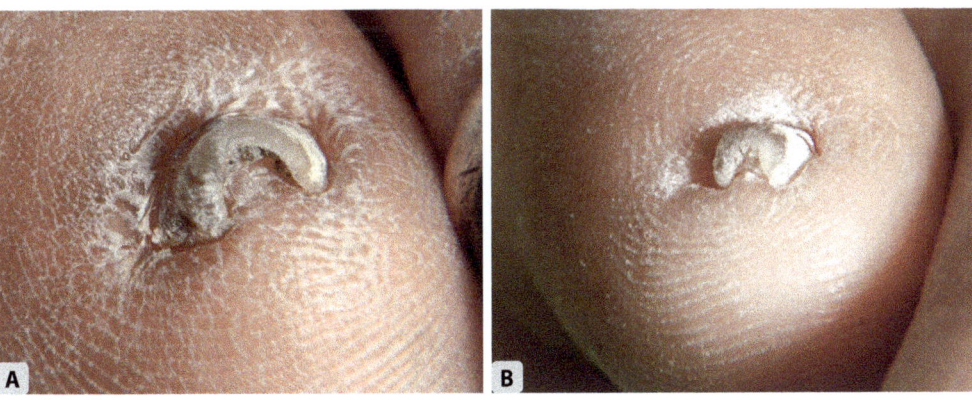

■ NAIL PLATE—PULP KISS SIGN

A: The distal nail plate bends downward and forward as if to kiss the pulp.
B: Similar nail plate changes as in A.
C: Similar sign.
D: (Left) second TN displaying the same feature.

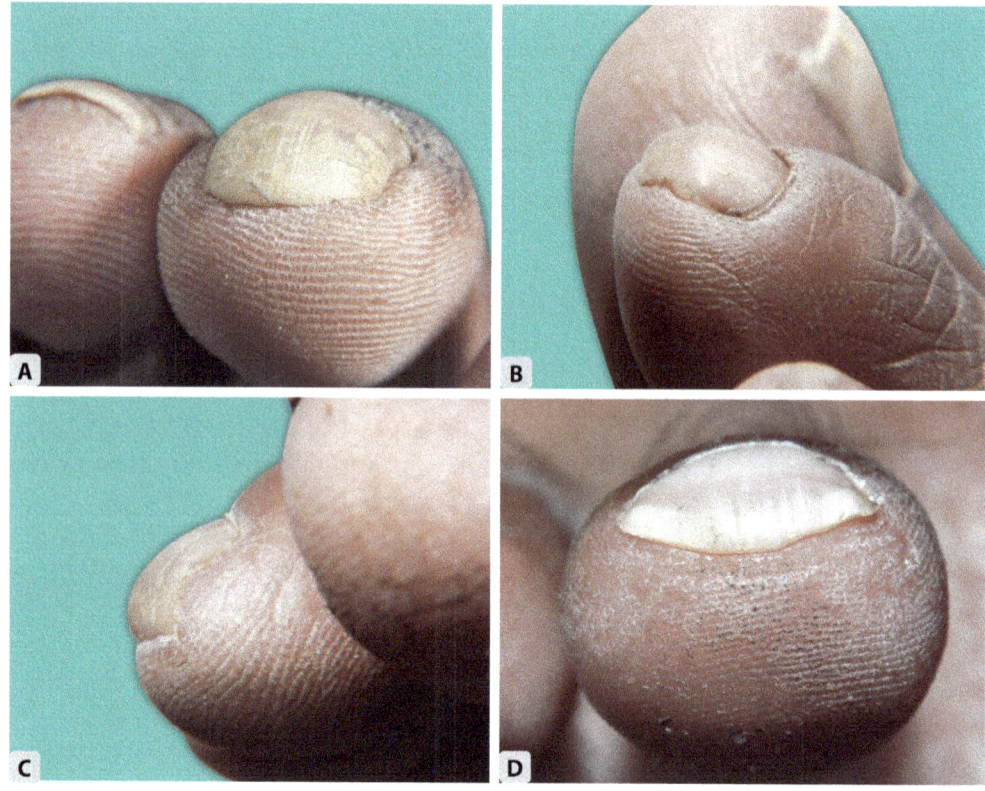

Color Atlas: Nail Abnormalities 183

LITTLE TOENAIL SPLIT

A: (Left) LTN typically splits into two unequal halves; the outer small piece is melanotic and inner bigger piece is usually amelanotic.

B: (Right) LTN with similar changes; psoriatic scaling in the periphery of the nail apparatus may also be noted.

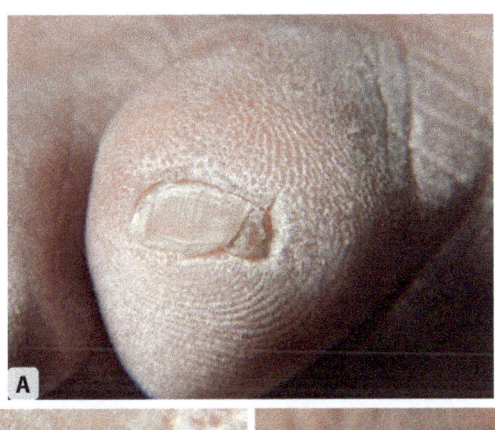
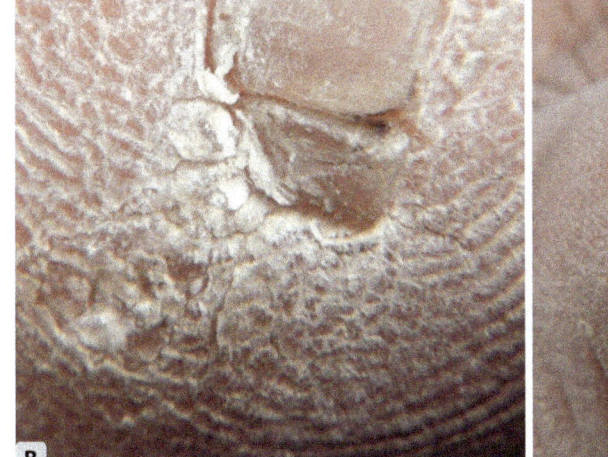
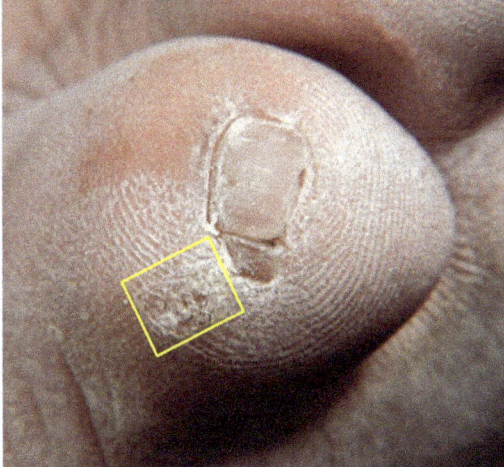

C to F: Display similar feature.

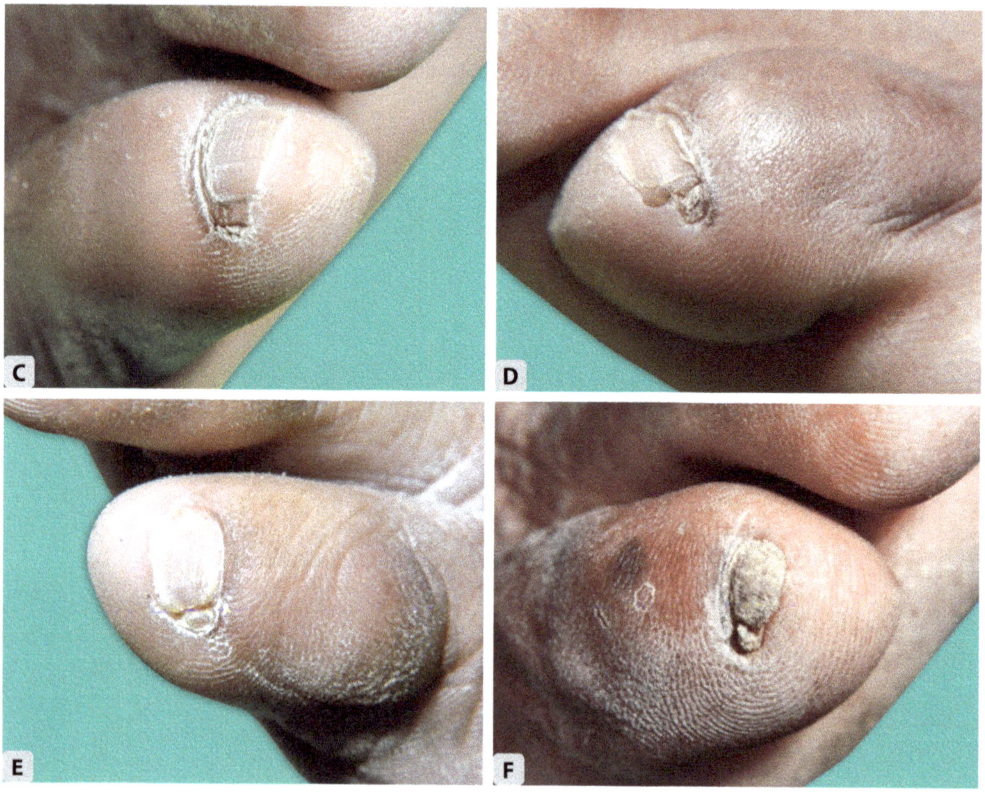

UNFOLDING CARPET ROLL-LIKE CURVATURE

A: This abnormality, though fairly rare, is a highly diagnostic clue for psoriasis (right) GTN.
B: (Left) fourth TN displaying similar feature.

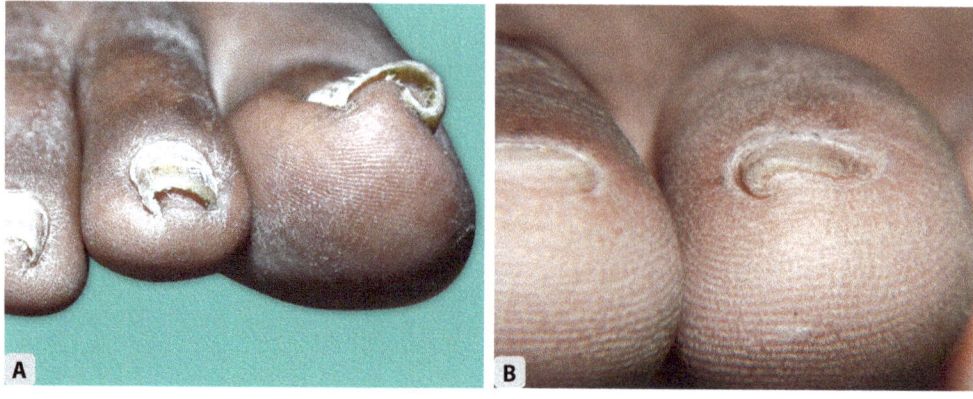

SHORT LITTLE TOENAIL

Short nail is a fairly rare finding and very interesting to note that it is observed only in little toe. Once this feature is noted, any puzzling dermatitis in question can be labeled as psoriasis. One may find some more clues elsewhere on the body to further substantiate the diagnosis.

A: (Right) LTN displays a very short nail.

B1 and B2: Another patient's feet display short LTNs in both feet.

C1 and C2: Similarly, another patient's feet displaying similar feature. Length of the nail depends on nail growth which in turn depends on nail matrix activity. Therefore, when trauma is significant enough to affect nail matrix activity, it may result in arrest of nail matrix activity.

Eventually a short nail results. Why only LTN is affected? As per my observations, GTN and LTN appear to be more prone to trauma than the middle toes.

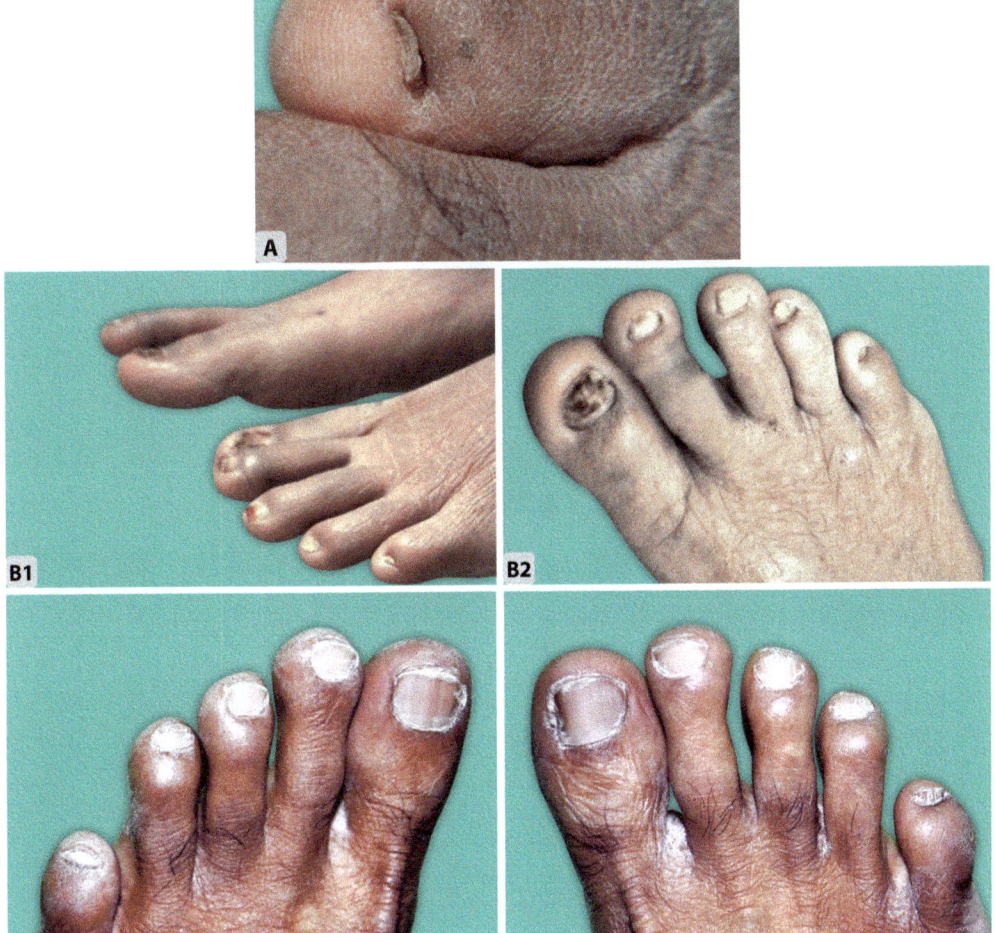

■ MORE THAN ONE IN A SINGLE FOOT

A: (Left) foot displays three clues: (1) TLE, (2) Asbestos sheet-shaped nail margin, and (3) Angulated free nail margin.

B: Overcurvature, angulation, SUHK, and band-like MLN may be noted in this foot. So, also psoriasiform scaling involving toe pads.

C: Angulation, SUHK, and overcurvature may be noted in (left) GTN, (left) second toe, and (left) third toe, respectively.

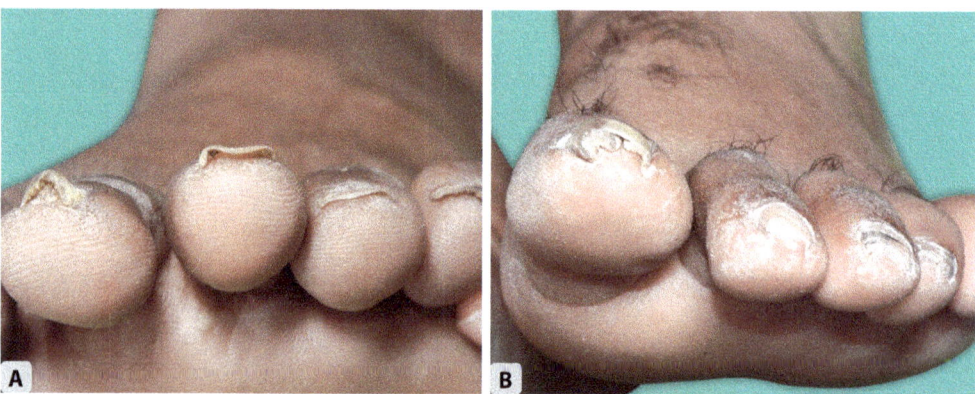

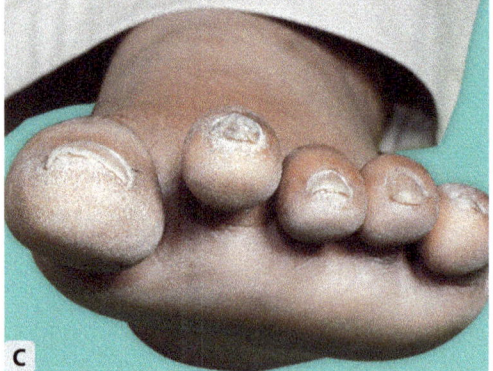

Index

Page numbers followed by *b* refer to box, *f* refer to figure, *fc* refer to flowchart, and *t* refer to table.

A

Acne vulgaris 16
Adherens junctions 131
   functions 131
Alpha-catenin 131
American Academy of
   Dermatology 15
Antecubital fossa 52
Antidandruff agents 21
Antifungal's cytostatic effect 24
Arch-like curvature 166
Asbestos sheet's shape 91, 147
   nail 164, 171

B

Basement membrane zone 140
Beard region 109
Beau's lines 143
Beta-catenin 131
Blaschko'slines pattern 149
Blood and nerve supply 140

C

Cadherin-catenin complex 131
Candida
   albicans 134, 145
   species 134, 143
Cave-like curvature 164, 181
Cell
   adhesion proteins, calcium-
      dependent 130
   kinetic studies 127
Cell-cell adhesions 127
Cetirizine 10
Chest, itchy lesions on 108
Child's hair 6
Child's scalp 6
Coalescent papules 78*f*
   scaly 90

Connexions 131
   components of 131
Corneocyte 125
Corona seborrheica 103*f*, 104*f*
Cutaneous sensory nerves 141
Cyclic adenosine
   monophosphate 133
Cystatin 129
Cytoplasmic plaque proteins
   131
Cytostatic drugs 141

D

Dandruff 4-6, 8-12, 19-21, 25,
   27, 59
   ameliorating 20, 24
   experience with 7
   history of 29, 39, 63, 73, 93,
      108, 112, 116
   itching 86
   meant 6
   moderate cases of 10
   moderate-to-severe cases
      of 10
   pathogenesis of 21
   persistent 43
   recurrent 37, 38
   relapses 20
   severity of 10
   suffering from 6
   treatment of 24
Darier disease 128
Dermal-epidermal basement
   membrane 132
Dermatitis 11, 13, 26, 52, 147
   chronic 13
   puzzling 147
Dermis 140
Dermoepidermal junction 132
Desmoplakin 130

Desmosomal cadherin
   desmoglein-3 128
Desmosomal proteins 129
Desmosomes 127, 130
   functions 130
Dome-shaped elevation 164,
   172
Dry nails 146
Dystrophic nail 146

E

Ear
   concha 103
   lobule, external 107
Earlobe 83
   external 93, 94, 112
   upper part of 29
Econazole 21
Eczema
   atopic 13, 144
   chronic 16, 144
   dyshidrotic 15
   hand 15
   seborrheic 7
   subacute 16
Eczematous
   eruption 101
   plaque 40
   psoriasis 15, 16
Elbow 11, 117
Envoplakin 129
Epidermal keratinocytes 132
Epidermal proliferation 13
Epidermal stem cells,
   interfollicular 128
Epidermis 138, 149
   hyperproliferation of 20
Epidermolytic hyperkeratosis
   127
Episodic dandruff, history of 55
Epithelia 137

Epithelial keratin 138
  genes 127
  normal 138
Erythema 11, 89, 93
  mild 79, 84, 101
Erythematous 94
  patches 112
  plaque 85
Erythematous scaly
  patch 81, 82
    large 81
  plaques 80, 82, 109
External auditory canals 36, 82, 90
Eye involvement, history of 116
Eyebrows 90
  medial 7, 103, 108
  scaling of 90

F

Face 61, 95
  diffuse 95
  dry 95
  history of itching of 74
  itching of 95
  itchy lesions on 108
Facial lesions 94f
Feet 11
  border 104, 153
    fissures 149
  dorsae of 7, 96
  epidermal abnormalities of 149
  first toe web 47
  single 186
Filaggrin 129
Fingernails 145
Fissures, depict linear 153
Follicular papules 7, 100
Follicular psoriasis 43f
Forefoot, medial border of 34
Forehead patch, history of 103
Frank psoriatic plaques, devoid of 25

G

Gap junctions 131
  functions 131
Genetic disease 14
Germinative matrix 138

Glabella 108
Glans penis 11
Granular cell 125, 126
Granular layer 129
Great toe
  dorsum of 161
  lateral aspect of 77, 149
  nail 30, 34, 41, 53, 109
    left 165
Groin psoriasis 11

H

Hailey-Hailey disease 130
Hair 4
  keratin genes 127
  parting 29, 58
  shafts 11, 31
Heel 49, 54
  fissures 149
  border 149
Hemidesmosomes 132
Hepatitis B infection 17
Hindfeet 102
Hyperkeratosis 10, 49, 134, 149
  subclinical 25
Hyperproliferative disorder 3, 27, 128
Hyponychium 137, 140

I

Idiopathic onycholysis 143
Impetus 3
Index finger 180
Inflammatory bowel disease 17
Inflammatory cells 13
Interfollicular papules 100f
Intertriginous hyperkeratosis 10
Involucrin 129
Irritable lesions 110f
Isthmus 139
Itching 25, 90, 114
  history of 53, 67, 69, 76, 92, 98, 114, 115
  of occasional 59
Itchy
  disease 13
  eruption, history of 84
  lesions 83, 108
    history of 109

patches 7, 9, 88
  rash 106
    chest 106
    history of 97
    face 1-6

K

Keratin 129, 141
  filaments 125
    intermediate 127
  pseudogenes 127
Keratinocytes 13, 126
Keratohyalin granules 129
Knees 11
Knockout mouse 126
Koebner phenomenon 23, 25
Koilonychia 146, 147, 164, 167

L

Lamellar granules 128, 133
Langerhans cells 138
Lateral nail
  dystrophy 164, 175
  fold hyperkeratosis 175
  plate dystrophy 147
Levocetirizine 10
Lichenified plaques 115f
Lipophilic yeasts 17
Loricrin 129
Lower lip, half of 78
Low-sulfur filamentous proteins 141

M

Malassezia 18, 19
  furfur 18
  globosa 17-19
  restricta 17, 18
  species 17
  sympodialis 17, 18
Malleoli 162
Matrix protein 125
Melanocytes 138
Melanonychia 164, 168
  complete 147
  partial 147
Merkel cells 139
Multiple scaly patches 65f
Murmurs 9
Mycobiome 17

N

Nail
  abnormalities 146, 164, 181
  anatomy of normal 137
  apparatus, homeostasis of 141
  bed 137, 140
  changes, nonspecific 143
  fold, proximal 137
  proximal fold stem cells 139
  split, median 164, 174
  wall 138
Nail growth 141
  arrest of 141
Nail matrix 137, 138
  cells in 138
Nail plate 139, 141, 164, 182
  abnormalities 143
  angulation of 147
  sheet-shaped 79
  thinning of 146
Nail psoriasis 142, 143
  diagnosis of 143
Nail unit 137
  affected by psoriasis 142
  components of 137
Nasolabial
  folds 81
  furrows 7
Natal cleft 11
  upper 113
Neck
  fold, anterior 110
  nape of 88, 106
Nongreasy scales 79f
North American Dermatology Clinics 15
Nostril rims 75
Nystatin 21

O

Occipital scalp 46f, 65f, 80f, 106f
Odland bodies 128, 133
Onychauxis 178
Onychocorneal band 141
Onychogryphosis 145
Onycholysis 143, 147, 164, 170

P

Palmoplantar psoriasis 9, 10
Papillae 13
Papular eruption 46f
Parakeratotic cells 25
Parietal scalp 46
Paronychia 11
  acute 143
  chronic 143
Perianal skin 110f
Pincer nail 32, 39, 41, 97, 146, 147, 164, 173
Pits 142
Pityriasis alba 61f
  lesion 61f
Pityriasis amiantacea 86f, 112f
Pityriasis capitis 6, 11, 12, 20
Pityriasis versicolor 18
  lesions 94
Pityrosporum orbiculare 18
Pityrosporum ovale 3, 18, 20, 23, 27
  infection 23
Plakoglobin 130, 131
Plantar psoriasis 82, 96
  chronic 88
Plaque type psoriasis 87
Plaque with fissures pattern 152
Plasmodium ovale 22
Polymorphous light eruption 14
Pompholyx 15
Postmitotic cells 128
Preclinical psoriasis 25
Prepubertal child 6
Proliferating cells 125
Protein kinase C 126
Protein-reinforced plasma membrane 125
Pruritus, cognizance of 13
Pseudomonas 143
Psoriasis 9-11, 13, 15, 16, 27, 142, 146, 149
  capitis 11
  clinical behavior of 15
  mild 21
  nail apparatus in 142
  photosensitive 14, 44
  scaly plaques of 88f
  subclinical 24
  toenail in 137
  vulgaris 10, 27, 147
Psoriatic fissures 154
Psoriatic lesion 83
  typical 116, 117
Psoriatic paronychia 164, 180
  chronic 143, 168
Psoriatic plaque 24, 41, 83, 111
Psoriatic scaling, displays 168, 178
Pulp 158
  kiss sign 164, 182

R

Retro ala nasi 89f, 112f
Retroauricular erythema 74t
Robust scientific logic 20, 24

S

Scales hair 5
Scaling scalp
  condition of 48
  history of 44, 58
Scalp 11, 36, 112
  displays 53
  hair 11, 59
  normal 61, 73
  occiput area of 33
  plus 9
  psoriasis 23
  region of 5
  scaling of 35, 40, 53, 57, 109, 114, 115
  surface 12
Scaly dermatitis 74f, 95f
Scaly erythema 51f
Scaly lesions 92
Scaly patches 94
Scaly plaques 93, 120
  thin 87
Scanty papulation 99f
Sebopsoriasis 11
Seborrhea 24, 26
Seborrheic dermatitis 7, 11, 12, 15, 16, 18, 19, 24, 27
  pathogenesis of 20

Seborrheic distribution 81
Seborrheic sites 74f
Sebum 24
Selenium sulfide 21
Sexually transmitted diseases 15
Shampoo regularly 4
Silvery scales 119f
Silvery white scales 115
　papules 80, 109
Skin 100
　dorsum of 149
　normal 11
　over frontal scalp 72
　submental 112
Soles 154
　fissures of 149
Spinous layer 128
Splinter hemorrhages 140, 143
Spongiosis 13, 15
Squirting papilla 13
Stem cells 127, 139
Stratum basale 127
Stratum corneum 13, 129
　functions of 129

Stratum lucidum 129
Streaks, yellowish to whitish 164, 177
Subungual hyperkeratosis 142, 143, 172
Suprabasal cells 126

T

Tent-like elevation 164, 179
Tight junctions 132
　functions 132
Tiny papules mimicking lichen nitidus 45
Toe
　foot, dorsum of second 115
　insteps under 49
　pads 157, 158
　pulps 157
　web 77
Toenail 146
　abnormalities 164
　fourth 39
　little 39, 111
　plate 147
　short little 185

split, little 164, 183
　third 165
Tonofilaments 126, 127
Tonsuration, history of 73
Tonsured scalp 65
Tortoise-shell pattern 151

U

Under toes 10
　foot 115
Upper lip 7, 75

W

Web spaces 159
White scaly plaques 119

Y

Yeasts 20
　in dandruff, role of 18
Yellow dots 165

Z

Zinc pyrithione 21

EU GSPR Authorised Reprsentative
Logos Europe, 9 rue Nicolas Poussin
1700, La Rochelle, France
Phone: +33 (0) 6 67 93 73 78
E-mail: contact@logoseurope.eu